Human Teeth - Key Skills and Clinical Illustrations

Edited by Zühre Akarslan and Farid Bourzgui

Published in London, United Kingdom

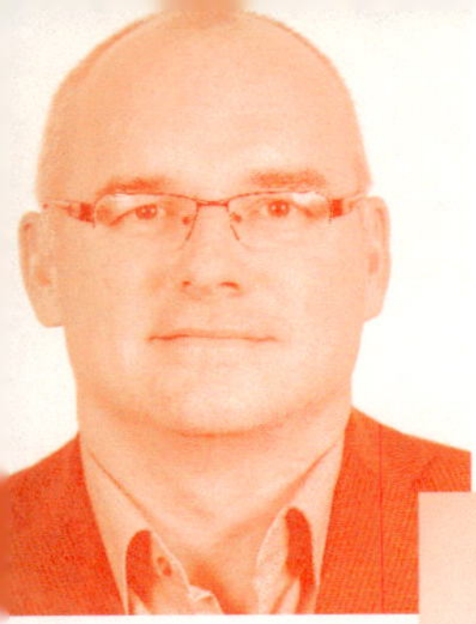
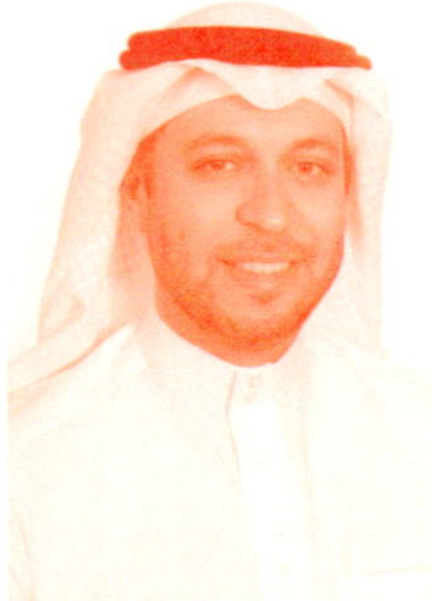
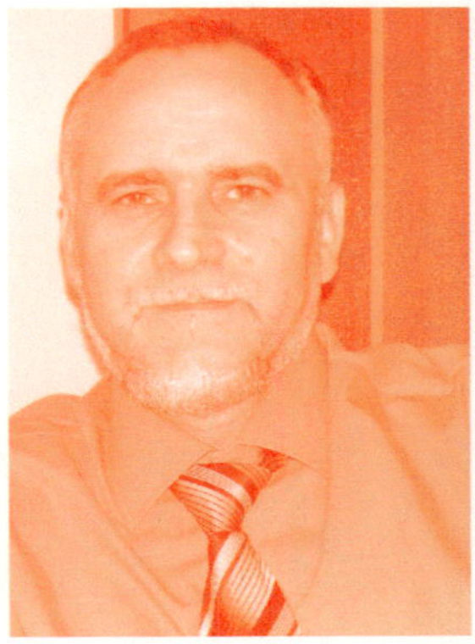
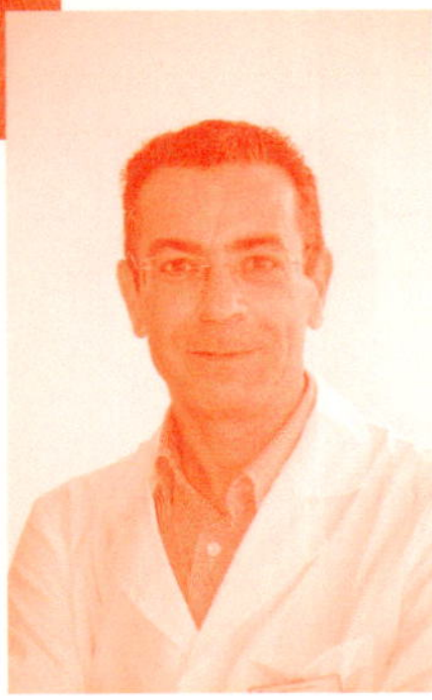
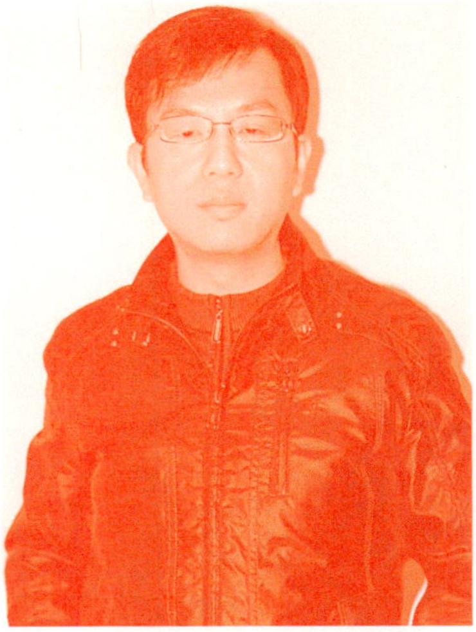
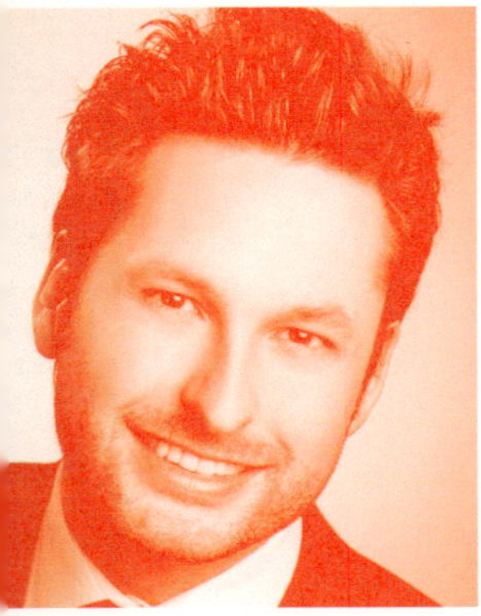
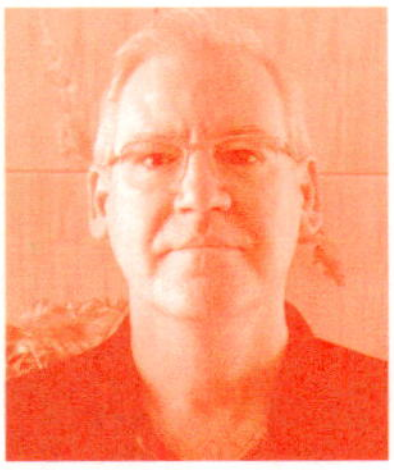

IntechOpen

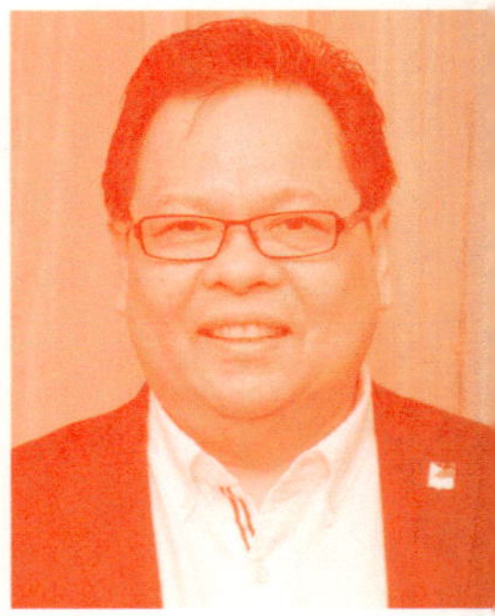
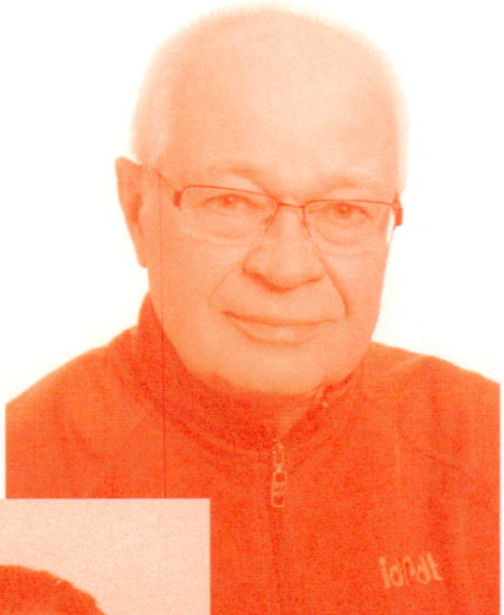
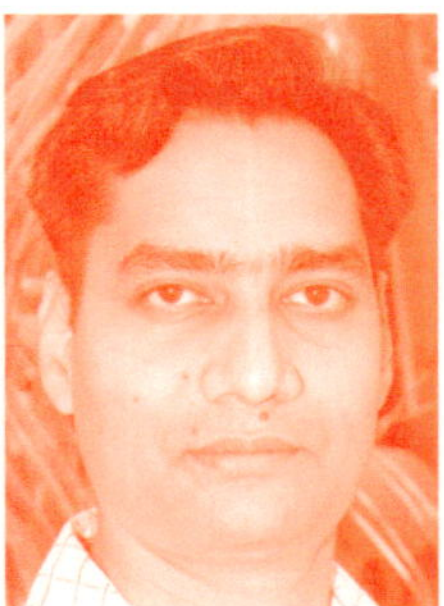
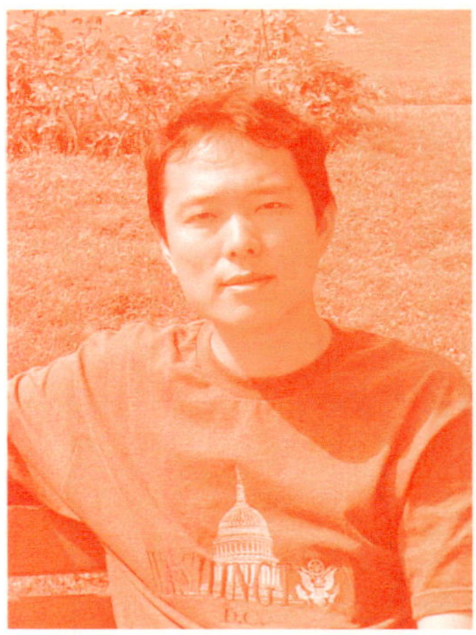
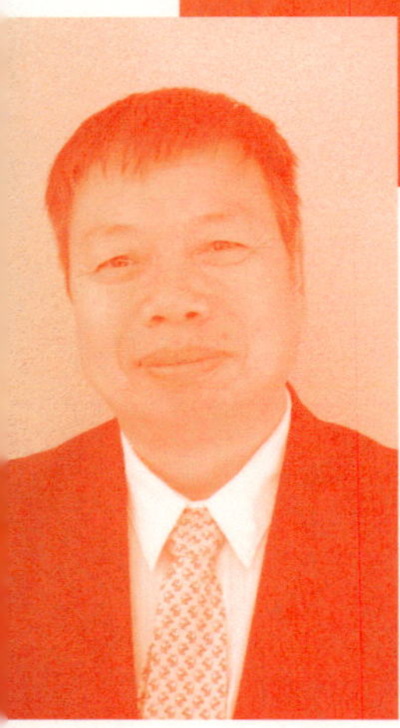
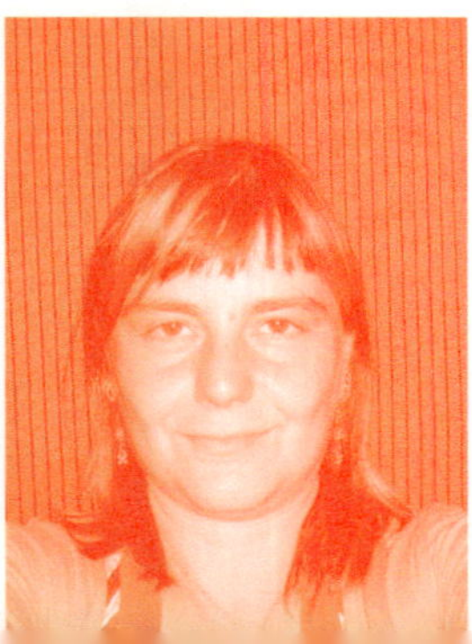

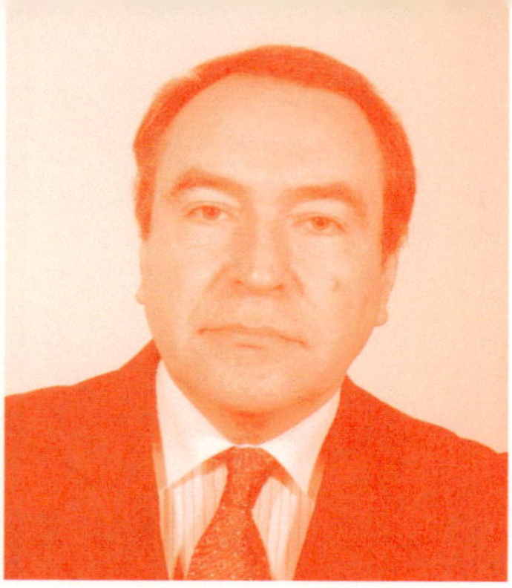
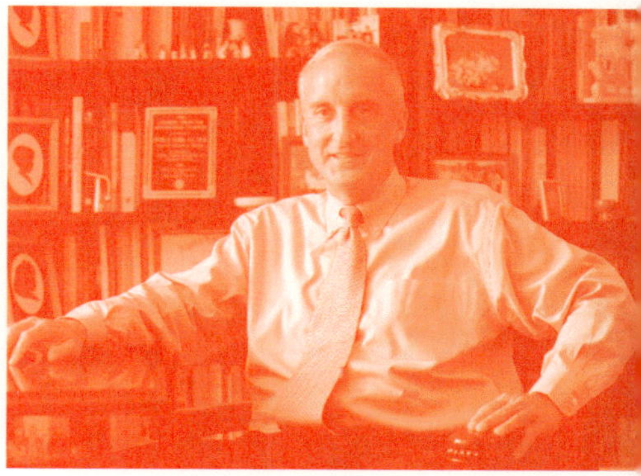
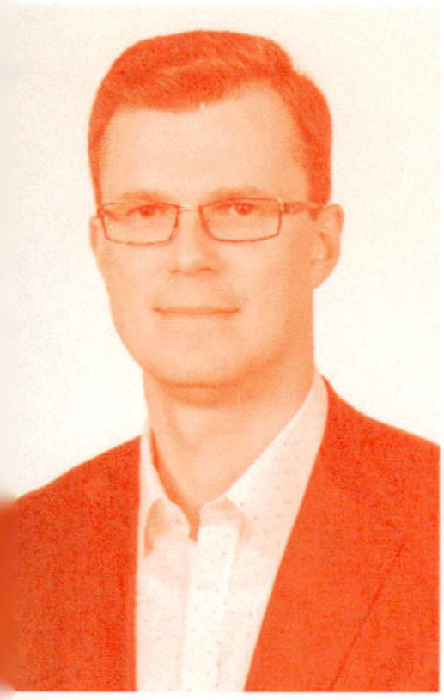
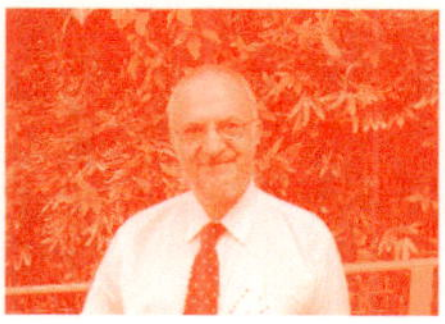
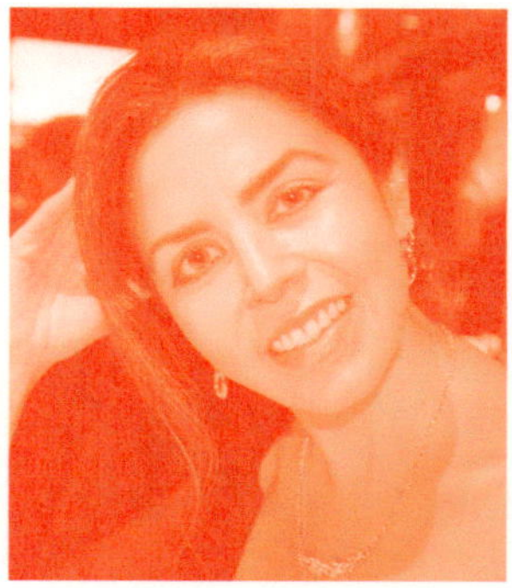

Supporting open minds since 2005

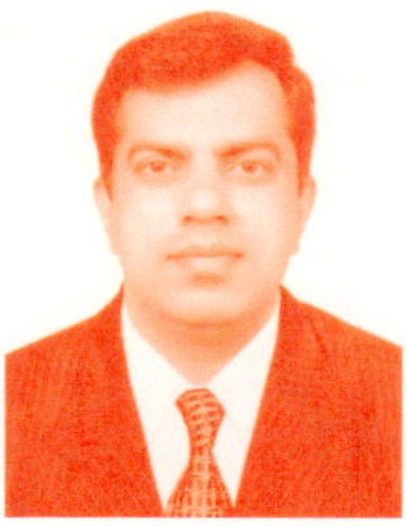
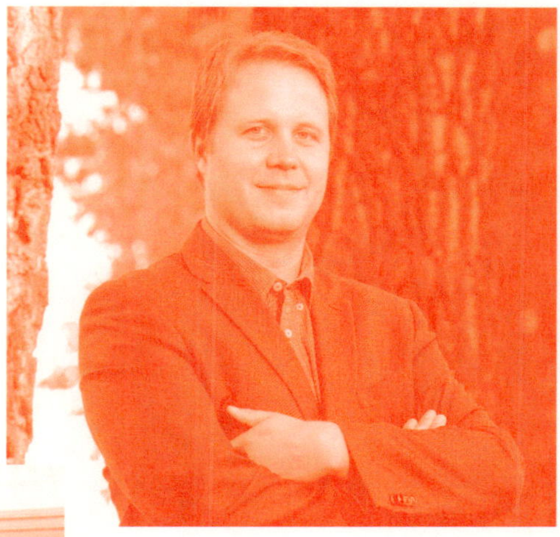
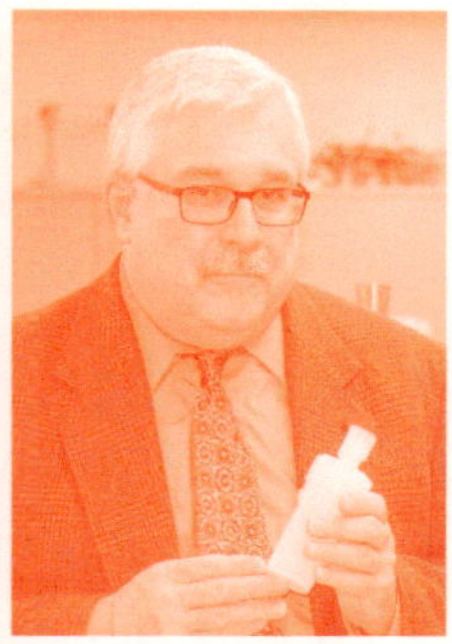
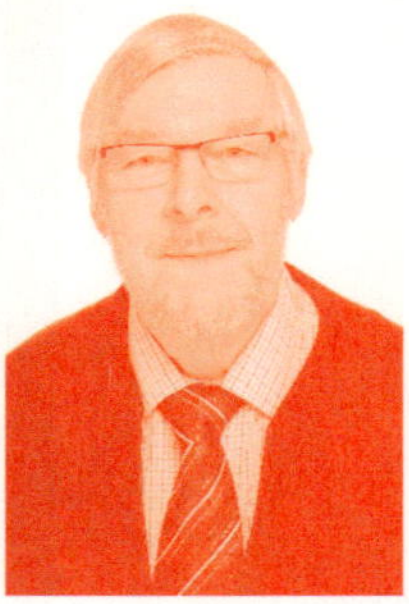
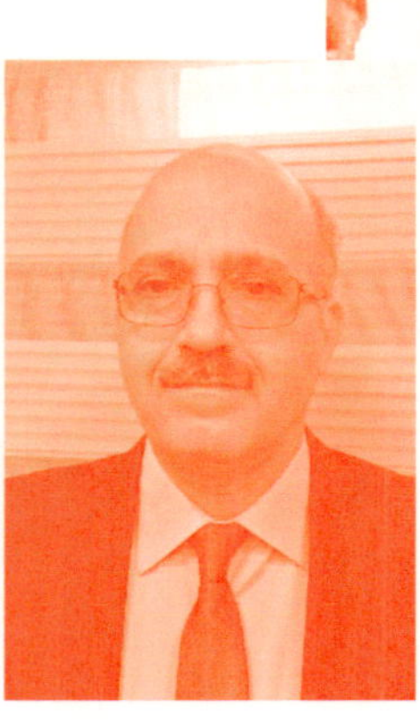
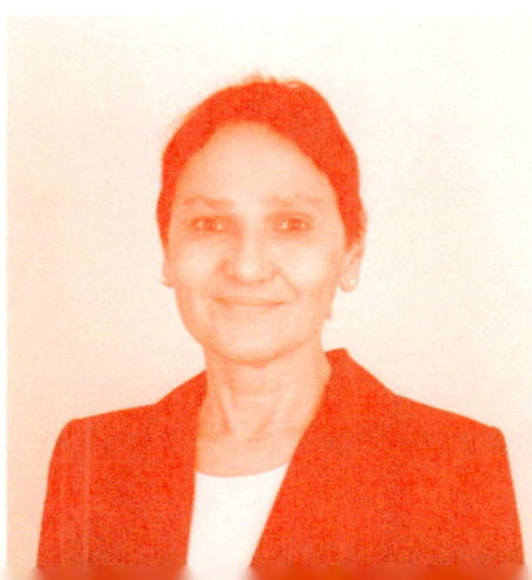
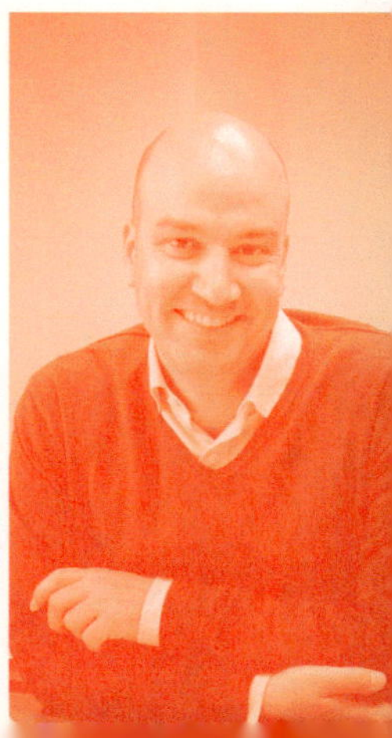

Human Teeth - Key Skills and Clinical Illustrations
http://dx.doi.org/10.5772/intechopen.81278
Edited by Zühre Akarslan and Farid Bourzgui

Part of IntechOpen Book Series: Dentistry, Volume 5
Book Series Editor: Zühre Akarslan

Contributors
Monika Wahi, Shatha ALHarthi, Abeer Alshami, Munirah Binshabaib, Amanda Valentim, Renata Furlan, Mariana Amaral, Fernanda Guimarães, Esra Pamukcu Guven, Ayşe Sümeyye Akay, Ahmed A. Madfa, Mohammed A. Aldawla, Abdulbaset A. Mufadhal, Haydar Barakat, Ammar Howijieh, Svetlana Razumova, Anzhela Brago, Hakima Aghoutan, Sanaa Alami, Amal El Aouame, Farid El Quars, Jesús Alejandro Quiñones Pedraza, Sana Alami, Samira El Arabi, Bouchra Bousfiha, Amal Chlyah, Bouchra Badre, Mouna Hamza, Maria Mtalsi, Hasna Saih, Fatiha Rhrich, Said Dhaimy, Imane Benkiran, Lamyae Bedida, Hafsa El Merini, Zühre Akarslan

First published in London, United Kingdom, 2020 by IntechOpen
IntechOpen is the global imprint of INTECHOPEN LIMITED, registered in England and Wales, registration number: 11086078, 7th floor, 10 Lower Thames Street, London, EC3R 6AF, United Kingdom
Printed in Croatia

British Library Cataloguing-in-Publication Data
A catalogue record for this book is available from the British Library

Additional hard and PDF copies can be obtained from orders@intechopen.com

Human Teeth - Key Skills and Clinical Illustrations
Edited by Zühre Akarslan and Farid Bourzgui
p. cm.
Print ISBN 978-1-78923-839-6
Online ISBN 978-1-78923-840-2
eBook (PDF) ISBN 978-1-78984-522-8
ISSN 2631-6218

For EU product safety concerns:
IN TECH d.o.o., Prolaz Marije Krucifikse Kozulić 3, 51000 Rijeka, Croatia,
info@intechopen.com or visit our website at intechopen.com.

IntechOpen Book Series
Dentistry
Volume 5

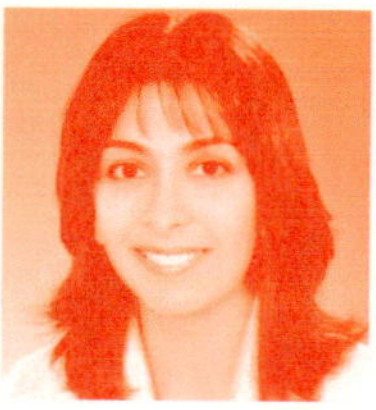

Zühre Akarslan was born in 1977 in Cyprus. She graduated from Gazi University Faculty of Dentistry, Ankara, Turkey, in 2000. She received her PhD degree from the Oral Diagnosis and Radiology Department of the same university in 2007. The department was recently renamed Oral and Dentomaxillofacial Radiology. She is working as a full-time professor in Gazi University. She has published research in various international and national journals, written book chapters, and served as editors of books and as an editorial board member and reviewer of several scientific journals. Her expertise areas are dental caries, cancer, dental fear and anxiety, gag reflex in dentistry, oral medicine, and dentomaxillofacial radiology. She is married and has two children.

Series Editor and Editor of Volume 5: Zühre Akarslan
Gazi University Faculty of Dentistry, Turkey

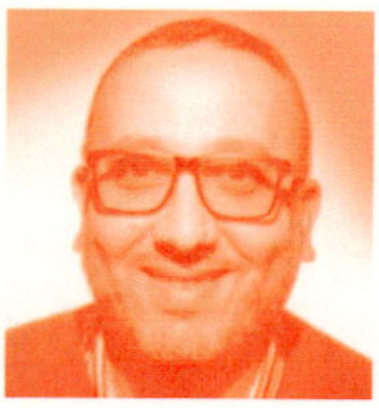

Pr. Bourzgui is a Professor of Orthodontics in the School of Dental Medicine at Casablanca Hassan II University, Morocco. He holds various certificates and diplomas: a Certificate of Higher Studies in Group A (major: Technology of Biomaterials used in Dentistry, 1996), a Certificate of Advanced Studies of Group B, (major: Dentofacial Orthopedics, 1997) from the Faculty of Dental Surgery at University Denis Diderot-Paris VII, France, a diploma of Higher Studies in Biocompatibility of Biomaterials from the Faculty of Medicine and Pharmacy of Casablanca (2002), a Certificate of Clinical Occlusal Odontology from the Faculty of Dentistry Casablanca (2004), and a university degree in Biostatistics and Perceptual Health Measurement from the Faculty of Medicine and Pharmacy of Casablanca in 2011. Farid Bourzgui is a former intern and resident of Casablanca University Hospital, Ibn Rushd in Casablanca. Pr. Bourzgui has published a number of articles and book chapters on various aspects of orthodontics. In addition to his educational qualifications, Pr. Bourzgui has been the Head of the Orthodontics and Dentofacial Orthopedics Department since 2013, and a member of the Casablanca Dental School Council. He is currently an expert evaluator at the Centre National pour la Recherche Scientifique et technique (CNRST) Rabat-Morocco.

Editor of Volume 5: Prof. Farid Bourzgui
University Hassan II, Faculty of dentistry, Casablanca, Morocco

Scope of the Series

Teeth are unique structures in the human beings. They are located in the oral cavity and play a key role in digestion, phonation, and aesthetics. There are two sets of teeth during the human lifecycle: deciduous teeth and permanent teeth. Deciduous teeth consist of incisors, canines, and molars. They are present in childhood and replaced with the permanent teeth during growth. Permanent teeth consist of incisors, canines, premolars, and molars. Although the majority of teeth have normal morphology and anatomy, developmental and environmental factors may lead to anomalies affecting the size, shape, number, and structure of teeth.
Knowledge of tooth morphology, anatomy, and anomalies is essential to succeed in restorative treatment, prosthodontics, periodontal treatment, orthodontics, endodontics, and oral surgery. Readers will find a current overview of tooth morphology, anatomy, and anomalies in this book. Hopefully, it will serve as a practical guide to dentistry.

Contents

Preface

This book is the outcome of the confluence of two initial projects: "Human Molars" led by Prof. BOURZGUI Farid and "Basics of Dental Morphology and Anatomy" by Prof. Zühre Akarslan. The experience of co-editing was very enriching for both editors and led to a final product that we hope will be very useful and valuable for our readers.

The book is divided into three sections:

1. *Basic Principles - Embryology and Development* examines the basic tenants of embryology and molar development. A particular focus was the relationship between oro-facial structures and tooth morphology.

2. *Background on Dental Anatomy and Morphology* investigates the internal and external anatomy of teeth, as well as their anatomical variants.

3. *Pathology and Clinical Considerations* reviews some pathologies and anomalies of the molars. The question addressed here is in case of extraction of these teeth, should the orthodontist orthodontically close their residual spaces or maintain them for prosthetic rehabilitation? In the case of the choice of the implant solution, a chapter on the evolution of implant shapes closes this section.

As a final note, we would like to express our thanks to the authors of the different chapters and their respective teams, as well as all those who contributed to the final outcome of this book.

Farid Bourzgui
Professor and Head of Orthodontics Department,
University Hassan II,
Faculty of dentistry,
Casablanca, Morocco

Zühre Akarslan
Professor,
Department of Oral and Maxillofacial Radiology,
Gazi University Faculty of Dentistry,
Ankara, Turkey

Section 1

Basic Principles - Embryology and Development

Chapter 1

Can Orofacial Structures Affect Tooth Morphology?

Amanda Valentim, Renata Furlan, Mariana Amaral and Fernanda Martins

Abstract

This chapter presents how orofacial muscles can affect teeth positioning, occlusion, and also the size/shape of teeth. Pressures exerted on teeth will be discussed in specific cases such as mouth breathing, chronic mastication disorders, oral habits, like thumb sucking or tongue thrust, and also when there is hyperfunction of masticatory muscles during sleep or wakefulness. In these situations, the imbalance of muscle forces brings undesirable consequences to the dentition. Each condition will be explained, showing which muscle is affected, how it changes, and what consequences to the teeth it brings. It is a chapter that shows how close the relationship is between dentistry and speech language pathology (orofacial myology).

Keywords: tooth, malocclusion, tongue, lip, cheek, bruxism, mastication

1. Introduction

Malocclusions are generally considered alterations in the normal field of craniofacial growth and morphology. Due to its different possibilities of etiological factors, it is often difficult to determine its specific cause [1].

There are four main structures that can cause malocclusions: the craniofacial skeleton, the teeth, the orofacial neuromuscular system, and other soft tissues. An example of how the musculature can generate malocclusion is the constantly open mandible in the mouth breathing leading to a constant anteriority of the tongue, which may force the incisors or prevent the eruption of the mandibular incisors [1]. Another example is that if a patient has a tongue with anterior posture during rest, the duration of this pressure, even if very light, may interfere with the eruption process or move the anterior teeth, resulting in an open bite [2]. There are also environmental influences, such as oral habits and balance between the orofacial musculature and the teeth, both at rest and during the functions [3]. Mouth breathing is one of these conditions. It causes muscle posture alteration that changes the balance in the oral cavity and modifies the forces exerted on teeth and bones, impacting facial growth and tooth positioning.

Other muscles that can influence tooth morphology are masseter and temporalis, which are jaw elevators. When they are active during rest or sleep, it is considered as bruxism, and may cause tooth wear.

2. Orofacial forces on the teeth

The teeth are structures of the stomatognathic system, classified as static [4]. These structures are subject to innumerable forces that balance [5].

There are four main factors responsible for the dental balance: intrinsic forces of the tongue, lips, and cheeks; extrinsic forces such as oral habits or orthodontic appliances; forces of the dental occlusion; and forces of the periodontal membrane, as for example, the eruption of teeth. Among these, the most important are the resting position of tongue and lips, in addition to the periodontal forces, since they have a long duration [1]. When one of these forces stands out, tooth movement occurs, and the teeth are susceptible to adaptations when subjected to some pressure or force [4].

The balance between the pressure of the tongue, lip, and cheek contributes to the maintenance of the teeth in their positions. The forces exerted by these structures are lighter than those of the masticatory function, but longer in duration. Even though the magnitude of force is low, it can cause a movement in the teeth when applied for a sufficient amount of time [6, 7].

The final position of the tooth, responsible for final shape of the dental arches, results from the balance between the perioral musculature represented by the mechanism of the buccinator and the intraoral pressure exerted by the musculature of the tongue [7].

A study of 3041 children [8] found that individuals without myofunctional disorders had significantly fewer malocclusions. In addition, a significantly larger number of children with anterior open bite were observed among those with functional alterations, and also the opposite, children with open bite had more functional disorders. Another study [9] found that children with occlusal alterations presented more myofunctional disorders such as lack of lip seal and altered tongue habitual position, compared to children with normal occlusion.

2.1 Tongue

The tongue is a mobile muscular organ that composes the stomatognathic system and is located on the mouth floor. This structure assists in the functions of chewing, swallowing, sucking, and speaking [10].

Eight pairs of muscles compose the tongue and they can be divided into intrinsic and extrinsic. The muscles denominated intrinsic are responsible for the alteration of their form: longitudinal superior, inferior longitudinal, transverse, and vertical. The extrinsic muscles originate in the proximal bony structures and are responsible for the movements of the tongue: genioglossus, styloglossus, palatoglossus, and hyoglossus [11].

Cheeks, lips, and tongue exert a great influence on the occurrence and persistence of malocclusions. In view of these facts, it is expected that the lingual structure exerts a certain force during its rest. When this structure is improperly positioned, its pressure can reach the teeth and promote inadequate occlusion.

Efforts to answer the question "what factors or combination of factors control physiologic movement of teeth" lead researchers to measure the magnitude of forces exerted by the relaxed tongue in the region of the mandibular canines. The conclusions were that the normal relaxed tongue produces a very low force against the lingual surfaces of the mandibular dentition [12].

One study [13] aimed to verify the force threshold that causes displacement of the maxillary central incisor teeth. Their findings indicated that the forces caused by the orofacial organs can initiate a dental displacement of the incisors.

Thus, gentle pressure, but continuous, exerted by the tongue against the teeth is able to move them, producing negative effects on the occlusion [14]. The resting tongue posture has a long duration, many hours during 1 day, which makes it

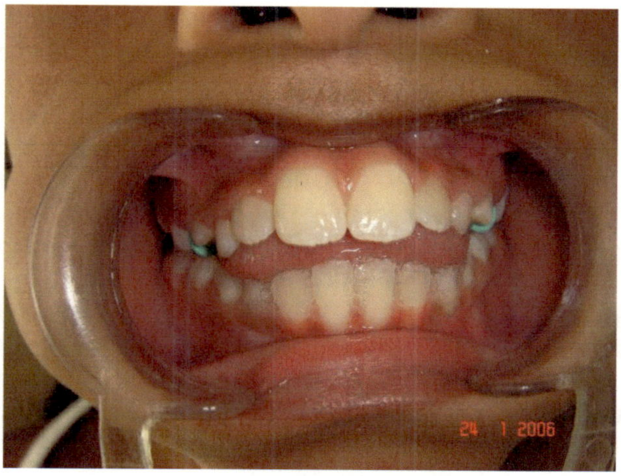

Figure 1.
Tongue rest in anterior position and open bite malocclusion.

clinically important, and can impede eruption of the incisors, causing and maintaining the anterior open bite [2].

Individuals who rest their tongue in anterior position may have the position of the teeth affected (**Figure 1**). On the other hand, the tongue interposition during swallowing has a very short duration to have an impact on dental position. In a typical swallowing, the pressure made by the tongue lasts about 1 second. Normal individuals swallow about 800 times a day when awake, which totals only a few minutes, which would be insufficient to affect the intraoral balance [15].

Furthermore, the low position of the tongue can promote the eruption of the back teeth and cause constriction of the upper arch in the absence of the tongue on the palate [16]. Some authors have confirmed that the inadequate position of the tongue is one of the main causes of the occurrence of oral recurrences with regard to the maintenance of occlusal stability [2, 17, 18].

Many clinicians feel that pressures exerted by tongue prevent teeth from erupting in patients with open bite malocclusion. This view amounts to an extension of the equilibrium theory to the vertical plane of space [19]. Lower lip resting pressure affects more the position of the upper incisors rather than the upper lip (**Figure 2**). In some studies, high lip line was shown as the reason behind the retroclined position of the upper incisors, while in others, the hyperactive lip or mentalis muscle were shown as the reason [20].

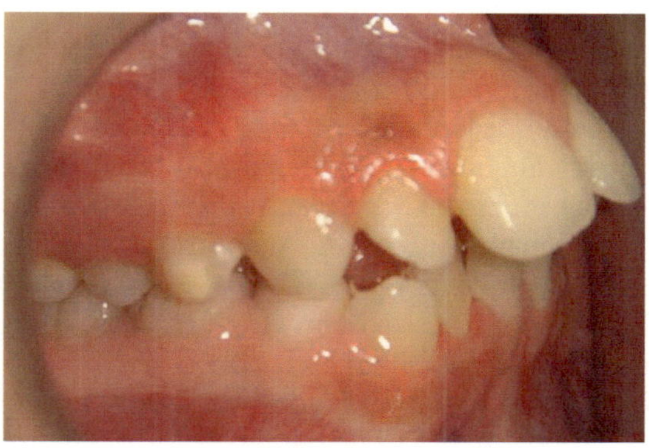

Figure 2.
Teeth position influenced by lower lip.

To test the hypothesis that an imbalance in buccolingual pressure plays a role in dental compensation of the molars and asymmetry in the mandibular dental arch, researchers [21] compared the pressure of cheek and tongue between the shifted and nonshifted side in 12 individuals with facial asymmetry. Asymmetry was defined as 4 mm or more deviation of the midline in the mandibular incisors. The results showed that regardless of the side, there were significant negative correlations between the buccolingual position of the mandibular first molars and cheek pressure and significant positive correlations between the buccolingual position of the first molars and tongue/cheek pressure ratio.

A study [22] compared a group of individuals with anterior open bite who did only orthodontic treatment and another group who did orthodontic treatment and orofacial myofunctional therapy. This therapy exercises the muscles and promotes modification on orofacial functions. They observed that participants who only did orthodontic treatment presented more occlusion recurrence compared to those who also did therapy. This finding indicates that when the form is altered, often the function will also be and that the correction of the former will not necessarily lead to the adequacy of the latter.

3. Different types of tooth have specific function on mastication

The teeth are structures that together with the gums, the tongue, the palate, the palatine tonsils, and the oral cavity form the oral region. Teeth have many different functions, like:

- cutting, reducing, and mixing food with saliva during mastication;
- helping their own support in the dental alveoli, assisting the development and protection of the tissues that sustain them; and
- participating as an articulator in speech [23].

Humans have two generations of teeth, the deciduous (primary) dentition and the permanent (secondary) dentition. There are 20 teeth in the deciduous dentition with 10 in each jaw. There are 32 teeth in the permanent dentition with 16 in each jaw [23].

The characteristics of teeth define their functions in the oral cavity. The incisors have fine cutting margins, the canines have single prominent, cusps, the premolars have two cusps and molars have three or more cusps [23].

Humans have four maxillary incisors and four mandibular incisors, two central and two lateral in each jaw. The mandibular incisors are very similar in form and are usually smaller than the maxillary incisors. The incisors cut food, aid in articulation of speech, and support the upper lip [24].

There are four canines, one left and one right in each jaw. They are located at the corners of the dental arch and are often referred to as fangs. They are the longest of all permanent teeth from root to crown tip and usually have a single long root. The canines are the teeth responsible for cutting and piercing food and they also help to guide the jaws to occlude correctly, therefore protecting the posterior teeth from horizontal forces. They also play a role in preventing the appearance of premature aging by supporting the lips and facial muscles [24].

There are four maxillary and four mandibular premolars, two right and two left in each jaw. They only appear in the permanent dentition. Their crowns are shorter (cervico-occlusally) than the anterior tooth and have two cusps. The premolars work along with the molars to grind food and also assist the canines with cutting and slicing through food. They play a role in preventing the appearance of premature aging by maintaining the vertical dimension of the face and supporting the corners of the mouth and the cheeks [24].

There are six molars in each jaw in the permanent dentition and eight molars in the deciduous dentition, four in each jaw. The molar most anteriorly positioned is designed the "first molar," the one behind it, the second molar. In the permanent dentition, the tooth most posteriorly positioned is the third molar. The main function of molars is to grind food and maintain the integrity of the dental arch to avoid the other teeth from moving out of alignment. Like premolars, they also play a role in preventing the appearance of premature aging [24].

A literature review [25] concluded that the contraction of the muscles involved in mastication stimulates bone growth. The effect of food consistency on orofacial development suggests that a diet with harder textures is partly responsible for enhancing muscle and bone growth. That can be seen in subjects with thin masseters which generally have longer faces, due to the lack of both bone and muscle volume, while subjects with a thick masseter have a short lower anterior face. According to studies in animals [26, 27] and humans [28], a diet based in liquid and puree consistencies results in a size reduction of masseter and temporal muscles. This theory is supported by an author [29] who suggests that modern, softer foods are responsible for a failing chewing function and the stress on the growth process is often insufficient, causing functional atrophies of masticatory muscles and bone and, consequently, malocclusions.

4. Impact of mouth breathing on the dentition

Nasal breathing is important to ensure a functional environment for the harmonious craniofacial growth [30]. When breathing occurs continuously through the mouth, the craniofacial growth changes its pattern, leading to consequences as high and narrow hard palate, convex facial profile [31], increased vertical facial height [32] and malocclusion. A study carried out on 3017 children verified that mouth breathing is closely related to increased or reduced overjet, anterior or posterior crossbite, open bite, and displacement of contact points [30]. In another study [33] with 401 mouth breathers, posterior crossbite was detected in almost 30% of the sample during primary and mixed dentitions and in 48% in permanent dentition. This prevalence is higher than in the general population [34, 35]. Anterior open bite and Class II malocclusion were also highly prevalent in children during mixed and permanent dentitions [33].

The causes of mouth breathing includes anatomical predisposition and several pathologies, such as palatine and pharyngeal tonsils hypertrophy, septal deviation, allergic rhinitis, and nasal turbinate hypertrophy, among others. The literature showed no association between the type of obstruction and the presence of malocclusion [33] and there seems to be a similar effect on mandibular growth irrespective of the etiology of mouth breathing [32]. However a study verified that children with adenotonsillar hypertrophy have a higher lower posterior facial height than the children with isolated adenoid hypertrophy. An explanation to this fact is that the palatine tonsils, when hypertrophied, could occupy a huge space in the pharynx. Thus, children protruded their mandible in order to breathe better, stimulating the growth of mandible and increasing their lower posterior facial height [32].

Mouth breathing leads to muscle changes including lip incompetence [31, 36, 37]; low position of the tongue in the mouth floor [36, 37]; and lack of force of lips, tongue, and mandibular elevator muscles [31, 36]. The lack of orofacial muscle force and the posture alterations are strictly related. The individual keeps the tongue low to allow airflow to pass and this habitual posture causes a decrease in tongue tone, which contributes even more to the lower position of the tongue. The same happens with the lips. Postural alterations in soft tissues change the equilibrium of the pressure that they exert on teeth and facial bones, thus altering these structures.

The muscles that depress the jaw to open the mouth exert a backward pressure upon it, which displaces the mandible distally and retards its growth, causing a Class II malocclusion and a skeletal Class II profile with increased overjet. The tongue has an anterior and low position to allow the airflow through the mouth while the buccinator muscles exert pressure on the buccal surface of molars, but there is no pressure of the tongue on the lingual surface, so the maxillary arch and the palate get narrow. There is also lip dysfunction, characterized by shorter upper lip, eversion of lower lip, and hypofunction of both, with no lip sealing, (**Figure 3**), which causes an imbalance especially when tongue exerts a forward pressure on the incisors. The lower lip sometimes forces up under the upper incisor, increasing the overjet [30].

Mouth breathing also impacts the other stomatognathic functions, such as mastication and swallowing, indirectly impairing dentition development. The mouth breather tends to prefer soft food, that is easy to chew. Also, they tend to ingest fluids during mastication in order to help the process. The mastication of the mouth breather has a shorter duration with less masticatory cycles, because of the necessity to liberate the mouth to breathe [38]. Swallowing usually occurs with an atypical pattern, involving tongue protrusion against the incisors or lip interposition which contributes to maintain the overjet [33].

An author [39] pointed out to the irrefutable evidence of a significant genetic influence in many dental and occlusal variables. According to him, phenotype is the result of both genetic and environmental factors. Other authors, who investigated prevalence of malocclusion in mouth breathers, agree with the primary role of heredity in malocclusion in sagittal plane, with mouth breathing as secondary etiological factor to Class II development. According to them, mouth breathers have unbalanced muscular forces, which are not enough to change a strong Class I or III pattern into a Class II. However, some children have genetic tendency to develop a Class II occlusion. These children, depending on environmental stimuli, can become Class I or, if there is a factor like mouth breathing, can develop Class II [33]. In the same way, vertical and transversal dental relationship also has heredity as the major determinant, but environmental factors such as mouth breathing work as secondary causes of anterior open bite or posterior crossbite [33].

Sometimes, changing the breath mode to nasal is not enough to avoid the consequences on occlusion. For this reason, we recommend an early intervention on etiological factors of mouth breathing to prevent the development or worsening of malocclusion.

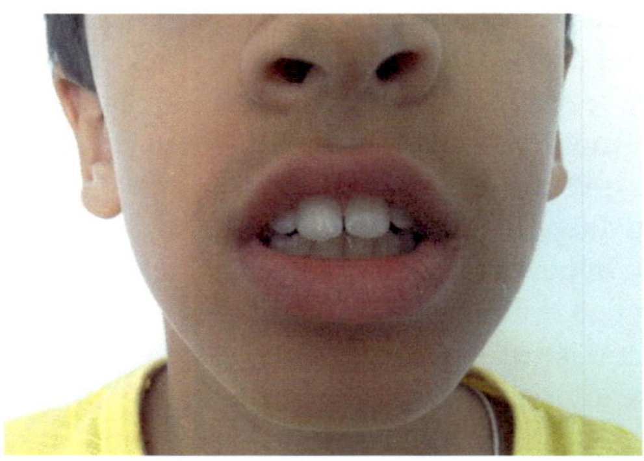

Figure 3.
Mouth breather with abnormal lip function, with no sealing.

5. Impact of oral habits on the dentition

Deleterious oral habits can interfere not only with the position of the teeth, but also with the normal skeletal growth pattern [30]. Pacifier sucking, bottle sucking, finger sucking, nail biting, and tongue thrusting are examples of deleterious oral habits which may result in long-term problems and can affect the stomatognathic system, leading to an imbalance between external and internal muscle forces. The most frequent occlusion alterations caused by oral habits are protrusion of the upper incisors [30], anterior open bite [30, 40], and posterior crossbite [40, 41]. The consequences are dependent on the nature, age of initiation, intensity, frequency and duration of habits, as well as individual biological and genetic features [30].

A study [40] concluded that children with non-nutritive sucking activity and accustomed to using a bottle had more than double the risk of posterior crossbite right from the primary dentition. The low position of the tongue due to sucking, with lack of thrust of the tongue on the palate and increased activity of the muscles of the cheeks, causes an alteration of muscle pressure on the upper arch resulting in the posterior crossbite [40]. Breastfeeding seems to have a protective effect on development of posterior crossbite. A study found a low prevalence of posterior crossbite in breastfed children, even when they have non-nutritive sucking activity [40]. This happens because the mechanism of sucking is different in these two methods of infant feeding. During breastfeeding, lips and tongue apex squeeze the areola where the lactiferous sinuses are located, the tongue compresses the soft breast nipple against the palate using a peristaltic-like motion. In bottle feeding, the tongue acts in a piston-like motion compressing the artificial teat against the palate, with higher force exerted by cheeks [40]. Breastfeeding has also a protective effect on development of artificial sucking habits [41].

Finger sucking generally results in anterior open bite and increased overjet with labial inclination of the upper incisors. The influence of finger sucking on teeth position depends on the position of the finger during the habit. There are two main types of finger sucking (**Figure 4**). The typical type is thumb sucking with the ventral side of the finger facing the palate and maxillary incisors. The thumb acts as a lever, forcing the maxilla forward. The second type, less common, is sucking with the dorsal side of the finger facing upward. In this case, the finger or fingers are passive and the effect is similar to that of the pacifier [42].

The use of pacifier before the teeth have erupted can hinder the full eruption of the primary incisors as well as the growth of the alveolar processes, resulting in anterior open bite, which can be worse at the time of eruption of the permanent incisors if the habit persists. When the pacifier is tied together with more pacifiers

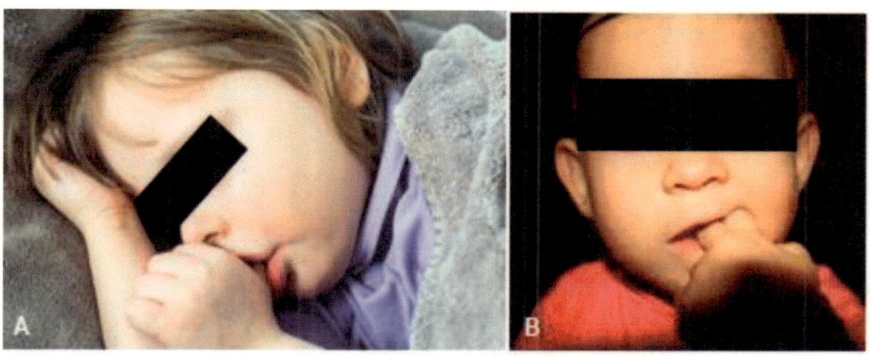

Figure 4.
(A) Child sucking with the ventral side of the finger. (B) Child sucking with the dorsal side of the finger.

or with other objects, the extra weight acts as a lever, affecting the dentition in a similar way as finger sucking [42].

If the pacifier is kept in the mouth for extend periods, the tongue will stay in a lower and anterior position, reducing the palatal support of the primary canines and molars against the pressure exerted by cheeks and increasing lateral pressure on the lower canines and first molars. This position can result in a narrower upper arch and wider lower arch, creating a posterior crossbite [41, 42].

A common question is whether spontaneous resolution of the malocclusion occurs when deleterious oral habits stop. This question, however, remains unanswered because each individual has a different genetic predisposition. On the other hand, some authors have found that anterior openbite and posterior crossbite were associated with habits in children with age 36 months or more. Sustained pacifier habits in children with 24–47 months of age were associated with anterior openbite and Class II molar relationships, while digit habits in children with 60 months of age or longer were associated with anterior openbite [43]. The author concluded that the risk for malocclusion appears to increase with longer habit duration, and that, while in some cases malocclusions resolve soon after the habits are discontinued, in other cases the malocclusions persist [43]. For this reason, we strongly recommend breastfeeding as a protection against the development of oral habits and, if they are already installed, an early intervention in order to decrease their frequency, intensity, and duration and finally to encourage the child to stop those oral habits.

6. Bruxism and tooth wear

Tooth wear (**Figure 5**) is a condition that leads to the loss of dental hard tissues (enamel and dentine) changing size and/or shape of tooth, with multifactorial causes. It can be divided into mechanical and chemical wear. Mechanical wear can happen with attrition of tooth-to-tooth contact made on mastication or bruxism, and it also happens with abrasion, made by oral hygiene procedures and habits such as nail-biting and biting objects. Chemical wear is the erosion that happens due to the action of extrinsic acids on the tooth [44].

Extensive tooth wear (TW) can be caused by chemical factors, mechanical factors, or a combination of both. The most common factors associated with TW were daily functions (e.g., chewing); oral habits (e.g., bruxism, nail biting); having a diet full of acid foods or some diseases that involve acids from the own body (e.g., gastric reflux); and also medicines, stress, and salivary dysfunctions [45].

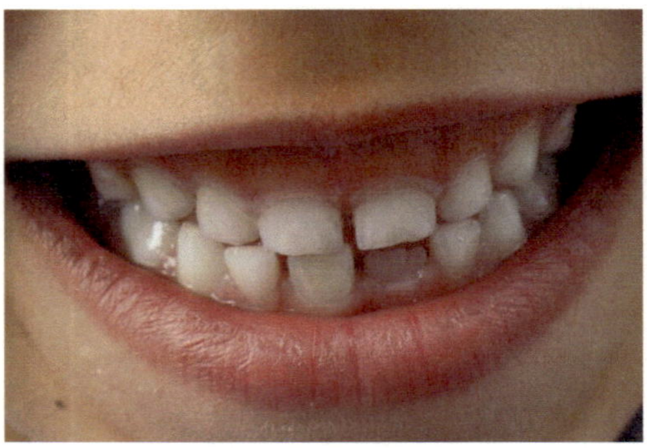

Figure 5.
Child with tooth wear.

TW has become more prevalent and severe in developed countries due to changes in lifestyle and nutritional habits, and also the population is aging and retaining teeth for longer time [45].

As mentioned above, tooth wear and bruxism have a close relationship. According to the international consensus on the assessment of bruxism, sleep bruxism is a rhythmic or non rythmic masticatory muscle activity during sleep. Awake bruxism is a masticatory muscle activity during wakefulness that is characterized by repetitive or sustained tooth contact and/or by bracing or thrusting of the mandible. Both cannot be considered as a movement or sleep disorder in otherwise healthy individuals. Bruxism is not a disorder in healthy individuals but might be defined as a motor behavior with multifactorial causes. It can be a risk factor for negative oral health consequences, but can also be a potential protective factor when associated with other clinical conditions (e.g., sleep apnea or other sleep disorders) or symptoms (e.g., xerostomia) without a cause-and-effect relationship. Or it can be harmless behavior (not risk or protective factor) in terms of consequences [46].

The main masticatory muscles are masseter and temporalis. They are responsible for elevating the jaw and pressing teeth against each other on the mastication function.

Non-instrumental approaches for assessing bruxism include self-report and clinical inspection. It is important to investigate the presence of sleep or awake bruxism, and how often it happens. Clinical signs of bruxism include masticatory muscle hypertrophy, indentations on the tongue or lip, and/or a linea alba on the inner cheek. However, these signs can also be present on orofacial myofunctional disorders, such as atypical swallowing. Damage to the dental hard tissues, repetitive failures of restorative work, or mechanical wear of the teeth may also be indicators of awake bruxism and sleep bruxism. Yet, it does not assure that it is still active. A bruxism in the past would have left the same signs on the teeth [46].

A study with 440 school children found prevalence of probable sleep bruxism in 40.0% of them. It was more prevalent between children with history of nail biting or biting objects [47].

A population-based study made in Brazil showed prevalence of possible bruxism in 8.1% of the adults, and it was associated with higher level of education and psychological stress [48].

A research investigated the correlation between the masseter electromyographic (EMG) activity during sleep and tooth wear in 41 healthy adults. The individuals underwent a two-night in-home evaluation of EMG activity of muscle masseter and a tooth wear evaluation. The canines and mandibular incisors were the teeth with the highest wear scores. No significant correlation was found between tooth wear and sleep masseter muscle activity. They discussed that even if tooth wear was a consequence of bruxism, it could not be used as a diagnostic tool for sleep bruxism, because the wear is irreversible and bruxism is an unstable phenomenon that may have happened in the past, but stopped [49].

A review was made to investigate the relationship between bruxism and occlusion. The conclusion was that neither occlusal interferences nor factors related to the anatomy of the orofacial skeleton had any evidence available to suggest their involvement in the etiology of bruxism. On the other side, psychosocial and behavioral factors were related as important in the etiology of bruxism [50].

Another review investigated to what extent bruxism is associated to musculoskeletal signs and symptoms. The data from the studies included were very heterogeneous, considering age of participants, type of bruxism (during sleep or wakefulness), and methodology of diagnosis. Most of the studies based the diagnosis of bruxism only on information given by self report, which is not the most reliable information. Besides that, it was concluded that bruxism is somehow associated with musculoskeletal symptoms. There is no support for a linear causal relationship, but the literature points more to a multifactorial relationship [51].

Besides bruxism, other factors can change tooth aspect and morphology. A systematic review with meta-analysis investigated if eating disorders increase the risk of tooth erosion. Fourteen papers from eight databases were included in the meta-analysis. It showed that patients with eating disorders had 12.4 times more risk of tooth erosion than controls, and patients with eating disorders who self-induced vomiting had 19.6 times more risk of tooth erosion than those patients who did not self-induce vomiting. So it is an important aspect that dentists should be aware of, to prevent disturbs that can be serious [52].

7. Conclusion

It is a fact that orofacial postural alterations can significantly influence the development of the occlusion. So, myofunctional and dentoocclusal changes are quite related. Thus, for the maintenance of correct dental positioning, the balance between orofacial muscular forces becomes primordial. The work of dentistry and speech therapy (orofacial myology) together brings more effective results, since the first professional will be responsible for the improvement of the occlusal structures and the second for the balance of the dynamic structures, especially the tongue, due to its great impact on the occlusion.

Author details

Amanda Valentim*, Renata Furlan, Mariana Amaral and Fernanda Martins
Federal University of Minas Gerais, Belo Horizonte, MG, Brazil

*Address all correspondence to: amandafvalentim@gmail.com

References

[1] Valentim AF. Avaliação da força sofrida pelos dentes com a ação de lábios e língua [dissertação]. Belo Horizonte (MG): Universidade Federal Minas Gerais; 2012

[2] Justus R. Correction of anterior open bite with spurs: Long-term stability. World Journal of Orthodontics. 2001;**2**(3):219-231

[3] Proffit WR, Fields HW Jr, Sarver DM. A Etiologia dos problemas ortodônticos. In: Proffit WR, Fields HW Jr, Sarver DM, editors. Ortodontia Contemporânea. 4th ed. Rio de Janeiro: Elsevier; 2007. pp. 121-153

[4] Douglas CR. Fisiologia geral do sistema estomatognático. In: Douglas CR, editor. Fisiologia aplicada à fonoaudiologia. 2nd ed. Guanabara Koogan: Rio de Janeiro; 2006. pp. 270-282

[5] Valentim AF, Furlan RMMM, Perilo TVC, Berbert MCB, Motta AR, Casas EBL. Evaluation of the force applied by the tongue and lip on the maxillary central incisor tooth. Codas. 2014;**26**(3):235-240

[6] Menezes LF, Neto AMR, Paulino CEB, Laureano Filho JR, Studant-Pereira LM. Pressão da língua em pacientes com má-oclusão classe II e III. Revista Cefac. 2018;**20**(2):166-174

[7] Silva Filho OG, Garib DG, Lara TS. Ortodontia interceptativa Protocolo de tratamento em duas fase. Artes médicas: São Paulo; 2013

[8] Stahl F, Grabowski R, Gaebel M, Kundt G. Relationship between occlusal findings and orofacial myofunctional status in primary and mixed dentition. Part II: Prevalence of orofacial dysfunctions. Journal of Orofacial Orthopedics. 2007;**68**(2):74-90

[9] Grabowski R, Kundt G, Stahl F. Interrelation between occlusal findings and orofacial myofunctional status in primary and mixed dentition part III: Interrelation between malocclusions and orofacial dysfunctions. Journal of Orofacial Orthopedics. 2007;**68**(6):462-476

[10] Motta AR, Duarte LIM, Migliorucci RR, TVC P. Vocabulário técnico científico em Motricidade Orofacial. In: Rahal A, Motta AR, Fernandes AG, Cunha DA, Migliorucci RR, Felix GB, editors. Manual de Motricidade Orofacial. 1st ed. São José, dos Campos: Pulso; 2014. pp. 77-122

[11] Hanson ML, Barret RH. Fundamentos da miologia orofacial. Rio de Janeiro: Enelivros; 1995

[12] Christiansen RL, Evans CA, Sue SK. Resting tongue pressures. The Angle Orthodontist. 1979;**49**(2):92-97

[13] Lear CSC, Flanagan JB, Moorrees CFA. The frequency of deglutition in man. Archives of Oral Biology. 1965;**10**(1):83-99

[14] Artese A, Drummond S, Nascimento JM, Artese F. Criteria for diagnosing and treating anterior open bite with stability. Dental Press Journal of Orthodontics. 2011;**16**(3):136-161

[15] Proffit WR, Ackerma JL, Sinclair PM, Thomas PM, Tulloch JFC. Ortodontia Contemporânea. 2nd ed. Rio de Janeiro: Guanabara Koogan; 1995

[16] Proffit WR. Equilibrium theory revisited: Factors influencing position of the teeth. The Angle Orthodontist. 1978;**48**(3):175-186

[17] Cheng CF, Peng CL, Chiou HY, Tsai CY. Dentofacial morphology and tongue function during swallowing. American Journal of Orthodontics and Dentofacial Orthopedics. 2002;**122**(5):491-499

[18] Mendes ACS, Costa AA, Nerm K. O papel da fonoaudiologia na ortodontia e na odontopediatria: avaliação do conhecimento dos odontólogos especialistas. Revista Cefac. 2005;**7**(1):60-67

[19] Wallen TR. Vertically directed forces and malocclusion: A new approach. Journal of Dental Research. 1974;**53**(5):1015-1021

[20] Partal I, Aksu M. Changes in lips, cheeks and tongue pressures after upper incisor protusion in class II division 2 malocclusion: A prospective study. Progress in Orthodontics. 2017;**18**:29

[21] Takada J, Takashi O, Myamato JJ, Yokota T, Moriyama K. Association between intraoral pressure and molar position and inclinatiom in subjects with facial asymmetri. European Journal of Orthodontics. 2010;**33**:243-249

[22] Smithpeter J, Covell D Jr. Relapse of anterior open bites treated with orthodontic appliances with and without orofacial myofunctional therapy. American Journal of Orthodontics and Dentofacial Orthopedics. 2010;**137**:605-614

[23] Moore KL, Dalley AF, Agur AMR. Anatomia orientada para a clínica. 7th ed. Rio de Janeiro: Guanabara Koogan; 2014. pp. 919-925

[24] Dental hygiene. In: Primal Pictures. London: Informa UK Limited; 2019. Available from: http://wwwanatomy-tv.ez27.periodicos.capes.gov.br/html5ui_2018/#/product/dental_hygiene/release/2018_04/

[25] Le Révérend BJ, Edelson LR, Loret C. Anatomical, functional, physiological and behavioral aspects of the development of masticaion in early childhood. The British Journal of Nutrition. 2014;**111**(3):403-414

[26] Ikeda K. Development of jaw muscles' function in rats fed a kneaded diet. Orthod Waves Journal of the Japanese Orthodontic Society. 1998;**57**:163-172

[27] Ciochon RL, Nisbett RA, Corruccini RS. Dietary consistency and craniofacial development related to masticatory function in minipigs. Journal of Craniofacial Genetics and Developmental Biology. 1997;**17**:96-102

[28] Larsson E. Orthodontic aspects on feeding of young children: 1. A comparison between Swedish and NorwegianSami children. Swedish Dental Journal. 1998;**22**:117-121

[29] Limme M. The need of efficient chewing function in young children as prevention of dental malposition and malocclusion. Archives de Pédiatrie. 2010;**17**:S213-S219

[30] Grippaudo C, Paolantonio EG, Antonini G, Saulle R, La Torre G, Deli R. Association between oral habits, mouth breathing and malocclusion. Acta Otorhinolaryngologica Italica. 2016;**36**:386-394

[31] Costa M, Valentim AF, Becker HMG, Motta AR. Findings of multiprofessional evaluation of mouth breathing children. Revista Cefac. 2015;**17**(3):864-878

[32] Sousa JBR, Anselmo-Lima WT, Valera FCP, Gallego AJ, Matsumoto MAN. Cephalometric assessment of the mandibular growth pattern in mouth-breathing children. International Journal of Pediatric Otorhinolaryngology. 2005;**69**:311-317

[33] Souki BQ, Pimenta GB, Souki MQ, Franco LP, Becker HMG, Pinto JA. Prevalence of malocclusion among mouth breathing children: Do expectations meet reality? International Journal of Pediatric Otorhinolaryngology. 2009;**73**:767-773

[34] Thilander B, Pena L, Infante C, Parada SS, Mayorga C. Prevalence of malocclusion and orthodontic treatment need in children and adolescents in Bogota, Colombia. An epidemiological study related to different stages of dental development. European Journal of Orthodontics. 2001;**23**:153-167

[35] Petren S, Bondemark L, Soderfeldt B. A systematic review concerning early orthodontic treatment of unilateral posterior crossbite. The Angle Orthodontist. 2003;**73**:588-596

[36] Valera FC, Travitzki LV, Mattar SE, Matsumoto MAN, Elias AM, Anselmo-Lima WT. Muscular, functional and orthodontic changes in preschool children with enlarged adenoids and tonsils. International Journal of Pediatric Otorhinolaryngology. 2003;**67**:761-770

[37] Cattoni DM, Fernandes FDM, Di Francesco RC, Latorre MRDO. Characteristics of the stomatognathic system of mouth breathing children: Anthroposcopic approach. Pró-Fono: Revista de Atualização Científica. 2007;**19**(4):347-351

[38] Silva MAA, Natalini V, Ramires RR, Ferreira LP. Comparative analysis of mastication in children with nasal and mouth breathing with first teething. Revista Cefac. 2007;**9**(2):190-198

[39] Mossey PA. The heritability of malocclusion. Part 2. The influence of genetics in malocclusion. British Journal of Orthodontics. 1999;**26**:195-203

[40] Viggiano D, Fasano D, Monaco G, Strohmenger L. Breast feeding, bottle feeding and non-nutritive sucking; effects on occlusion in deciduous dentition. Archives of Disease in Childhood. 2004;**89**:1121-1123

[41] Larsson E. Sucking, chewing and feeding habits and the development of crossbite: A longitudinal study of girls from birth to 3 years of age. The Angle Orthodontist. 2001;**71**:116-119

[42] Larsson E, Bishara S. Pacifier- and digit-sucking habits. The Canadian Journal of Dental Hygiene. 2007;**41**:23-29

[43] Warren JJ, Slayton RL, Bishara SE, et al. Effects of nonnutritive sucking habits on occlusal characteristics in the mixed dentition. Pediatric Dentistry. 2005;**27**:445-450

[44] Wetselaar P, Lobbezoo F. The tooth wear evaluation system: A modular clinical guideline for the diagnosis and management planning of worn dentitions. Journal of Oral Rehabilitation. 2016;**43**(1):69-80

[45] Hammoudi W, Trulsson M, Smedberg J, Svensson P. Phenotypes of patients with extensive tooth wear—A novel approach using cluster analysis. Journal of Dentistry. 2019;**82**:22-29

[46] Lobezoo F, Kato T, Ahlberg J, et al. International consensus on the assessment of bruxism: Report of a work in progress. Journal of Oral Rehabilitation. 2018;**45**:1-8

[47] Drumond CL, Ramos-Jorge J, Vieira-Andrade RG, Paiva SM, Serra-Negra JMC, Ramos-Jorge ML. Prevalence of probable sleep bruxism and associated factors in Brazilian schoolchildren. International Journal of Paediatric Dentistry. 2018;**29**(2):221-227

[48] Pontes LDS, Prietsch SOM. Sleep bruxism: Population based study in people with 18 years or more in the city of Rio Grande, Brazil. Revista Brasileira de Epidemiologia. 2019;**22**:e190038

[49] Manfredini D, Lombardo L, Visentin A, Arreghini A, Siciliani G. Correlation between sleep-time masseter muscle activity and tooth wear: An electromyographic study. Journal of

Oral & Facial Pain and Headache. 2019;**33**(2):199-204

[50] Lobbezoo F, Ahlberg J, Manfredini D, Winocur E. Are bruxism and the bite causally related? Journal of Oral Rehabilitation. 2012;**39**(7):489-501

[51] Baad-Hansen L, Thymi M, Lobbezoo F, Svensson P. To what extent is bruxism associated with musculoskeletal signs and symptoms? A systematic review. Journal of Oral Rehabilitation. 2019;**46**(9):845-861

[52] Hermont AP, Oliveira PAD, Martins CC, Paiva SM, Pordeus IA, Auad SM. Tooth erosion and eating disorders: A systematic review and meta-analysis. PLoS One. 2014;**9**(11):e111123

Chapter 2

Embryological Development of Human Molars

Fatiha Rhrich and Hakima Aghoutan

Abstract

Dental development is a complex process by which teeth from embryonic cells grow and erupt into the mouth. It is governed by epithelio-mesenchymal interactions. The biological mechanism is the same for all teeth; however, epithelial signaling and homeogenous combinatorics are different from one type of tooth to another. The primary dental blade splits into the vestibular and primary dental blades opposite to the mesenchymal condensation. During dental development, three successive stages are described: bud, cup, and bell. The secondary dental blade responsible for the formation of germs in permanent teeth is formed from the primary dental blade in the bell stage. For the central incisor, lateral incisor, canine, first temporary molar, and second temporary molar, each primary dental blade gives rise to a single secondary dental blade for the corresponding permanent tooth. On the other hand, the primary dental blade of the second temporary molar will cause the formation of four secondary dental blades that will cause the formation of permanent germs of the second premolar, the first permanent molar, the second permanent molar, and the third permanent molar. The objective of this chapter is to focus on the cellular and molecular mechanisms explaining the normal development of molars by presenting the different current data and theories of science illustrating the human molar embryological development.

Keywords: tooth development, molar, morphological appearance, molecular regulation, epithelial-mesenchymal interaction

1. Introduction

Teeth are a topic of interest to paleontologists because they are very well preserved. As a matter of fact, the dental remains have made it possible to study the evolution of mammals by analyzing their morphology. In developmental biology, the mouse model is an interesting model for studying dental development.

Humans have two dentitions (temporary and permanent) and different types of teeth, incisor, canine, premolar, and molar with different morphologies, whereas mice only have two types (incisor and molar) separated by a diastema from which the incisors have unlimited growth. Despite these differences, the dental development process is similar in humans and mice, and regulatory phenomena have been maintained over the evolution.

Teeth, such as mammary glands, hair, and feathers, develop from two adjacent tissues: the epithelium and the mesenchyme, although they all have different morphologies. Indeed, during development, the specific shape of each organ is defined in relation to epithelial-mesenchymal proliferation and to all the changes that the epithelium undergoes [1].

The embryological aspect of the molars was addressed in order to clarify the etiopathogenic aspect and to adapt therapeutic attitudes according to the diagnosis.

The objective of this chapter is to address the embryology of human molars by focusing on its molecular and morphological characteristics.

2. Phylogenetic aspects

Teeth represent a new morphological feature of mammals [2, 3]. Molars are complex teeth able to become occluded. Interlocking intercuspation between upper and lower molars allows food to be crushed [4]. Evolutionary dietary radiations are related to the great diversity of the current mammalian molars. They are clarified in the fossil record, where new molar organizations are often related to significant line diversifications. Several theories have been advanced to explain the evolution of molars. Like all primates, Man is a placental mammal, and the ancestor of contemporary humans is *Homo sapiens*. For 200 million years, in Therian mammals, the molars have trigonodontal morphology; in other words, the three tubercles are arranged in a triangle [5].

In 1965, the discovery of a fossil of a lower molar made it possible to show that on this Therian branch around 135 million years ago, these molars already existed. They were called tribosphenic by Simpson in 1936 [6]. These mandibular molars have six tubercles, three of which are pointed, high, sharp, and are arranged in a triangle and distal position. The three others tubercles are lower and are arranged in a central basin to receive the main palatal tubercle of the opposite teeth that have only three cusps. The fact of having six tubercles is of physiological interest when taking food.

Nearly 110 million years ago, the oldest placental mammals had a dental formula with 52 teeth, including 3 molars in a decreasing series, the first being the largest. This primitive disposition is found in modern man.

Around 75 million years ago, with the dinosaurs extinction, other species invaded space, and the dental formula was reduced to 44 teeth for all placental mammals including the man.

In the Catarrhini, the loss of one incisor and two premolars leads to a dental formula with 32 teeth found in monkeys of the ancient world (Afro-Eurasia), the Hominids, and the contemporary Men. It has been recognized for 45 million years [7].

In the genus Homo, the 32-teeth morphology does not differ much from the modern men, except for the great variability in size. Root morphology may vary from one group to another. The reduction in the number of cusps observed in humans can be considered as a specialization trait and not as a step backward. However, the reduction in the dental formula in the placentals and primates mainly affected the incisors, premolars, and even canines but not the molars.

Wisdom tooth agenesis, especially mandibular agenesis, is often considered as a sign of evolution. On the other hand, the presence of supernumerary teeth or hypergenesis is explained as a return to ancestral forms

3. Morphological aspects

3.1 Formation of the odontogenic epithelium

The odontogenic epithelium is formed from the oral epithelium that lines the primary oral cavity called the "stomodeum." It appears as a localized thickening of the oral epithelium, and it is formed by several cellular layers resulting from a series of localized mitoses affecting the oral epithelium. The mitotic spindle of dividing cells is oriented perpendicular to the basal membrane that separates the epithelium from the ectomesenchyma.

3.2 Placement of the vestibular and primary dental blades

Epithelial thickening continues to proliferate and sinks into the underlying ectomesenchymal tissue forming a plunging wall (also called a primitive dental blade). This latter splits into two blades: vestibular and dental. The vestibular blade determines the formation of the buccal vestibule, which is the space between the cheek/lip and the dental arch.

3.3 Evolution of dental placodes

In humans, as in rats and mice, the dental blade will give birth to the dental placodes that will be at the origin of the formation of future dental germs. Dental placodes are cellular clusters attached to the dental blade by a net of epithelial cells called the primary dental blade. Each dental arch initially contains 10 dental placodes. From the primary dental blade develops the secondary dental blade, which is at the origin of the 16 permanent teeth per arch.

Each placode will undergo morphological changes that are described as three successive stages: bud stage, cup stage, and bell stage [1].

4. Placement of molar dental germs

Since the three molars are not preceded by temporary teeth, they evolve from the distal end of the initial dental blade, which proliferates in a posterior direction. The primary dental blade of the second temporary molar will cause the formation of four secondary dental blades. For each half of the arch, starting from the anterior area toward the posterior area, each of these four secondary dental blades will give the permanent germ of the following teeth: the first permanent molar, the second permanent molar, and the third permanent molar.

The secondary dental blades that are at the origin of the formation of the 1st and 2nd molar will orient themselves vertically as long as they have space that allows them to orient themselves in the mesenchyma. On the other hand, in most cases for the 3rd molar, orientation problems arise because there is not enough space for its secondary dental blade to be parallel to the other two blades [8].

All dental buds, with the exception of the second and third permanent molars, are present and begin to develop before birth [9]. The chronology of the appearance of molar germs remains variable according to the authors; however, it is often found that the germ of the first molar appears around the 4th or 5th month of intrauterine life. The one of the second molar appears around the 9th month or 1 year after birth.

The germ of the third molar does not appear until around 4 or 5 years of age. Mineralization begins between 7, 9, and 10 years, and the crown is completed between 12 and 16 years. The emergence in the oral cavity is between 17- and 21-year-olds; the tooth will then slide along the distal surface of the second molar to reach the occlusion level. Root building ends between the ages of 18 and 25 years. The place it has depends on the growth in the posterior region of the arch. The main activity of the dental blade is spread over a period of about 5 years. However, the dental blade near the third molar continues to be active until about 15 years of age [9].

A number of anomalies can occur during the development of the tooth. The development of excess dental blade can lead to an increase in the number of dental buds, resulting in too many teeth (supernumerary). A deficient dental blade can lead to a reduction in the number of teeth (hypodontia) [9].

5. Root formation

Molars are multiradiculated teeth. Indeed, the vast majority of the first maxillary molars have three roots. The second maxillary molar has more frequent variations in the number of roots than the first maxillary molar, and the first mandibular molar and the second have two roots in the majority.

Root formation or radiculogenesis or rhizagenesis is the development of the root pulpo-dentinary organ in close relationship with cemenesis, the outline of the dentoalveolar ligament and the construction of the alveolar bone. It begins when the final dimensions are acquired. The Hertwig epithelial sheath is at the origin of root formation, depending on their number, shape, and size [10].

As for the crown, root development is governed by interactions involving the Hertwig epithelial sheath, basement membrane, mesenchymal papilla, and dental follicle.

5.1 Formation of the Hertwig epithelial sheath

The Hertwig epithelial sheath originates from the reflection zone or cervical loop which is the place where the external and internal adamantin epitheliums (EAE and EAI) meet to form a double epithelial layer. Hertwig epithelial sheath has an annular structure surrounded by a basal membrane that separates it from the pulpal and follicular mesenchyma. This basement membrane has anchoring fibrils on the pulp side. The internal epithelium faces the papilla and the external epithelium faces the dental follicle. The Hertwig epithelial sheath will emit tongues in the centripetal direction that will fuse in the central region of the papilla and form rings from which the roots can be identified. The number of strips emitted is proportional to the number of roots that each molar can have. For example, for the molar which will have two roots, two tongues are formed, and after fusion of two rings, each of the two will be at the origin of the formation of a root. These two leaves remain attached and progress in the underlying connective tissue in the apical direction defining the future shape of the dental root [11].

Root elongation and tissue formation are related to the coordinated proliferation of sheath epithelial cells and surrounding mesenchymal cells [12].

5.2 Formation of root dentin, cement, and apex

Root dentin forms in parallel with the proliferation in the apical direction of the Hertwig sheath. The latter gradually induces odontoblastic differentiation. The pulp parenchyma cells close to the anchor fibrils differentiate into odontoblasts. These odontoblasts produce preentine, which mineralizes to form dentin. The cells of the outer dental epithelium forming the outer layer of the sheath do not differentiate into ameloblasts as is the case for the crown. Then, the basement membrane degrades, and the epithelial blade involutes and gradually dissociates.

Developmental defects of the Hertwig sheath at the apical third of the root are at the origin of the formation of the lateral canals following a stop of dentinogenesis at this site due to the nondifferentiation of pulp fibroblasts into odontoblasts.

The cells of the sheath can undergo three spells: some can form the "Malassez epithelial debris," others can die by apoptosis, while others can undergo epithelial-mesenchymal transformation.

As the sheath disintegrates, follicular cells near the surface of the root dentin differentiate into cementoblasts. These synthesize and deposit the cement matrix in contact with the dentin.

As the root development progresses, the epithelial ring forming the Hertwig epithelial sheath gradually shrinks as a result of a reduction in mitosis, thereby reducing the size of the root tube. This narrowing allows the development of one or more orifices (or foramina), which are the place where vascular and nervous elements intended for the pulp to pass through.

The development of the root ends with the construction of the apex, which is a slow process. In humans, for example, for the 1st permanent molar, this operation is performed until the age of 9–10 years. In the case of permanent teeth, this phenomenon lasts longer and requires more time than the development of the root itself.

6. Molecular aspects

6.1 Epithelial-mesenchymal interactions

In humans, dental development includes the morphogenesis of crowns and roots and results in the formation of the enamel organ, odontoblastic, ameloblastic, and cementoblastic differentiation. Huge advances in research have made it possible to understand the phenomena of molecular regulation of dental development.

Dental development follows a precisely controlled and regulated genetic program. The dental organ consists of an epithelial part that derives from the ectoderm and a mesenchymal part that derives from mesodermal cells on the one hand and cells from neural ridges on the other hand [13–16].

The dental organ develops from a communication between the epithelium and the underlying mesenchyma. The communication language has been preserved throughout the evolution. This communication between the epithelium and the mesenchyma is done through signaling molecules and growth factors [17–19].

The studies carried out on the mouse molar have enabled us to gather a body of knowledge with many similarities to those of humans. However, the experimental data obtained in animals can be extrapolated relatively reliably to understand what is actually happening in humans.

Several families have been described, including:

- TGF-beta (transforming growth factor beta) including BMP (bone morphogenetic proteins) activins and follistatin;

- FGF (Fibroblast growth factors);

- Hedgehog (only Sonic hedgehog (Shh) is known for its role in odontogenesis);

- Wnts [20–24].

These molecules send their message to the nucleus through the signaling pathways and receptors on the cell membrane surface. Transcription factors will then modulate the expression of different target genes and induce changes in cell response and behavior (**Figure 1**) [25].

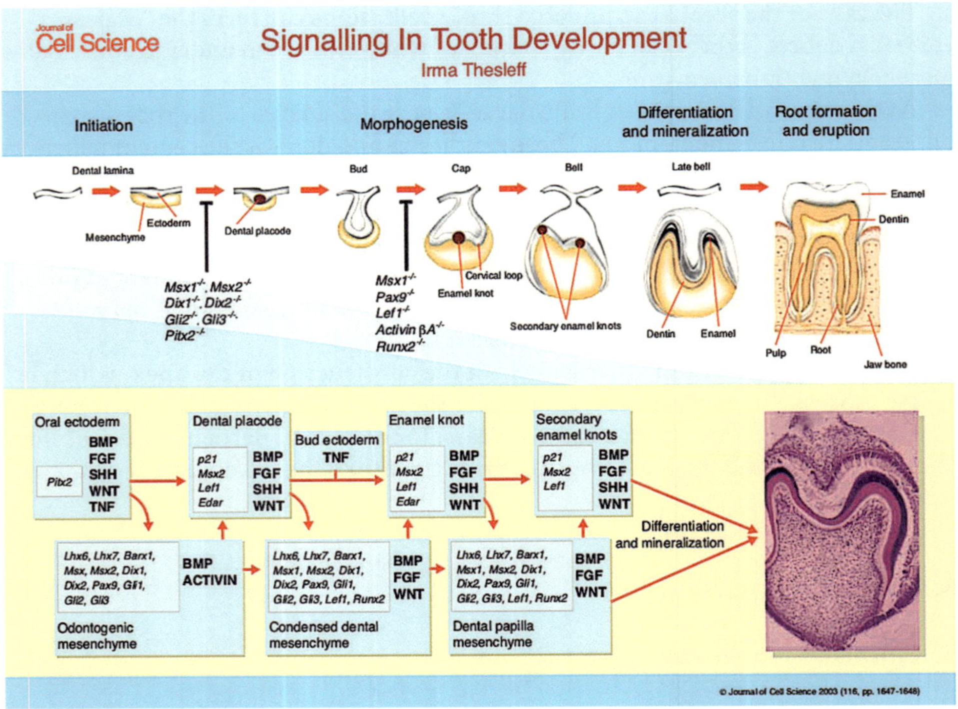

Figure 1.
Signaling in tooth development [25].

Genes represented in "light blue" colored squares or rectangles are responsible, when inactivated, for stopping dental development.

6.2 Determination of the dental region

It should be remembered that the odontogenic epithelium is formed at the first gill arch. The latter undergoes pharyngeal regionalization, resulting in the expression of Fgf8 and 9 (fibroblast growth factors 8 and 9) and Lhx-6 and -7 (LIM homeobox 6 and 7) in the oral part (rostral) and Gsc (goosecoid) in the aboral part (caudal). Indeed, the expression of Fgf8 in the odontogenic epithelium in the oral part of the first pharyngeal arch causes the expression of Lhx-7 in the underlying ectomesenchyma. In the aboral region, there is an important expression of Gsc in the ectomesenchyma. Gsc expression in the caudal region is not responsible for inhibiting Lhx-7 expression in this area; however, Lhx-7 expression in the rostral region will result in blocking Gsc gene expression in this.

In addition to Fgf8, a second BMP4 signaling molecule (bone morphogenetic protein 4) is expressed in the epithelium in the distal and therefore in the median region of the 1st arc.

The activation and inhibition of transcription factors allows the delimitation of the odontogenic territory by BMP4 and Fgf8a double signalling. (**Figure 2**) [19].

6.3 Determination of dental identity

Mammalian teeth are meristic series. The determination of different morphology was explained by two theories:

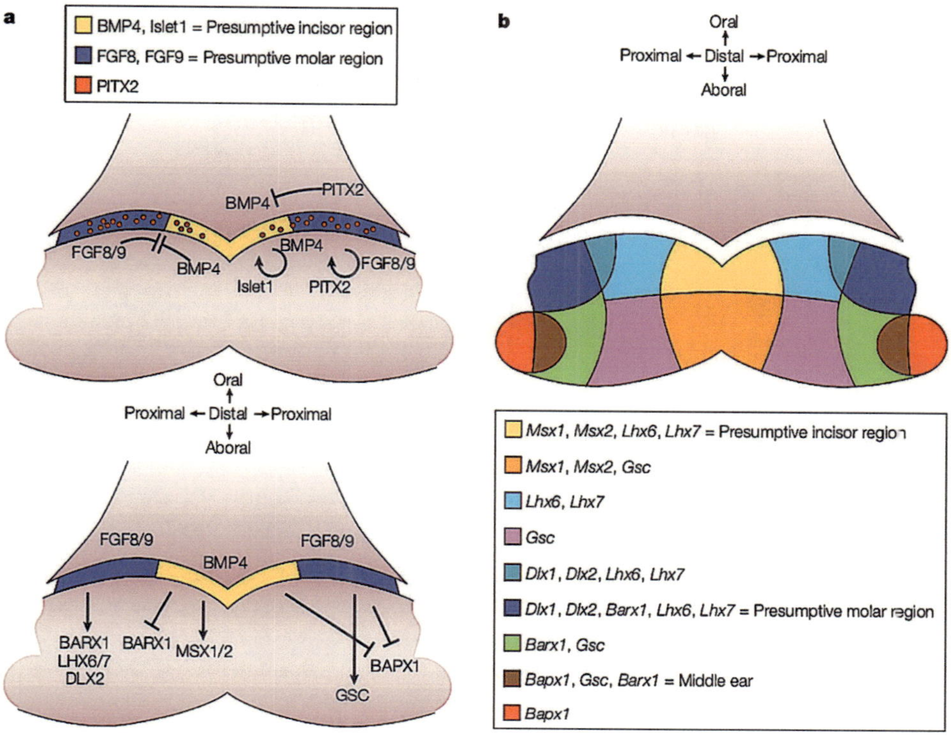

Figure 2.
Pattern of gene expression in the developing tooth [19]. (a) Signaling within the epithelium and between the epithelium and the mesenchyme at embryonic day (E) 10.5. The diagram shows an isolated mandibular arch. Positive autoregulatory loops and mutual repression within the epithelium lead to the formation of strict boundaries of gene expression, which sets up the presumptive incisor and molar fields. Members of the bone morphogenetic protein (BMP) and fibroblast growth factor (FGF) families of protein in the epithelium induce and inhibit the expression of various homeobox genes. This results in a complex pattern of gene expression in the mesenchyme, across both the proximal–distal and oral–aboral/rostral–caudal axes. (b) The odontogenic homeobox code model of dental patterning. The nested expression pattern of homeobox genes in the mandible produces a homeobox code that defines tooth type. Bapx1 (bagpipe homeobox gene 1 homolog); Barx1 (BarH-like homeobox 1); Dlx (distalless homeobox); Gsc (goosecoid); Lhx (LIM homeodomain genes); Msx (homeobox, msh-like); Pitx (paired-related homeobox gene).

- The gradient theory proposed by Butler [26] which stipulates the presence of morphogenetic fields and that the determination of the shape of the tooth is a function of its position in the field independent of local factors.

- The theory of clones proposed by Osborn [27] which stipulates that ectomesenchyma is already differentiated into three cellular clones, incisal, canine, and molar clones, before its migration. The proposal of this second concept suggested that the two theories are competing.

In 1995, the theory of odontogenic homeocode was developed by Sharpe [22], which represents a synthesis of the two theories: gradients and clones and shows that the latter two are complementary. These two concepts were explained in the light of the discovery of new genes and signaling molecules (**Figure 3**) [26–28].

The identity of each tooth, including the molars, is characterized by its homeocode, which represents the combination of homeogens that defines the position and identity of the tooth. Indeed, different homeogens are expressed by the neural crest cells of the ectomesenchyma under the instructive induction of the oral epithelial cells. These homeogens are divergent and therefore of the nonhox type.

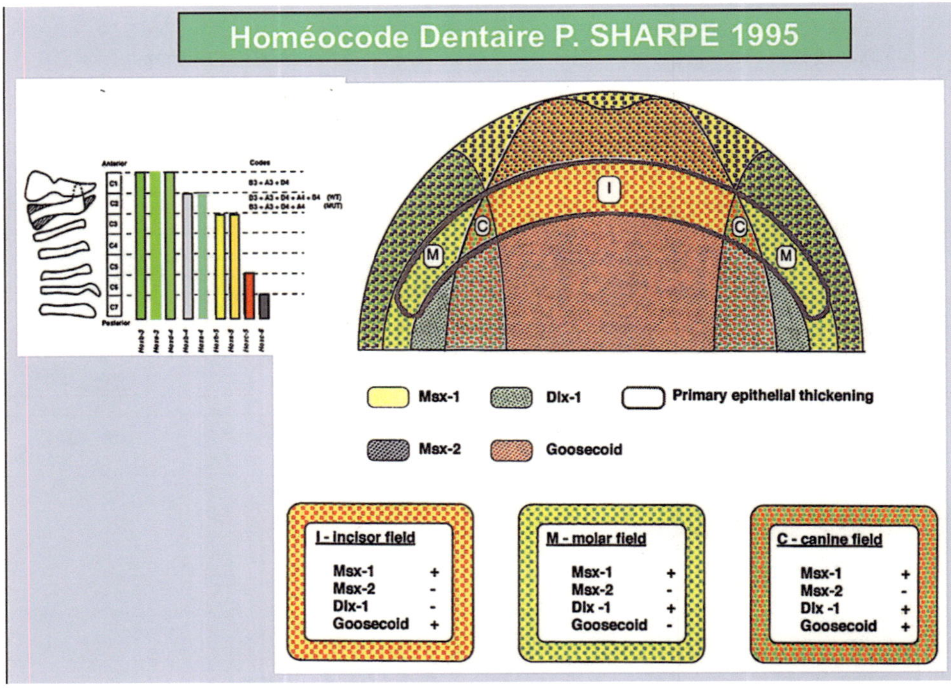

Figure 3.
(A) Regional field theory. (B) Clone theory. (C) Homeobox [26–28].

This odontogenic homeocode theory involves four homogenous genes: muscle segment homeodomain-homeobox 1 (Msx-1), muscle segment homeodomain-homeobox 2 (Msx-2), distal-less homeobox 1 (Dlx1), and goosecoide. In the molar sector, Msx-1 and Dlx-1 are expressed and Msx-2 and goosecoide are not expressed. In the canine sector, Msx-1, Msx-2, and goosecoide are expressed, and Dlx-1 is not expressed; in incisal sector, Msx-1 and goosecoide are expressed, Msx-2 and Dlx-1 are not expressed.

In the concept of morphogenetic fields, the consideration of various genetic factors and their epigenetic modulation influences dental development [29].

According to Mitsiadis' work in 2006, the three models, gradients, clones, and homeocodes, could be grouped into a single model to explain dental identity. Indeed, dental identity, including molars, is given by the presence of morphogenetic fields defined by the diffusion of growth factors. The odontogenic epithelium expresses gradients of signaling molecules that are mainly Fgf, Bmp, Shh, and Wint that will diffuse to the underlying mesenchymal tissue containing neural peak cells. Depending on the location and instruction received by these cells, they will express a set of divergent genes in relation to concentrations of signaling molecules. The locally defined tooth type is related to the locally expressed divergent homeogen combinatorics of these ridge cells (**Figure 4**) [30].

The Mitsiadis model combines the three concepts: morphogenetic fields, clone, and odontogenic homeocode.

These three models should be viewed as complementary rather than contradictory and propose that this unifying view can be extended into the clinical setting using findings on dental patterning in individuals with missing teeth. The proposals are compatible with the unifying etiological model developed by Brook in 1984 based on human epidemiological and clinical findings. Indeed, this new synthesis can provide a sound foundation for clinical diagnosis, counseling, and management of patients with various anomalies of dental development, as well as suggesting hypotheses for future studies.

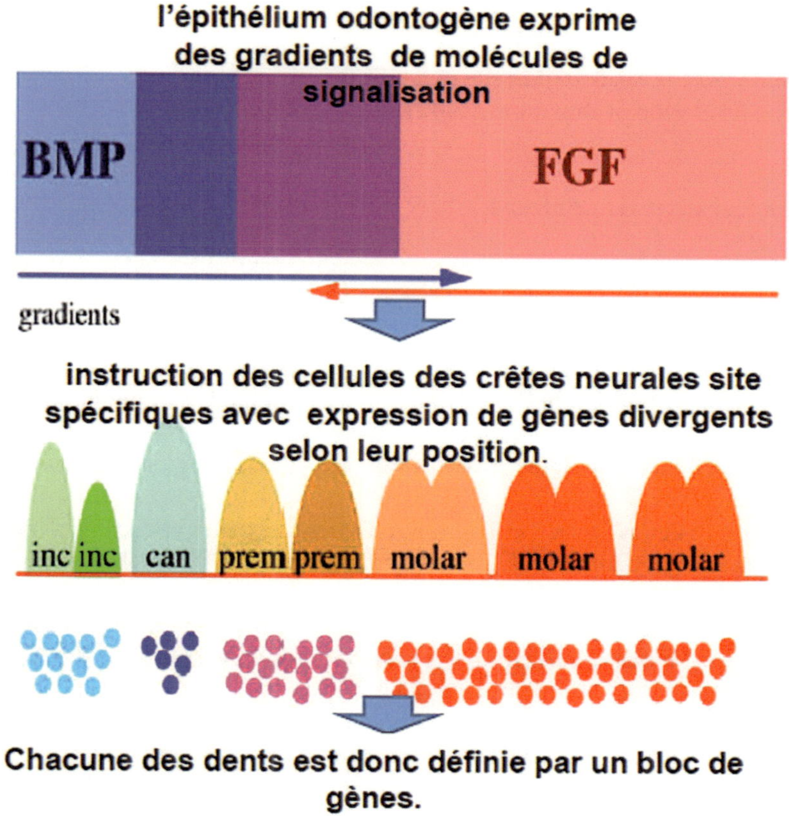

Figure 4.
Dental identity determination (adapted from Ref. [30]).

6.4 Molecular factors involved in root formation

The root development process involves a set of signaling cascades. Various growth factors, including BMPs (bone morphogenetic proteins), EGF (epidermal growth factor), IGF (insulin-like growth factor), FGF (fibroblast growth factor), transcription factors Msx1, Msx2, Runx-2, Sonic Hedgehog (Shh), enamel proteins (secreted by HGH cells), and other proteins such as follistatin and activin A, are involved in the root development process. Indeed, they are involved in the growth and/or differentiation of odontoblasts and cementoblasts and/or in the mineralization of dentin and/or cementum [21, 31–36].

7. Signaling center (primary and secondary enamel knots)

Dental morphology is controlled by an epithelial signaling center called the enamel node. The node of the enamel is a particular and transient histological structure formed by a cellular cluster that appears at the basal part of the internal dental epithelium. The node of the primary enamel is present in the dental germs of all types of teeth including incisors.

Because the enamel nodes link cell differentiation to morphogenesis, Thesleff suggests that the latter can be considered as central regulators of dental development [37].

During molar development, the node of the secondary enamel is formed during the bell stage at the location of future cusp areas. At this point, the expression of signaling molecules precedes the folding and growth of the dental epithelium [38, 39].

The Slit1 gene is expressed in the nodes of the primary and secondary enamel during the formation of molar cusps [40].

8. Genes and dental problems

The approaches provided by Line and Mitsiadis have advanced the clinic's understanding of dental identity establishment based on gradient, clone, and homeocode theories [29, 30].

The multifactorial model involving genetic, epigenetic, and environmental determinants has provided better explanations and helped to understand missing and supernumerary teeth in monozygotic twins [41].

In humans, dental problems are observed during pathologies of dental development or syndromes.

Mutations in genes known as divergent homeobox genes encoding transcription factors such as MSX1 and PAX9 (paired domain box gene 9) are at the origin of oligodontia. Indeed, a mutation in the homeobox of the MSX1 gene (substitution of an arginine by a proline in the homeodomain region) is associated with the agenesis of third molars, indicating the involvement of MSX1 in the dentition pattern [42–44].

Also, mutations in the PAX9 gene cause oligodontia characteristic of molars [45–48]. The severity of dental agenesis appears to be correlated with the ability of the mutated PAX9 protein to bind to DNA [49].

A misdirection mutation during the sequencing of the PAX9 gene may explain a different phenotype of hereditary oligodontia observed in humans, which affects not only molars but also other tooth lines; and is characterized by tooth small size in both types of dentition. This mutation is characterized by a replacement of the amino acid arginine by tryptophan in a region entirely preserved in all genes of the matched sequenced box [50].

In humans, Pitx2 expression deficiency associated with Rieger syndrome is characterized by oligodontia [51].

9. Conclusion

The biological process is the same for all teeth, including molars, regardless of their identity, but epithelial signaling and homeogenic combination differ from one tooth type to another.

The study of first molar of the mouse has allowed us to better understand and follow the stages of dental development in humans. The general pattern remains the same, unlike the training time, the complexity of the dental system, the presence of two types of teeth in humans, and unlimited incisors growth in mice.

The multidisciplinary approach between fundamental and clinical research is essential to clarify the relationship between molecular involvement and clinical manifestations.

Understanding the molecular mechanisms of dental anomalies, including those affecting human molars, helps to propose diagnostic hypotheses and thus to improve patient management.

Future research should focus on synergizing molecular and genetic approaches to further analyze the action mechanisms of key genes involved in the development of human molars.

Conflict of interest

The authors declare that they have no conflicts of interest with the contents of this article.

Author details

Fatiha Rhrich[1*] and Hakima Aghoutan[2]

1 Faculty of Dentistry, Department of Biology and Basic Subjects, Hassan II University, Casablanca, Morocco

2 Faculty of Dentistry, Dento-Facial Orthopedic Department, Hassan II University, Casablanca, Morocco

*Address all correspondence to: fatiharhrich@hotmail.com

References

[1] Pispa J, Thesleff I. Mechanisms of ectodermal organogenesis. Developmental Biology. 2003;**262**:195-205. DOI: 10.1016/S0012-1606(03)00325-7

[2] Tims HWM. The evolution of the teeth in the mammalia. Journal of Anatomy and Physiology. 1903;**37**(2):131-149. PMC1287046

[3] Luo ZX. Transformation and diversification in early mammal evolution. Nature. 2007;**450**(7172):1011-1019. DOI: 10.1038/nature06277

[4] Reisz RR. Origin of dental occlusion in tetrapods: Signal for terrestrial vertebrate evolution? Journal of Experimental Zoology Part B: Molecular and Developmental Evolution. 2006;**306B**(3):261-277. DOI: 10.1002/jez.b.21115

[5] Kermack DM, Kermack KA, Mussett F. The Welsh pantothere *Kuehneotherium praecursoris*. Journal of the Linnean Society of London, Zoology. 1968;**47**(312):407-423. DOI: 10.1111/j.1096-3642.1968.tb00519.x

[6] Kermack KA, Lees PM, Musset F. *Aegialodon dawsoni*, a new trituberculosectorial tooth from the Lower Wealden. Proceedings of the Royal Society of London—Series B: Biological Sciences. 1965;**162**(989):535-554. DOI: 10.1098/rspb.1965.0055

[7] Franzen JL et al. Complete primate skeleton from the middle eocene of Messel in Germany: Morphology and paleobiology. PLoS One. 2009;**4**(5):e5723. DOI :10.1371. John Hawks, University of Wisconsin

[8] Cohen-Lévy J, Cohen N. Permanent molar eruption anomalies: Differential diagnosis and radiographic investigations. Revue d'Orthopédie Dento-Faciale. 2015;**49**(3):217-230. DOI: 10.1051/odf/2014054

[9] Zohrabian VM, Poon CS, Abrahams JJ. Embryology and anatomy of the jaw and dentition. Seminars in Ultrasound, CT and MRI. 2015;**36**(5):397-406. Elsevier

[10] Ten Cate JM, Imfeld T. Dental erosion, summary. European Journal of Oral Sciences. 1996;**104**:241-244. DOI: 10.1111/j.1600-0722. 1996.tb00073.x

[11] Luan X, Ito Y, Diekwisch TG. Evolution and development of Hertwig's epithelial root sheath. Developmental Dynamics. 2006;**235**:1167-1180. DOI: 10.1002/dvdy.20674

[12] Cho MI, Garant PR. Development and general structure of the periodontium. Periodontology 2000. 2000;**24**:9-27. DOI: 10.1034/j.1600-0757.2000.2240102.x

[13] Chai Y, Jiang X, Ito Y, Bringas P Jr, Han J, Rowitch DH, et al. Fate of the mammalian cranial neural crest during tooth and mandibular morphogenesis. Development. 2000;**127**:1671-1679

[14] Cho SW, Hwang HJ, Kim JY, Song WC, SongHitoshi Yamamoto SJ, Jung HS. Lineage of non-cranial neural crest cell in the dental mesenchyme: Using a lacZ reporter gene during early tooth development. Journal of Electron Microscopy. 2003;**52**(6):567-571. DOI: 10.1093/jmicro/52.6.567

[15] Miletich I, Sharpe PT. Neural crest contribution to mammalian tooth formation. Birth Defects Research, Part C Embryo Today. 2004;**72**(2):200-212. DOI: 10.1002/bdrc.20012

[16] Rothová M, Feng J, Sharpe PT, Peterková R, Tucker AS. Contribution of mesoderm to the developing

dental papilla. The International Journal of Developmental Biology. 2011;**55**: 59-64. DOI: 10.1387/ijdb.103083mr

[17] Peters H, Balling R. Teeth. Where and how to make them. Trends in Genetics. 1999;**15**(2):59-65. DOI: 10.1016/S0168-9525(98)01662-X

[18] Thesleff I, Aberg T. Molecular regulation of tooth development. Bone. 1999;**25**:123-125. DOI: 10.1016/S8756-3282(99)00119-2

[19] Tucker A, Sharpe P. The cutting-edge of mammalian development; how the embryo makes teeth. Nature Reviews. Genetics. 2004;**5**(7):499-508. DOI: 10.1038/nrg1380

[20] Cobourne MT, Sharpe PT. Sonic hedgehog signaling and the developing tooth. In: Schatten GP, editors. Current Topics in Developmental Biology. 1st ed. 2005; 65: 255-287. ISBN: 9780080457833. Hardcover ISBN: 9780121531652

[21] Dassule HR, Lewis P, Bei M, Maas R, McMahon AP. Sonic hedgehog regulates growth and morphogenesis of the tooth. Development. 2000;**127**(22):4775-4785. PMID: 11044393

[22] Hardcastle Z, Hui CC, Sharpe PT. The Shh signaling pathway in early tooth development. Cellular and Molecular Biology. 1999;**45**(5):567-578. PMID: 10512189

[23] Nie X, Luukko R, Kettunen P. BMP signalling in craniofacial development. The International Journal of Developmental Biology. 2006;**50**:511-521. DOI: 10.1387/ijdb.052101xn

[24] Nie X, Luukko R, Kettunen P. FGF signalling in craniofacial development and developmental disorders. In: Scully C, editors. Oral Diseases. 2006;**12**(2):77-215. DOI: 10.1111/j.1601-0825.2005.01176.x

[25] Thesleff I. Epithelial-mesenchymal signalling regulating tooth morphogenesis. Journal of Cell Science. 2003;**116**:1647-1648. DOI: 10.1242/jcs.00410

[26] Butler PM. Dental merism and tooth development. Journal of Dental Research. 1967;**46**(5):845-850. DOI: 10.1177/00220345670460053801

[27] Osborn JW. Morphogenetic gradients: Fields versus clones. In: Butler PM, Joysey KA, editors. Development, Function and Evolution of Teeth. London: Academic Press; 1978. pp. 171-201

[28] Sharpe PT. Homeobox genes and orofacial development. Connective Tissue Research. 1995;**32**:1-4. DOI: 10.3109/03008209509013701

[29] Line SRP. Molecular morphogenetic fields in the development of human dentition. Journal of Theoretical Biology. 2001;**211**:67-75. DOI: 10.1006/jtbi.2001.2333

[30] Mitsiadis TA, Smith MM. How do genes make teeth to order through development? Journal of Experimental Zoology. Part B, Molecular and Developmental Evolution. 2006;**306**(3):177-182. DOI: 10.1002/jez.b.21104

[31] Aberg T, Wozney J, Thesleff I. Expression patterns of bone morphogenetic proteins (Bmps) in the developing mouse tooth suggest roles in morphogenesis and cell differentiation. Developmental Dynamics. 1997;**210**(4):383-396. DOI: 10.1002/(SICI)1097-0177(199712)210:4<383::AID-AJA3>3.0.CO;2-C

[32] Yamashiro T, Tummers M, Thesleff I. Expression of bone morphogenetic proteins and Msx genes during root formation. Journal of Dental

Research. 2003;**82**(3):172-176. DOI: 10.1177/154405910308200305

[33] Yamashiro T, Tummers M, Thesleff I. Modulation of epithelial cell fate of the root in vitro. Journal of Dental Research. 2007;**86**(11):1063-1067. DOI: 10.1177/154405910708601108

[34] Hammerschmidt M, Brook A, McMahon AP. The world according to to hedgehog. Trends in Genetics. 1997;**13**(1):14-21. DOI: 10.1016/S0168-9525(96)10051-2

[35] Koyama E, Wu CS, Shimo T, et al. Development of stratum intermedium and its role as a sonic hedgehog-signaling structure during odontogenesis. Developmental Dynamics. 2001;**222**(2):178-191. DOI: 10.1002/dvdy.1186

[36] Nakao A, Kajiya H, Fukushima H, et al. PTHrP induces notch signaling in periodontal ligament cells. Journal of Dental Research. 2009;**88**(6):551-556. DOI: 10.1177/002202203450509337899

[37] Thesleff I, Keranen S, Jernvall J. Enamel knots as signaling centers linking tooth morphogenesis and odontoblast differentiation. Advances in Dental Research. 2001;**15**:14-18. DOI: 10.1177/08959374010150010401

[38] Jernvall J, Kettunen P, Karavanova I, Martin LB, Thesleff I. Evidence for the role of the enamel knot as a control center in mammalian tooth cusp formation: Non-dividing cells express growth stimulating Fgf-4 gene. The International Journal of Developmental Biology. 1994;**38**:463-469

[39] Matalova E, Antonarakis GS, Sharpe PT, Tucker AS. Cell lineage of primary and secondary enamel knots. Developmental Dynamics. 2005;**233**:754-759. DOI: 10.1002/dvdy.20396

[40] Løes S, Luukko K, Kvinnsland IH, Kettunen P. Slit1 is specifically expressed in the primary and secondary enamel knots during molar tooth cusp formation. Mechanisms of Development. 2001;**107**(1-2):155-157. DOI: 10.1016/S0925-4773(01)00454-3

[41] Townsend G, Harris EF, Lesot H, Clauss F, Brook A. Morphogenetic fields within the human dentition: A new, clinically relevant synthesis of an old concept. Archives of Oral Biology. 2009;**54**(Suppl 1):S34-S44. DOI: 10.1016/j.archoralbio.2008.06.011

[42] Vastardis H, Karimbux N, Guthua SW, Seidman JG, Seidman CE. A human MSX1 homeodomain missense mutation causes selective tooth agenesis. Nature Genetics. 1996;**13**:417-421. DOI: 10.1038/ng0896-417

[43] Vastardis H. The genetics of human tooth agenesis: New discoveries for understanding dental anomalies. American Journal of Orthodontics and Dentofacial Orthopedics. 2000;**117**:650-656. DOI: 10.1016/S0889- 5406(00)70173-9

[44] Nieminen P, Kotilainen J, Aalto Y, Knuutila S, Pirinen S, Thesleff I. MSX1 gene is deleted in Wolf-Hirschhorn syndrome patients with oligodontia. Journal of Dental Research. 2003;**82**(12):1013-1017. DOI: 10.1177/154405910308201215

[45] Das P, Stockton DW, Bauer C, Shaffer LG, D'Souza RN, Wright TJ, et al. Haploinsufficiency of PAX9 is associated with autosomal dominant hypodontia. Human Genetics. 2002;**110**(4):371-376. DOI: 10.1007/s00439-002-0699-1

[46] Mostowska A, Biedziak B, Trzeciak WH. A novel mutation in PAX9 causes familial form of molar oligodontia. European Journal of Human Genetics. 2006;**14**:173-179

[47] Nieminen P, Arte S, Tanner D, Paulin L, Alaluusua S, Thesleff I, et al. Identification of a nonsense mutation in the PAX9 gene in molar oligodontia. European Journal of Human Genetics. 2001;**9**:743-746. DOI: 10.1038/sj.ejhg.5200715

[48] Stockton DW, Das P, Goldenberg M, D'Souza RN, Patel PI. Mutation of PAX9 is associated with oligodontia. Nature Genetics.2000 ;24 :18-19. DOI:10.1007/s00439-002-002-0699-1

[49] Wang Y, Wu H, Wu J, Zhao H, Zhang X, Mues G, et al. Identification and functional analysis of two novel PAX9 mutations. Cells Tissues Organs, 2009;**189**(1-4):80-87. DOI: 10.1159/000151448

[50] Lammi L, Halonen K, Pirinen S, Thesleff I, Arte S, Nieminen P. A missense mutation in PAX9 in a family with distinct phenotype of oligodontia. European Journal of Human Genetics. 2003;**11**:866-871. DOI: 10.1038/sj.ejhg.5201060

[51] O'Dwyer EM, Jones DC. Dental anomalies in Axenfeld-Rieger syndrome. International Journal of Paediatric Dentistry. 2005 Nov;**15**(6):459-463. DOI: 10.1111/d.1365-263X.2005.00639

Section 2

Background on Dental Anatomy and Morphology

Chapter 3

Prologue: Tooth Anatomy and Morphology

Zühre Akarslan

1. Introduction

Knowledge of tooth morphology and anatomy is important in dentistry. Crown morphology is essential in restorative treatment and prosthodontic treatment. External root morphology influences the success of oral surgery, periodontal treatment, orthodontic treatment, and prosthodontic treatment. The knowledge of root canal anatomy is important in endodontics. There can be various root canal configurations affecting the success of root canal treatment [1–3]. The size of teeth crowns, number of roots, and morphology of occlusal surfaces, including cusps, interconnecting depressions, grooves, or pits, may differ among populations and genders [4–9].

There are two sets of teeth during lifetime, the deciduous teeth and the permanent teeth. The deciduous teeth are present in childhood and replaced with the permanent teeth. There are 20 deciduous teeth. Ten of these are located at the maxillae, and 10 of them are located at the mandible. They are consisted of incisors, canines, and molars. There are 32 permanent teeth. Sixteen of these teeth are located in the maxillae, and 16 are located in the mandible. They are consisted of incisors, canines, premolars, and molars. The main difference between the deciduous and permanent dentition is that the permanent dentition has the premolar teeth. There are four premolars in the maxillae and four premolars in the mandible [10].

The permanent incisors are placed in front of the oral cavity. There are total eight incisors, four at the maxillae, and four at the mandible. The function of these teeth is cutting food. Their crowns are flattened and they usually have a single root. The incisors are consisted of the central and lateral teeth. The mandibular central incisor is the smallest tooth in the mouth, but the buccolingual dimension of its root is very large [11–13].

The permanent canines are placed after the lateral incisors. There are two canines in the maxillae and two canines in the mandible. The canines tear and shred food. The canine has a single root and root canal. Its root is longer compared to the incisors [12].

The premolar teeth are located between the canines and the molars. There are four premolars in the maxillae and four premolars in the mandible. The premolars are the transitional teeth. They are only present in the permanent dentition. They guide food from the front of the mouth back to the molars. They can have two or more cusps on their crown [10]. The second maxillary premolar tooth in the maxillae and the first and second premolar tooth in the mandible have one root and root canal. Different from these, the first maxillary premolar tooth has two roots and root canals, one located in the buccal and the other in the palatal area. In some cases there can be extra roots and root canals in these teeth [3].

The permanent molars are located in the posterior region in the oral cavity. The molars are placed after the premolars in the permanent dentition. There are six molars in the maxillae and six molars in the mandible. The functions of these teeth are to crush and grind food. They have multiple cusps on their crown [10]. The root configuration and number differ among these teeth. The maxillary molars usually have three separate roots; mesiobuccal, distobuccal, and palatal. Sometimes there can be one, two, or four roots [14]. On the other hand, the mandibular molars usually have two roots: mesial and distal. However, rarely these teeth can have one or three roots [15].

The teeth may be affected from various anomalies. These anomalies can change the structure, color, shape, and form of the teeth. The anomalies are named as concrescence, fusion, germination, taurodontism, dilaceration, enamel pearls, dens invaginatus, dens in dente, dilated odontoma, dens evaginatus, talon cusp, amelogenesis imperfecta, dentinogenesis imperfecta, osteogenesis imperfecta, dentin dysplasia, regional odontodysplasia, and Turner's hypoplasia. Dentists should have knowledge about these anomalies and the possible complications they can lead during dental treatment [16].

The aim of this book is to provide the readers information about dental morphology, anatomy, and anomalies.

2. Overview of the chapters of this book

Second chapter: "Tooth Morphology Overview" written by Abeer Alshami, Shatha Alharthi, Munirah bin Shabeeb, and Monika Wahi. The authors start with the nomenclature and continue with tooth numbering systems in this chapter. They give details about the Fédération Dentaire Internationale (FDI) system, tooth morphology and anatomy, and stages of tooth formation. They end the chapter with the hypotheses accepted nowadays about formation of the tooth. The authors provide useful information and rich illustrations for the readers.

Third chapter: "Root Canal Morphology and Anatomy" written by Esra Güven Pamukçu. This chapter gives the readers beneficial information about root canal anatomy and morphology of maxillary and mandibular incisors, canines, premolars, and molars. A novel tooth morphology classification respecting tooth number, number of roots, and root canal configuration types is presented. A summary of dental anomalies can be found at the end of the chapter.

Fourth chapter: "External and Internal Anatomy of Mandibular Permanent Incisors" written by Mohammed A. Aldawla, Abdulbaset A. Mufadhal, and Ahmed A. Madfa. In this chapter detailed information is given about the external root morphology, the internal root anatomy, and the dental anomalies which can be seen in permanent mandibular incisor teeth. The chapter is written according to a rich literature review which is particularly informative.

Fifth chapter: "External and Internal Anatomy of Maxillary Permanent First Molars" written by Abdulbaset A. Mufadhal, Mohammed A. Aldawla, and Ahmed A. Madfa. This chapter provides the readers useful information about external root morphology, internal root anatomy, variations, and anatomical anomalies of permanent maxillary first molars. The chapter is written according to a rich literature review in an elucidative manner.

Sixth chapter: "Can Orofacial Structures Affect Tooth Morphology?" written by Amanda Valentim, Renata Furlan, Mariana Amaral, and Fernanda Guimarães. This chapter focuses on the role of orofacial forces on the teeth. The authors give information about all factors related in detail. They emphasize the role of the orofacial muscles, oral habits, and hyperfunction of masticator muscles on the occlusion and size and shape of the teeth according to a rich literature review.

Seventh chapter: "Evolution of Dental Implant Shapes and Today's Custom Root Analogue Implants" written by Ayse Sumeyye Akay. The author provides information about root morphology of teeth. Evolution and the fabrication procedures and clinical predictability of root-shaped dental implants are explained in the chapter. The readers can benefit from the advantages of the root-shaped implants for immediate placement.

Author details

Zühre Akarslan
Department of Oral and Maxillofacial Radiology, Faculty of Dentistry, Gazi University, Ankara, Turkey

*Address all correspondence to: dtzuhre@yahoo.com

References

[1] Sanson G. Cutting food in terrestrial carnivores and herbivores. Interface Focus. 2016;**6**:20150109. DOI: 10.1098/rsfs.2015.0109

[2] Brook AH, Jernvall J, Smith RN, Hughes TE, Townsend GC. The dentition: The outcomes of morphogenesis leading to variations of tooth number, size and shape. Australian Dental Journal. 2014;**59**:131-142. DOI: 10.1111/adj.12160

[3] Mohammadi Z, Shalavi S, Jafarzadeh H. Extra roots and root canals in premolar and molar teeth: Review of an endodontic challenge. The Journal of Contemporary Dental Practice. 2013;**14**:980-986

[4] Felemban NH, Manjunatha BS. Prevalence of the number of cusps and occlusal groove patterns of the mandibular molars in a Saudi Arabian population. Journal of Forensic and Legal Medicine. 2017;**49**:54-58. DOI: 10.1016/j.jflm.2017.05.013

[5] Dholia B, Manjunatha BS. Occlusal morphology of permanent mandibular first and second molars in Gujarati population. Journal of Forensic Dental Sciences. 2015;**7**:137-141. DOI: 10.4103/0975-1475.146368

[6] Mallineni SK, Panampally GK, Chen Y, Tian T. Mandibular talon cusps: A systematic review and data analysis. Journal of Clinical and Experimental Dentistry. 2014;**6**:e408-e413. DOI: 10.4317/jced.51476

[7] Khraisat A, Taha ST, Jung RE, Hattar S, Smadi L, Al-Omari IK, et al. Prevalence, association, and sexual dimorphism of Carabelli's molar and shovel incisor traits amongst Jordanian population. Odonto-Stomatologie Tropicale. 2007;**30**:17-21

[8] Filipovic G, Kanjevac T, Cetenovic B, Ajdukovic Z, Petrovic N. Sexual dimorphism in the dimensions of teeth in Serbian population. Collegium Antropologicum. 2016;**40**:23-28

[9] Martins JNR, Marques D, Francisco H, Caramês J. Gender influence on the number of roots and root canal system configuration in human permanent teeth of a Portuguese subpopulation. Quintessence International. 2018;**49**:103-111. DOI: 10.3290/j.qi.a39508.

[10] Yavuzyılmaz H. Diş Morfolojisi ve Anatomisi. [Tooth Morphology and Anatomy]. 6th ed. Beşevler Ankara Türkiye: Gazi Kitapevi; 2013. pp. 27-191

[11] Ozaki T, Satake T, Kanazama E. Morphological significance of root length variability in comparison with other crown dimensions. The Journal of Nihon University School of Dentistry. 1987;**29**:233-240

[12] Yamanaka A, Iwai H, Uemura M, Goto T. Patterning of mammalian heterodont dentition within the upper and lower jaws. Evololution and Development. 2015;**17**:127-138. DOI: 10.1111/ede.12116

[13] McGowan S. Characteristics of teeth: A review of size, shape, composition, and appearance of maxillary anterior teeth. The Compendium of Continuing Education in Dentistry. 2016;**37**:164-171

[14] Alrahabi M, Sohail Zafar M. Evaluation of root canal morphology of maxillary molars using cone beam computed tomography. Pakistan Journal of Medical Sciences. 2015;**31**:426-430. DOI: 10.12669/pjms.312.6753

[15] Akpınar KE, Ay S, Er K, Köşger HH. Türk toplumunda alt molar dişlerin kök ve kanal sayıları [The number of roots and canals in mandibular molars of a Turkish sub-population]. Ondokuz Mayis Universitesi Dis Hekimliği Fakültesi Dergisi. 2004;**5**:123-127

[16] Lam EWN. Dental anomalies. In: White SC, Pharoah MJ, editors. Oral Radiology Principles and Interpretation. 6th ed. St. Louis, Missouri: Mosby, Elsevier; 2009. pp. 295-323

Chapter 4

External and Internal Anatomy of Mandibular Permanent Incisors

Mohammed A. Aldawla, Abdulbaset A. Mufadhal and Ahmed A. Madfa

Abstract

A clear understanding of dental root anatomy, external and internal, is an essential prerequisite to all dental procedures. In periodontology, the external root morphology has been proven to have a clinical significance in the predisposing factors of periodontal diseases. Orthodontic literature shows the importance of radicular anatomy in orthodontic mechanics through the concept of anchorage. The significance of internal root anatomy has been emphasized by studies demonstrating that variations in canal geometry before cleaning, shaping, and obturation procedures had a greater effect on the outcome than the techniques themselves. The mandibular central incisor is the smallest tooth in the mouth, but the buccolingual dimension of its root is very large. This tooth is usually single-rooted; however, the root canal system of this group is unpredictable. The incidence of two canals has been reported as low as 0.3% and as high as 45.3%. The wide range of variation reported in literature regarding the prevalence of a second canal has been related to methodological and racial differences. This chapter will summarize the morphological aspects of the root canal anatomy published in the literature of the anterior mandibular teeth. This will provide precious knowledge regarding root canal morphology and its variation among populations.

Keywords: morphology, mandibular incisors, variation, root canal

1. External root morphology

The mandibular central and lateral incisors have a single conical root. The root dimensions of both incisors vary corresponding to the crown. They are narrow in mesiodistal dimension and wide in labiolingual dimension and taper uniformly on both proximal sides from the CEJ to the apex. The apical end may curve slightly to the distal. Longitudinal root depressions can be seen in both incisors from the mesial and distal views. Multiple comparisons revealed that, among all permanent teeth, mandibular central incisor has the shortest root. Furthermore, in contrary to maxillary incisors, the root of mandibular lateral incisor is longer than that of mandibular central incisor [1]. It has been reported that the average lengths of mandibular central incisor and lateral incisor roots are 12.6 mm (7.7–17.9) and 13.5 (9.4–18.1), respectively [2]. Kim et al. [3] measured the mandibular incisor root lengths using CBCT in Korean population and found that no significant differences in crown and root lengths were noted between the CBCT-based and direct measurements. The R/C ratios were higher for the mandibular lateral incisors (1.4 ± 0.1) than mandibular central incisors (1.3 ± 0.1) [4]. Therefore, crown lengthening may not be possible in the case of traumatic fracture or iatrogenic orthodontic extrusion due to the short root length in these teeth. Variations in root length between males and females have been reported. According to Zorba et al. [5], it was observed that root length was greater in males than in females. Haghanifar et al. [6] found similar results when comparing crown and root lengths between males and females. He found that females had longer crowns while males had longer roots.

Many authors reported that the external crown and root morphology of mandibular central and lateral incisors are similar [2, 7, 8]. Mandibular incisors usually have a single root, which is wider buccolingually than mesiodistally and tapers toward the apex. The lateral incisor root is larger than that of the central incisor in mesiodistal and labiolingual directions [8, 9]. Variation in number of roots has not been reported in literature. However, Loushine et al. [10] have found two rooted mandibular lateral incisors. However, the shape may vary from conical to round in different populations. Sexual variation in the number and shape of roots has not been reported [9]. Mandibular incisor roots are commonly reported to be straight and in rare occasions curved in the apical region. Curvature can be in the mesial, distal, labial, or lingual direction [9].

2. Internal anatomy

2.1 Introduction

Orban stated that the shape of the root canal "to a large degree, conforms to the shape of the root. A few canals are round and tapering, but many are elliptical, broad and thin" [11].

The internal anatomy of permanent mandibular incisors does not usually reproduce the simplicity of external anatomy. Its internal anatomy is complicated by the presence of lingual canals, lateral canals, isthmus, and apical deltas [12]. The pulp cavity is the central cavity within a tooth and is entirely enclosed by dentin except at apical foramen. It is divided into coronal portion (pulp chamber) and radicular portion. The pulp chamber is wide and ovoid labiolingually and it tapers incisally. The size of the pulp chamber is not constant throughout life. It decreases in size with aging as a result of secondary dentin deposition [13]. The pulp horn is well developed in this tooth. The root canal systems of these single-rooted teeth often have a single root with a single root canal. However, studies have shown that the root canal anatomy of these teeth is not simple. It may not be single and straight as it appears on the periapical radiograph. Indeed, these teeth have a high prevalence of bifurcation, second canals, lateral canals, and apical deltas which would complicate surgical and nonsurgical endodontic treatment. Mandibular incisor's anatomy presents a challenge when an endodontic access is made, because of its small size and high prevalence of two canals. The main reason for failure in endodontic treatment of mandibular incisors is the inability to detect the presence of a second canal which can then not be prepared and filled during treatment [14]. In literature, the incidence of mandibular incisor teeth with more than one canal has been reported to range from 11 to 68% [15–19]. The differences between these morphology studies may be related to variations of examination methods, classification systems, sample sizes, and ethnic background of tooth sources. Many researchers have studied the prevalence of a second canal in mandibular permanent incisors on different populations and showed that the root canal morphology varies with race, sex, and age [20–24].

2.2 Shape and size of pulp cavity in permanent mandibular incisors

Routine clinical radiographs may mislead clinicians to be under an impression that all root canals are round in shape. A high prevalence of oval root canals in human teeth was reported [25, 26].

The pulp canal of the permanent mandibular central incisor is wider bucco-lingually than mesiodistally [9]. These dimensions are not constant along the root from the orifice till the apex. Oval canals and long oval canals are the most common canal shape seen in the coronal and middle third [27]. As we approach the apex, the canal shape becomes more rounded [28]. This canal shape morphology corresponds to the shape of the root.

2.3 Number of canals in permanent mandibular incisors

The root canal morphology of mandibular central and lateral incisors is very similar. Although they have only one root and a high prevalence of Type 1 root canal morphology, surgical and nonsurgical root canal treatment may fail in these teeth if there is a lack of awareness in their internal anatomy which is complicated by the presence of the lingual canal, bifurcation, lateral anatomy, and isthmus [17, 29]. The morphological characteristics of the root canal system were studied using a number of techniques [18, 27, 30]. The prevalence of a second canal in mandibular permanent incisors is different between populations. Vertucci [18] reported that the incidence of the presence of a second canal was 25.7% among American population, whereas the incidence in Chinese population for the mandibular central and lateral incisors was 5.71 and 27.36%, respectively [31], 30% in Saudi population [32], 26.2% in north Jordanian population [33], and 36.25% in North-East Indian population [34]. In Iranian population, the incidence of mandibular central and lateral incisors having two canals was 27.3 and 29.4%, respectively [35]. The highest incidence (63%) of a second canal in mandibular incisors has been reported in a study in Turkish population [19].

Rankine-Wilson and Henry [36] filled the root canals of mandibular anterior teeth with radio-opaque material, sectioned them in a horizontal plane, and exposed radiographs. They reported two canals in 40.5% of mandibular incisors. Later, Vertucci [18] studied the root canal morphology of 300 extracted mandibular anterior teeth using the clearing technique. In 30% of mandibular central incisors and in 25% of mandibular lateral incisors, there was a second canal. On the other hand, higher prevalence of a second canal in Chinese population was reported in lateral mandibular incisors 25.5% compared with 10.9% in central mandibular incisors [37].

Many researches have shown that root canal systems also vary according to gender. In Turkish population, Sert and Bayirli [19] reported the incidence of second canal in central incisors in females (70%) was higher than in males (65%). Also in Turkish population, Arslan et al. [38] found the frequency of mandibular incisors with a second root canal in males (63%) was higher than in females (35%). The differences among both studies may be due to the fact that Sert and Bayirli examined the root canal morphology in vitro, whereas Arslan et al. studied the root canal anatomy in vivo. In Chinese population, Zhengyan et al. [30] found a significant difference between sex. The result of his study showed that 9.4% of the mandibular lateral incisors in males had a second canal, whereas this value was 11.9% in females. Among Iranian population, Haji et al. [39] reported that there was no significant difference between males and females in the incidence of a second canal in mandibular incisors.

2.4 Canal configurations in permanent mandibular incisors

It has become clear that teeth have complicated root canal systems rather than simplified canals [40]. Most investigators have shown that the root canal systems for most, if not all, permanent teeth are complex and canals may branch, divide, and rejoin. In addition to the complexity of root canal anatomy, root canal morphology varies from tooth to tooth. Concerning root canal treatment, these variations in root canal morphology of permanent teeth may result in missing root canals, nonsurgical endodontic treatment failure, and a need for surgical procedures. Weine et al. [41] classified root canal systems into four basic types, but Vertucci [18] subsequently classified them into eight configurations. The Vertucci classification may give consideration to the complex reality of canal systems in a way that the Weine et al. system did not.

Weine [42] described each of the canal types as below:

Type I: Single canal from pulp chamber to apex.

Type II: Two canals leaving the chamber and merging to form a single canal short of the apex.

Type III: Two separate and distinct canals from chamber to apex.

Type IV: One canal leaving the chamber and dividing into two separate and distinct canals.

Vertucci [24] classified canal configurations into eight types as described below:

Type 1: A single canal from the pulp chamber to apex [1].

Type II: Two separate canals leaving the pulp chamber before joining short of the apex to form one canal [2-1].

Type III: One canal leaving the pulp chamber before dividing into two in the root and then merging to exit as one canal [1-2].

Type IV: Two distinct canals that extended from the pulp chamber to the apex [2].

Type V: One canal leaving the pulp chamber and dividing short of the apex into two separate distinct canals with different apical foramina [1-2].

Type VI: Two separate canals leaving the pulp chamber, merging in the body of the root, and re-dividing short of the apex to exit as two distinct canals [2-1-2].

Type VII: One canal leaving the pulp chamber, dividing and then rejoining in the body of the root, and finally re-dividing into two distinct canals short of the apex [1-2-1-2].

Type VIII: Three separate, distinct canals that extended from pulp chamber to apex [3].

Although mandibular incisors are usually single-rooted teeth, their root canal system cannot be predicted not only between different populations but also between the same population, with respect to the Vertucci's configuration. Studies reported that Vertucci's Type I configuration has the highest prevalence among the other Vertucci configurations [43–45]. When a second canal is present, Vertucci's Type III configuration is the most common for central and lateral incisors. Scarlatescu [46] found Type III has higher incidence than Type II, of 25 and 6.3% respectively in a Romanian population. de Almeida [47] reported that Vertucci's Type I and III configurations represented 92% of the sample. Leoni investigated the root canal anatomy of mandibular central (n = 100) and lateral (n = 100) incisors and founded that Vertucci's Type I (50 and 62%, respectively) and Type III (28%) were the most prevalent canal configurations in incisors [48]. However, researchers found high prevalence of Vertucci's Type II than Vertucci's Type III when a second canal is present. For example, Al-Qudah and Awawdeh [33] reported that the most common root canal configurations were Vertucci's Type I, II, III, IV, and V with a prevalence of 73.8, 10.9, 6.7, 5.1, and 3.6% of mandibular central and lateral incisors respectively in a Jordanian population. Another study done in an Iranian population conducted by Yazdi and Jafari [49] using in vitro radiography, staining, and sectioning technique reported 88, 3.5, 0.5, and 8% prevalence of canal types I, II, IV, and V respectively in mandibular incisors. A similar study done by Miyashita et al. [17] among Japanese population founded central and lateral incisors with prevalence of Vertucci's Type I, II, III and IV as 87.6, 9.3, 1.4, and 1.7% respectively. These configurations may have an implication in endodontic treatment outcome. A properly executed root canal treatment will lead to success in Type I, II, IV, and VIII canal configurations while the same treatment might lead to unfavorable treatment outcome in Type III canal configuration. Apically dividing systems like Type V, VI, and VII are the most difficult systems to prepare and obturate and may have an influence on the outcome of root canal treatment. Miyashita et al. [17] studied the relationship between canal configuration and external dimension, and found that Type II and III root canal configurations of mandibular incisors were larger in tooth length, and crown width labiolingually and mesiodistally. In cases of nonsurgical root canal procedure, disinfection and obturation of Type I and IV canal systems are relatively simple owing to that each of these configurations having definite canals with separate orifice and apex. Contrarily, Type II, III, and V systems are different because there are areas in the root where the two canals share space and others where the canals are separate. This requires an individualized procedure for preparation and filling in each of these conditions to obtain the most desirable results. Although the incidence of two separate canals is low, ribbon-like canals are detected in cases that were classified as Type I (simple root canal) based on their canal configuration, and this results in enabling the file to touch a large area of the canal walls.

2.5 Lateral canals in permanent mandibular incisors

Lateral canals are accessory canals located in the coronal or middle third of the root, extending horizontally from the main canal to the external surface of the root. Their formation is due to the entrapment of periodontal vessels in Hertwig's epithelial root sheath or when blood vessels running from the dental sac through the dental papilla persist during calcification [50]. Lateral canals communicate with the periodontal ligament space and this increases risk of spread of periodontal disease into the pulp canal. According to their location, Vertucci classified lateral canals into coronal, middle, apical, or furcation. He observed lower occurrence of canal ramifications in the middle 11.4% and coronal 6.3% thirds compared to the apical 73.5% third [18, 24]. Recent micro-CT studies on root canal morphology of mandibular anterior teeth reported that lateral canals are rare [48, 51]. Miyashita et al. [17] reported that out of mandibular incisors with lateral branches, single lateral branch had the highest prevalence (82.2%) and multiple branches were extremely narrow. Al-Qudah and Awawdeh [33] found that there was an increasing prevalence of lateral canals toward the apical third of the root with approximately 64% occurring in the apical part of the roots. On the other hand, other studies reported that lateral canals were frequently found in the middle of the canal [34, 46]. Clinically, lateral canals are not usually visible in preoperative radiographs, but its presence can be suspected when there is a localized thickening of the periodontal ligament or a lesion on the lateral surface of the root [50]. It is also important to note that lateral canals cannot be instrumented. Its contents can only be neutralized by the action of effective irrigation with appropriate tissue dissolvent properties and antimicrobial activity solution or with the addition of use of intracanal medications.

2.6 Apical deltas in permanent mandibular incisors

Apical deltas are defined as an intricate system of spaces within the root canal that allows free passage of blood vessels and nerves from the periapical compartment to the pulp tissue [52, 53]. The apical delta is different from the accessory canal in which the main pulp canal is still distinguishable. The prevalence of apical deltas in human permanent teeth varies among populations, and the type and locations of tooth and methods of study. High prevalence of apical deltas is found in maxillary second premolars, mandibular lateral incisors, and mandibular second premolars [22]. Among American population, Vertucci [18] reported that the incidence of apical deltas was 5, 6, and 8% in the mandibular central incisors, lateral incisors, and canines, respectively. However, Çalişkan et al. [22] reported that the prevalence of apical deltas in those teeth was 9.8, 23.5 and 7.8% in a Turkish population. Apical deltas have been reported to be of great importance in endodontics because they are difficult to be instrumented during chemical-mechanical preparation. Furthermore, their long vertical extension may cause failure of the apical surgery if not involved during apical resection [54]. Gao et al. [55] reported that the median vertical distance of the apical delta was 1.87 mm with 13% of them more than 3 mm. Therefore, resection of the apical 3 mm of a root may include the whole apical delta and residual microorganisms from 87% of roots with apical delta.

2.7 Intercanal anastomosis in permanent mandibular incisors

A thin communication can occur between two or more canals in the same root or between vascular elements in tissues [56]. Green [23] described this corridor as a "ribbon shaped passage." He found this corridor in 22% of mandibular incisors. An isthmus is formed when an individual root projection is unable to close itself off. Any root that contains two root canals has the potential to contain an isthmus [57]. It may contain tissue remnants and necrotic debris, which participate in microorganisms' growth resulting in root canal treatment failure [58]. Therefore, knowledge of the root canal anatomy is essential for complete cleaning of the root canal and successful endodontic treatment [11]. Isthmus classification was described by Hsu and Kim et al. [59]. They classified isthmus into five types: Type I—two canals with no notable communication; Type II—a hair-thin connection between the two main canals; Type III—differs from Type II because of the presence of three canals instead of two; Type IV—an isthmus with extended canals into the connection; and Type V—there is a true connection or wide corridor of tissue between two main canals. Mauger reported that isthmus was present in 20% of the teeth at the 1-mm level, 30% at 2 mm, and 55% at 3 mm [27]. Estrela et al. [60] demonstrated high prevalence of both partial and complete isthmii in mandibular lateral incisors (47.6%) compared with mandibular central incisors (33.3%). On the other hand, Arslan et al. [38] found a low incidence (3.7%) of intracanal communication among Turkish population. A similar study done by Haghanifar [61] found the prevalence of complete isthmus in the mandibular anterior teeth ranged from 3 to 5%.

2.8 Anatomy, number, and position of apical foramina in permanent mandibular incisors

As a result of large width of the root canal buccolingually than mesiodistally, mandibular incisors have oval and flattened canals [25]. The overall prevalence of long oval root canals in the apical region in mandibular incisors is >50% [25]. When using rotary files, these oval-shaped canals are a challenge for proper shaping of the canal. This is because rotary instrumentation cannot touch all the canal walls, leaving behind untouched area. To improve mechanical apical debridement, the use of instruments up to an ISO size 100 is required to avoid leaving untouched area on the buccal and/or lingual walls of the canal [62]. However, using files with large taper or tip may cause lateral or apical perforation of the root as the root has a narrower diameter in the mesiodistal direction. Therefore, it stresses the use of good chemical disinfection protocol on these teeth. Canals are considered as oval, long oval, and flattened when the ratio between the maximum and the minimum cross-sectional diameter is <2:1, 2–4:1, and >4:1, respectively. Apical foramina are the main apical opening of the root canal. It is the main exit of the root canal onto the external root surface. Variation in the number and position of apical foramina is especially seen in mandibular incisors with two canals. The apical foramen coincides with the anatomical apex in 17–52.2% of the cases [19, 22, 33, 57, 63].

A number of studies (17.33%) reported that the position and the number of the apical foramen vary according to the race. Al-Qudah and Awawdeh [33] reported that more than half of the roots (52.2%) had centrally located foramina and 47.8% had laterally located foramina. Apical deltas were observed in only eight teeth (1.8%), and among mandibular incisors with two canals, single foramen was more prevalent than two apical foramina. Miyashita et al. [17] reported that only 3% of the mandibular incisors containing two canals had two foramina. He also found that 67.9% of mandibular incisors with curved root had eccentrically located foramina toward the labial direction and none of the canals were curved lingually.

According to Walker [63], the distance between the apical foramen and the most apical end of the root ranges between 0.2 and 2.0 mm. The diameter of the apical foramen of mandibular incisors has been reported to be as 262.5 μm.

2.9 Anomalies in permanent mandibular incisors

Anomaly (Gk, anomalos; irregular) is a deviation from what is regarded as normal [64]. These abnormalities may occur, in terms of size or shape, to either crown or root. WHO listed the following dental anomalies: concrescence, fusion, gemination, dens evaginatus, dens in dente, dens invaginatus, enamel pearls, macrodontia, microdontia, peg-shaped teeth, taurodontism, and tuberculum paramolare [65]. Anomalies of permanent mandibular incisors regarding the crown and root shape are extremely rare. However, few case reports have registered anomalies associated with mandibular incisors. As an example, dens invaginatus, a deep surface invagination of the crown or root, which is lined by enamel and resulting from the invagination of the enamel organ into the dental papilla during odontogenesis, can be seen in these teeth [66]. Dens invaginatus has been classified into three categories according to the depth of invagination and communication with the periapical tissue or periodontal ligament [67].

Type 1: The invagination ends as a blind sac confined to the crown.

Type 2: The invagination extends apically beyond the external CEJ, ending as a blind sac and never reaching the periapical tissues.

Type 3: The invagination extends beyond the CEJ and a second "apical foramen" is found in either the periapical tissues or the periodontal ligament.

The prevalence of this anomaly has been found to range from 0.25 to 5.1% of the population [66]. More commonly, dens invaginatus occurs in the maxillary permanent lateral incisors. Also, it may occur in maxillary central incisors, premolars, canines, and molars. It usually occurs unilaterally, but bilateral cases have also been reported [68]. Occurrence of dens invaginatus in mandibular teeth is very rare. When it occurs in mandibular incisors, the central incisor has a higher incidence compared with lateral incisor [69, 70].

Talon cusp is also a rare developmental anomaly defined as an additional cusp that projects predominantly from the labial or lingual surface of primary or permanent anterior teeth [71]. Mellor and Ripa [72] named this anomaly "talon cusp" as it resembles the shape of an eagle's talon. Talon cusp was classified by Hattab [73] as follows:

Type 1: True talon cusp—this is a morphologically well-delineated additional cusp that prominently projects from the palatal surface of a primary or permanent anterior tooth and extends at least half the distance from the CEJ to the incisal edge.

Type 2: Semi talon cusp—this is an additional cusp of size a millimeter or more but extending less than half the distance from the CEJ to the incisal edge.

Type 3: Trace talon—this is enlarged or prominent cingula and their variations (i.e., conical, bifid, or tubercle-like).

Radiographically, the talon cusp may appear typically as a V-shaped radiopacity, starting from the cervical third of the crown. Most of the talon cusps occur in the maxillary lateral incisors (55%), followed by maxillary central incisors (32%) and maxillary canines (9%) [71]. Although it is rarely seen in mandibular teeth [74], Gündüz and Celenk [43] studied the site distribution of talon cusp among Turkish population and found only 3% of talon cusp was seen in the mandibular right central incisors.

Another rare developmental anomaly that has been reported to occur in mandibular central incisor is "Gemination" [75]. It is a rare anomaly that arises when the tooth bud of a single tooth attempts to divide. The structure most often presents as two crowns, either totally or partially separated, with a single root and one root canal [76]. In the anterior region, gemination can cause poor esthetic appearance due to irregular morphology. In addition, these teeth are more susceptible to periodontal disease and caries, if deep groove is present [77, 78].

Fusion is another developmental anomaly which can occur in these teeth. Contrary to gemination, fusion is defined as the union of two or more separately developing tooth germs during odontogenesis, when the crown is not yet mineralized at the dentinal level, yielding a single large tooth [79]. Depending on the stage of development at the time of union, the pulp might be merged or separated [80]. Fusion is more frequently seen in primary dentition, but it may occur in both dentitions. If it occurs in permanent dentition, the vast majority of permanent teeth fusion cases are seen in maxillary teeth. Although, the incidence of fusion of mandibular incisors is rare, mandibular central incisors have been reported to fuse with a supernumerary tooth [81] and bilaterally with the adjacent lateral incisor [82].

It should be emphasized that special attention is required during root canal treatment owing to the abnormal morphology of the crown and the complexity of the root canal system in fused teeth.

3. Clinical recommendation relevant to the mandibular incisors' anatomy

Mandibular incisors are prone to endodontic treatment as a result of several reasons. Due to their location in the jaw, they are prone to traumas that result in tooth fracture which may necessitate root canal therapy. Moreover, their proximity to the opening of the sublingual and submandibular ducts increases the incidence of dental caries as a result of lingual deposition of calculus. Therefore, an accurate knowledge of the external and internal anatomy of these teeth is an essential prerequisite to carry out root canal treatment. They often have two canals that are buccolingually located and the lingual canal usually is missed. Therefore, the dentist should extend the access preparation in lingual direction to locate the lingual canal which is usually below the cingulum. In case of two canals, Type II canal is the most prevalent configuration where the buccal canal is the most straight and easiest to be located. Consequently, it is recommended to instrument and fill these canals till the apex whereas the lingual canal merges with the labial canal. Presence of an isthmus may complicate the root canal disinfection as it may contain tissue remnants and necrotic debris, hence irrigation and activation are very essential to overcome these anatomical difficulties.

Author details

Mohammed A. Aldawla[1*], Abdulbaset A. Mufadhal[1] and Ahmed A. Madfa[1,2]

1 Department of Conservative Dentistry, Faculty of Dentistry, Sana'a University, Sana'a, Yemen

2 Department of Conservative Dentistry, Faculty of Dentistry, Thamar University, Dhamar, Yemen

*Address all correspondence to: mohdaldawla@gmail.com

References

[1] Ozaki T, Satake T, Kanazama E. Morphological significance of root length variability in comparison with other crown dimensions. The Journal of Nihon University School of Dentistry. 1987;**29**(4):233-240

[2] Scheid RC, Weiss G. Woefel's Dental Anatomy. 8th ed. Philadelphia: Lippincott Williams & Wikins; 2012

[3] Kim S-Y, Lim S-H, Gang S-N, Kim H-J. Crown and root lengths of incisors, canines, and premolars measured by cone-beam computed tomography in patients with malocclusions. The Korean Journal of Orthodontics. 2013;**43**(6):271-278

[4] Choi S-H, Kim J-S, Kim C-S, Yu H-S, Hwang C-J. Cone-beam computed tomography for the assessment of root–crown ratios of the maxillary and mandibular incisors in a Korean population. The Korean Journal of Orthodontics. 2017;**47**(1):39-49

[5] Zorba E, Vanna V, Moraitis K. Sexual dimorphism of root length on a Greek population sample. HOMO. 2014;**65**(2):143-154

[6] Haghanifar S, Moudi E, Bijani A, Ghanbarabadi MK. Morphologic assessment of mandibular anterior teeth root canal using CBCT. Acta Medica Academica. 2017;**46**(2):85-93

[7] Berman LH, Hargreaves KM, Cohen SR. Cohen's Pathways of the Pulp Expert Consult. 10th ed. New York: Elsevier Health Sciences; 2010

[8] Nelson SJ. Wheeler's Dental Anatomy, Physiology, and Occlusion. 10th ed. St. Louis: Elsevier Health Sciences; 2015

[9] Ngassapa D, Hassanali J, Amwayi P, Guthua S. Essentials of Orofacial Anatomy. Dar es Salaam: Dar es Salaam University Press; 1996. p. 98-129

[10] Loushine RJ, Jurcak JJ, Jeffalone DM. A two-rooted mandibular incisor. Journal of Endodontics. 1993;**19**(5):250-251

[11] Ingle JI, Baumgartner JC. Ingle's Endodontics. USA: PMPH; 2008

[12] White SC, Pharoah MJ. Oral Radiology-E-Book: Principles and Interpretation. St Louis: Elsevier Health Sciences; 2014

[13] Morse DR. Age-related changes of the dental pulp complex and their relationship to systemic aging. Oral Surgery, Oral Medicine, and Oral Pathology. 1991;**72**(6):721-745

[14] Cantatore G, Berutti E, Castellucci A. Missed anatomy: Frequency and clinical impact. Endodontic Topics. 2006;**15**(1):3-31

[15] Madeira MC, Hetem S. Incidence of bifurcations in mandibular incisors. Oral Surgery, Oral Medicine, and Oral Pathology. 1973;**36**(4):589-591

[16] Kartal N, Yanıkoğlu FÇ. Root canal morphology of mandibular incisors. Journal of Endodontics. 1992;**18**(11):562-564

[17] Miyashita M, Kasahara E, Yasuda E, Yamamoto A, Sekizawa T. Root canal system of the mandibular incisor. Journal of Endodontics. 1997;**23**(8):479-484

[18] Vertucci FJ. Root canal anatomy of the mandibular anterior teeth. The Journal of the American Dental Association. 1974;**89**(2):369-371

[19] Sert S, Bayirli GS. Evaluation of the root canal configurations of the mandibular and maxillary permanent teeth by gender in the Turkish

population. Journal of Endodontics. 2004;**30**(6):391-398

[20] Kaffe I, Kaufman A, MM L, Lazarson A. Radiographic study of the root canal system of mandibular anterior teeth. International Endodontic Journal. 1985;**18**(4):253-259

[21] Bellizzi R, Hartwell G. Clinical investigation of in vivo endodontically treated mandibular anterior teeth. Journal of Endodontics. 1983;**9**(6):246-248

[22] Çalişkan MK, Pehlivan Y, Sepetçioğlu F, Türkün M, Tuncer SŞ. Root canal morphology of human permanent teeth in a Turkish population. Journal of Endodontics. 1995;**21**(4):200-204

[23] Green D. Double canals in single roots. Oral Surgery, Oral Medicine, Oral Pathology, Oral Radiology. 1973;**35**(5):689-696

[24] Vertucci FJ. Root canal anatomy of the human permanent teeth. Oral Surgery, Oral Medicine, and Oral Pathology. 1984;**58**(5):589-599

[25] Wu M-K, R'oris A, Barkis D, Wesselink PR. Prevalence and extent of long oval canals in the apical third. Oral Surgery, Oral Medicine, Oral Pathology, and Oral Radiology. 2000;**89**(6):739-743

[26] Gani O, Visvisian C. Apical canal diameter in the first upper molar at various ages. Journal of Endodontics. 1999;**25**(10):689-691

[27] Mauger MJ, Schindler WG, Walker WA. An evaluation of canal morphology at different levels of root resection in mandibular incisors. Journal of Endodontics. 1998;**24**(9):607-609

[28] Ch U, Ramachandran S, Indira R, Shankar P. Canal and isthmus morphology in mandibular incisors–an in vitro study. Endodontology. 2004;**16**

[29] Funato A, Funato H, Matsumoto K. Mandibular central incisor with two root canals. Dental Traumatology. 1998;**14**(6):285-286

[30] Zhengyan Y, Keke L, Fei W, Yueheng L, Zhi Z. Cone-beam computed tomography study of the root and canal morphology of mandibular permanent anterior teeth in a Chongqing population. Therapeutics and Clinical Risk Management. 2016;**12**:19

[31] Han T, Ma Y, Yang L, Chen X, Zhang X, Wang Y. A study of the root canal morphology of mandibular anterior teeth using cone-beam computed tomography in a Chinese subpopulation. Journal of Endodontics. 2014;**40**(9):1309-1314

[32] Al-Fouzan KS, AlManee A, Jan J, Al-Rejaie M. Incidence of two canals in extracted mandibular incisors teeth of Saudi Arabian samples. Saudi Endodontic Journal. 2012;**2**(2):65

[33] Al-Qudah A, Awawdeh L. Root canal morphology of mandibular incisors in a Jordanian population. International Endodontic Journal. 2006;**39**(11):873-877

[34] Boruah LC, Bhuyan AC. Morphologic characteristics of root canal of mandibular incisors in north-east Indian population: An in vitro study. Journal of Conservative Dentistry. 2011;**14**(4):346

[35] Aminsobhani M, Sadegh M, Meraji N, Razmi H, Kharazifard MJ. Evaluation of the root and canal morphology of mandibular permanent anterior teeth in an Iranian population by cone-beam computed tomography. Journal of Dentistry. 2013;**10**(4):358

[36] Rankine-Wilson R, Henry P. The bifurcated root canal in lower anterior teeth. The Journal of the

American Dental Association. 1965;**70**(5):1162-1165

[37] Lin Z, Hu Q, Wang T, Ge J, Liu S, Zhu M, et al. Use of CBCT to investigate the root canal morphology of mandibular incisors. Surgical and Radiologic Anatomy. 2014;**36**(9):877-882

[38] Arslan H, Ertas H, Ertas ET, Kalabalık F, Saygılı G, Capar ID. Evaluating root canal configuration of mandibular incisors with cone-beam computed tomography in a Turkish population. Journal of Dental Sciences. 2015;**10**(4):359-364

[39] Haji-Hassani N, Tofangchiha M, Bakhshi M, Mostafaei FS. Evaluation of root canal morphology of mandibular incisor using cone beam computed tomography. Journal of International Oral Health. 2016;**8**(2):167

[40] Hess W, Zurcher E. The Anatomy of Root Canals of the Teeth of the Permanent and Deciduous Dentitions. New York: William Wood & Co; 1925

[41] Weine FS, Healey HJ, Gerstein H, Evanson L. Canal configuration in the mesiobuccal root of the maxillary first molar and its endodontic significance. Oral Surgery, Oral Medicine, and Oral Pathology. 1969;**28**(3):419-425

[42] Weine FS, Pasiewicz RA, Rice RT. Canal configuration of the mandibular second molar using a clinically oriented in vitro method. Journal of Endodontics. 1988;**14**(5):207-213

[43] Gündüz K, Celenk P. Survey of talon cusps in the permanent dentition of a Turkish population. The Journal of Contemporary Dental Practice. 2008;**9**(5):84-91

[44] Monsarrat P, Arcaute B, Peters OA, Maury E, Telmon N, Georgelin-Gurgel M, et al. Interrelationships in the variability of root canal anatomy among the permanent teeth: A full-mouth approach by cone-beam CT. PLoS One. 2016;**11**(10):e0165329

[45] Martins J, Marques D, Mata A, Caramês J. Root and root canal morphology of the permanent dentition in a Caucasian population: A cone-beam computed tomography study. International Endodontic Journal. 2017;**50**(11):1013-1026

[46] Scarlatescu S, Didilescu AC, Stratul S-I, Rusu D, Grigore M, Greabu M, et al. Root canal morphology of mandibular central incisors in a south-eastern Romanian population: Endodontic and periodontal implications. Timisoara Medical Journal. 2010;**60**(4):280-283

[47] de Almeida MM, Bernardineli N, Ordinola-Zapata R, Villas-Bôas MH, Amoroso-Silva PA, Brandao CG, et al. Micro–computed tomography analysis of the root canal anatomy and prevalence of oval canals in mandibular incisors. Journal of Endodontics. 2013;**39**(12):1529-1533

[48] Leoni GB, Versiani MA, Pécora JD, de Sousa-Neto MD. Micro–computed tomographic analysis of the root canal morphology of mandibular incisors. Journal of Endodontics. 2014;**40**(5):710-716

[49] Yazdi KA, Jafari A. Study of the internal anatomy of the mandibular incisor teeth. Journal of Dentistry of Tehran University of Medical Sciences. 2004;**1**(4):43-47

[50] Ricucci D, Siqueira JF Jr. Fate of the tissue in lateral canals and apical ramifications in response to pathologic conditions and treatment procedures. Journal of Endodontics. 2010;**36**(1):1-15

[51] Versiani M, Pécora J, Sousa-Neto M. Microcomputed tomography analysis of the root canal morphology of single-rooted mandibular canines.

International Endodontic Journal. 2013;**46**(9):800-807

[52] Takahashi K, Kishi Y, Kim S. A scanning electron microscope study of the blood vessels of dog pulp using corrosion resin casts. Journal of Endodontics. 1982;**8**(3):131-135

[53] Takahashi K. Session IV: Hemodynamics of the dental pulp—M. Meyer, chairman: Vascular architecture of dog pulp using corrosion resin cast examined under a scanning electron microscope. Journal of Dental Research. 1985;**64**(4):579-584

[54] Gilheany PA, Figdor D, Tyas MJ. Apical dentin permeability and microleakage associated with root end resection and retrograde filling. Journal of Endodontics. 1994;**20**(1):22-26

[55] Gao X, Tay FR, Gutmann JL, Fan W, Xu T, Fan B. Micro-CT evaluation of apical delta morphologies in human teeth. Scientific Reports. 2016;**6**:36501

[56] Weller RN, Niemczyk SP, Kim S. Incidence and position of the canal isthmus. Part 1. Mesiobuccal root of the maxillary first molar. Journal of Endodontics. 1995;**21**(7):380-383

[57] Vertucci FJ. Root canal morphology and its relationship to endodontic procedures. Endodontic Topics. 2005;**10**(1):3-29

[58] Kim S. Color Atlas of Microsurgery in Endodontics. Philadelphia: WB Saunders Company; 2001

[59] Y-y H, Kim S. The resected root surface. The issue of canal isthmuses. Dental Clinics of North America. 1997;**41**(3):529-540

[60] Estrela C, Rabelo LEG, de Souza JB, Alencar AHG, Estrela CR, Neto MDS, et al. Frequency of root canal isthmi in human permanent teeth determined by cone-beam computed tomography. Journal of Endodontics. 2015;**41**(9):1535-1539

[61] Haghanifar S, Moudi E, Madani Z, Farahbod F, Bijani A. Evaluation of the prevalence of complete Isthmii in permanent teeth using cone-beam computed tomography. Iranian Endodontic Journal. 2017;**12**(4):426

[62] Versiani MA, Pécora JD, de Sousa-Neto MD. Flat-oval root canal preparation with self-adjusting file instrument: A micro–computed tomography study. Journal of Endodontics. 2011;**37**(7):1002-1007

[63] Walker R. The root canal anatomy of mandibular incisors in a southern Chinese population. International Endodontic Journal. 1988;**21**(3):218-223

[64] Mosby I. Mosby's Medical Dictionary. St. Louis: Mosby; 2006

[65] Organization WH. International Statistical Classification of Diseases and Related Health Problems. 2nd ed. Geneva: World Health Organization; 2004

[66] Hülsmann M. Dens invaginatus: Aetiology, classification, prevalence, diagnosis, and treatment considerations. International Endodontic Journal. 1997;**30**(2):79-90

[67] Oehlers F. Dens invaginatus (dilated composite odontome): I. Variations of the invagination process and associated anterior crown forms. Oral Surgery, Oral Medicine, and Oral Pathology. 1957;**10**(11):1204-1218

[68] Mupparapu M, Singer S. A rare presentation of dens invaginatus in a mandibular lateral incisor occurring concurrently with bilateral maxillary dens invaginatus: Case report and review of literature. Australian Dental Journal. 2004;**49**(2):90-93

[69] Siraci E, Gungor HC, Cehreli ZC. Dens invaginatus and talon cusp co-occurring in a mandibular central incisor: A case report. Journal of Dentistry for Children. 2008;**75**(2):177-180

[70] Nagaveni NB, Umashanikara KV, Vidyullatha B, Radhika NB. Permanent mandibular incisor with multiple anomalies-report of a rare clinical case. Brazilian Dental Journal. 2011;**22**(4):346-350

[71] Davis P, Brook A. The presentation of talon cusp: Diagnosis, clinical features, associations and possible aetiology. British Dental Journal. 1986;**160**(3):84-88

[72] Mellor JK, Ripa LW. Talon cusp: A clinically significant anomaly. Oral Surgery, Oral Medicine, and Oral Pathology. 1970;**29**(2):225-228

[73] Hattab F. Talon cusp in permanent dentition associated with other dental anomalies: Review of literature and reports of seven cases. Journal of Dentistry for Children. 1996;**6**:368-376

[74] Tulunoglu O, Cankala D, Ozdemir R. Talon's cusp: Report of four unusual cases. Journal of the Indian Society of Pedodontics and Preventive Dentistry. 2007;**25**(1):52

[75] Beltrán V, Leiva C, Valdivia I, Cantín M, Fuentes R, BELTRÁN V, et al. Dental gemination in a permanent mandibular central incisor: An uncommon dental anomaly. International Journal of Odontostomatology. 2013;**7**(1):69-72

[76] Alvarez I, Creath C. Radiographic considerations for supernumerary tooth extraction: Report of case. ASDC Journal of Dentistry for Children. 1995;**62**(2):141-144

[77] Grover P, Lorton L. Gemination and twinning in the permanent dentition. Oral Surgery, Oral Medicine, and Oral Pathology. 1985;**59**(3):313-318

[78] Türkaslan S, Gökçe HS, Dalkız M. Esthetic rehabilitation of bilateral geminated teeth: A case report. European Journal of Dentistry. 2007;**1**(3):188

[79] Velasco LFL, FBd A, Ferreira ES, LEL V. Esthetic and functional treatment of a fused permanent tooth: A case report. Quintessence International. 1997;**28**(10):677-680

[80] Brook A, Winter G. Double teeth. A retrospective study of 'geminated' and 'fused' teeth in children. British Dental Journal. 1970;**129**(3):123

[81] Sachdeva G, Malhotra D, Sachdeva L, Sharma N, Negi A. Endodontic management of mandibular central incisor fused to a supernumerary tooth associated with a talon cusp: A case report. International Endodontic Journal. 2012;**45**(6):590-596

[82] Prabhakar AR, Kaur T, Nadig B. Bilateral fusion of permanent mandibular incisors with Talon's cusp: A rare case report. Journal of Oral and Maxillofacial Pathology. 2009;**13**(2):93

Chapter 5

Tooth Morphology Overview

Abeer ALShami, Shatha ALHarthi, Munerah Binshabaib and Monika Wahi

Abstract

This chapter provides an overview of tooth morphology, including a review of tooth anatomy, tooth development, and associated nomenclature and numbering systems. First, basic tooth morphology nomenclature is presented. Next, various tooth numbering systems are described and discussed, and the Federation Dentaire Internationale (FDI) system is detailed. Third, tooth surfaces and ridges are explained along with terminology, followed by an explanation of tooth crown and root anatomy. Fourth, the stages of tooth formation are described, starting with the bud stage, and followed by the cap stage, bell stage, and maturation. Annotated diagrams are presented for clarity. Finally, two currently accepted hypotheses explaining tooth formation are presented.

Keywords: tooth, tooth components, odontogenesis

1. Introduction

In order to understand tooth morphology, it is necessary to understand the anatomy of the structures within the tooth. In order to understand these, it is helpful to understand tooth development. Therefore, this chapter will cover tooth development and explain the tissues and structures involved in tooth growth. Because teeth take a variety of forms, it is necessary to enumerate them with numbering systems and apply nomenclature; these will be described as well.

To be most understandable, this chapter will begin by presenting the nomenclature associated with tooth morphology. Next, tooth numbering systems will be described and presented. Third, the anatomy of the crown and root of the tooth will be covered, and an explanation of tooth surfaces and ridges presented. Finally, an overview of tooth development will be provided, following the tooth through the bud stage, cap stage, bell stage, and maturation. Finally, two hypotheses behind tooth formation will be explained.

2. Nomenclature

In order to understand tooth morphology, it is important to understand both the nomenclature and the associated anatomy. To begin, the human jaw consists of two parts: the maxillary, referring to the upper jaw, and the mandibular, referring to the lower jaw (see **Figure 1**) [1]. The maxillary is divided into two quadrants called the upper left quadrant and the upper right quadrant. The mandibular is divided into the lower left quadrant and the lower right quadrant.

Humans have two sets of teeth during their lifetime. The first set is called the primary teeth (also called deciduous dentition), and are the first teeth to appear in the mouth. The primary teeth are replaced later on in childhood with permanent teeth (also referred to as succedaneous teeth) [1]. **Figure 1** shows a diagram of an adult human jaw with complete teeth.

Adult humans have four types of teeth: molars, premolars, canine teeth, and incisors (see **Figure 2**). As seen in **Figure 2**, in the adult jaw, there are a total of 32 teeth [1]. Both the mandibular and the maxillary have two front teeth, and these are called the central incisors. On either side of the pair of central incisors is a lateral incisor [1]. The lateral incisor on each side is followed by one canine tooth, which is followed by two premolars, which are then followed by three molars. In primary teeth, there are a total of 20 teeth [2]. Like with adults, primary teeth have the same central incisors, lateral incisors, and canines [2]. However, in primary teeth, the canines are followed by a first molar and second molar [2]. The first molar will eventually be exfoliated and replaced by the two premolars, and the second molar will eventually be exfoliated and replaced by the three molars [2].

As seen in **Figure 1**, the jaw is divided into quadrants. The teeth are numbered by quadrant using the Federation Dentaire Internationale (FDI) system, which will be explained in the next section.

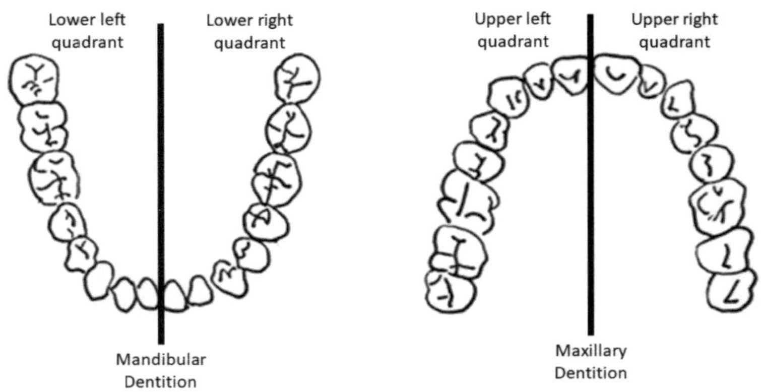

Figure 1.
Adult human jaw with quadrants.

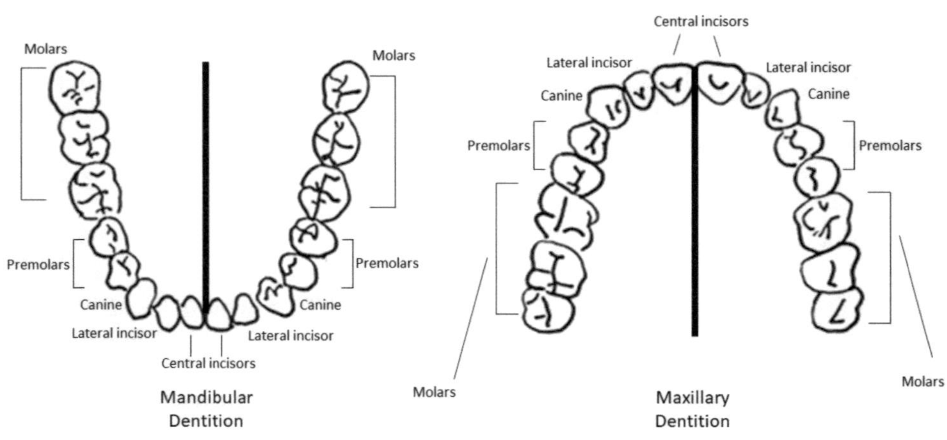

Figure 2.
Adult human jaw with tooth types.

2.1 Tooth numbering systems

Several systems are used in clinical practice for dental notation. In the late 1800s, the Zsigmondy-Palmer system, which is an "eight numerical quadrant system," came into use [3]. However, the coding involved complex symbols and was hard to adopt [3]. Next, the Universal System was proposed, and has been adopted by the American Dental Association (ADA) since 1975 [3]. Unfortunately, this system has the weakness of lacking an anatomic reference, so matching teeth and quadrants can be confusing [3].

In 1966, the FDI System was introduced [3]. Unlike the previous systems, it is simple and accurate while still being easy to memorize and apply [3]. Hence, it was adopted in 1970 by the FDI and later in 1994 by the International Standard Organization (ISO) [3, 4]. The main drawback of the FDI system is that with respect to primary teeth, it can be confusing and challenging to memorize [3]. However, this chapter will focus mainly on adult tooth morphology, so we will use the terminology from the FDI system.

2.1.1 The FDI system for primary teeth

Figure 3 shows the FDI numbering system for primary teeth. Each tooth is assigned a two-digit number. The first digit refers to the quadrant, with five representing the maxillary right quadrant, six representing the maxillary left quadrant, and seven and eight representing the mandibular right and left quadrants, respectively [4]. The second digit in the number represents the tooth number [4]. As an example, tooth 62 represents the maxillary left lateral incisor, and tooth 85 represents the mandibular right second molar. The pronunciation of the numbers is by digits; so tooth 62 is pronounced as "six, two," not "sixty-two," and tooth 85 is pronounced as "eight, five," not "eighty-five."

		Upper Right					Upper Left		
55	54	53	52	51	61	62	63	64	65
85	84	83	82	81	71	72	73	74	75
		Lower Right					Lower Left		

Figure 3.
FDI system for primary teeth.

2.1.2 The FDI system for permanent teeth

Figure 4 shows the FDI system for permanent teeth. As with primary teeth, the first digit represents the quadrant, so one represents the maxillary right quadrant, two represents the maxillary left quadrant, and three and four represent the mandibular right and left quadrants, respectively [4]. The second digit in the number represents the tooth number; so tooth 35 would be the mandibular left second premolar and tooth 17 would be the maxillary right second molar.

			Upper Right								Upper Left				
18	17	16	15	14	13	12	11	21	22	23	24	25	26	27	28
48	47	46	45	44	43	42	41	31	32	33	34	35	36	37	38
			Lower Right								Lower Left				

Figure 4.
FDI system for permanent teeth.

2.2 Tooth surfaces and ridges

Permanent teeth are divided into two groups: anterior teeth and posterior teeth. Anterior teeth include the teeth toward the front of the mouth, including the central incisors, the lateral incisors, and the canines, while posterior teeth, or the teeth toward the back of the mouth, include the premolars and molars [1]. The difference between these types of teeth will be described in the next section.

The crown is the part of the tooth that is visible in the oral cavity. The crowns of anterior teeth have four surfaces and one ridge, while posterior teeth only have surfaces [1] (see **Figure 5**). The surface of a tooth that is facing an adjacent tooth is referred to as a proximal surface. The area of the tooth that contacts the adjacent tooth is called the contact area [1]. In order to determine which proximal surface is being described, imagine a vertical line drawn down the center of the face. The proximal surface closest to that line would be considered as the mesial surface, and the one furthest from the line as the distal surface.

Another way to think about mesial and distal proximal surfaces is to consider them in relation to the palate. The palate refers to the upper portion of the mouth, where the maxillary dentition is housed. The surfaces facing the palate are referred to as palatal surfaces. On both anterior and posterior teeth, the distal surface is the surface facing away from the midline of the palate, and the mesial surface is the surface facing toward the midline of the palate [1].

As shown in **Figure 5**, the surfaces of anterior teeth facing the lips are referred to as labial surfaces, while the surfaces of posterior teeth facing the buccal mucosa are called buccal surfaces. Surfaces of posterior teeth which occlude opposing posterior surfaces are called occlusal surfaces. For example, in **Figure 5**, the occlusolingual line angle is likely on an occlusal surface. In anterior teeth, this situation is referred to as incisal surfaces [1]. In **Figure 5**, the incisocervical dimension would likely be an incisal surface.

In **Figure 5**, on the anterior tooth, a proximal surface would be near the mesiolabial line angle, and the distolingual and distolabial line angles would be away from the proximal surface. On the posterior tooth diagram in **Figure 5**, the mesiobuccal line angle and mesiodistal dimensions would be more likely to be on the proximal surface, while the distolingual and distobuccal line angles would be away from the proximal surface.

2.3 Crown and root anatomy

Each permanent tooth consists of a crown and root (see **Figure 6**). The crown is the part of the tooth that is visible in the oral cavity, while the root is the portion that is firmly embedded in the alveolar bone. The crown and root join at a surface

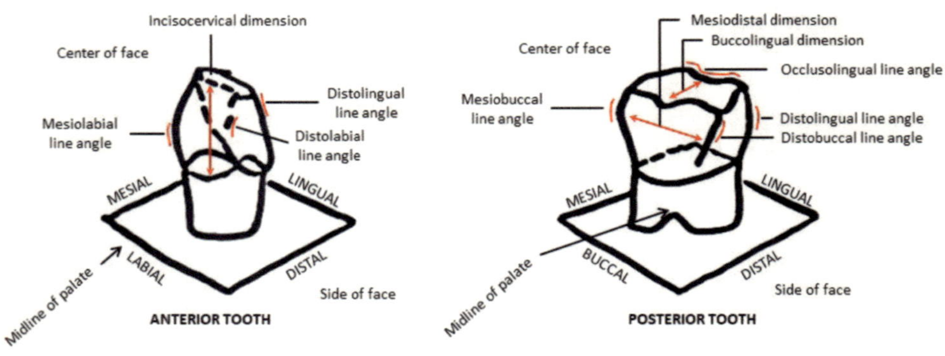

Figure 5.
Surfaces of anterior and posterior teeth.

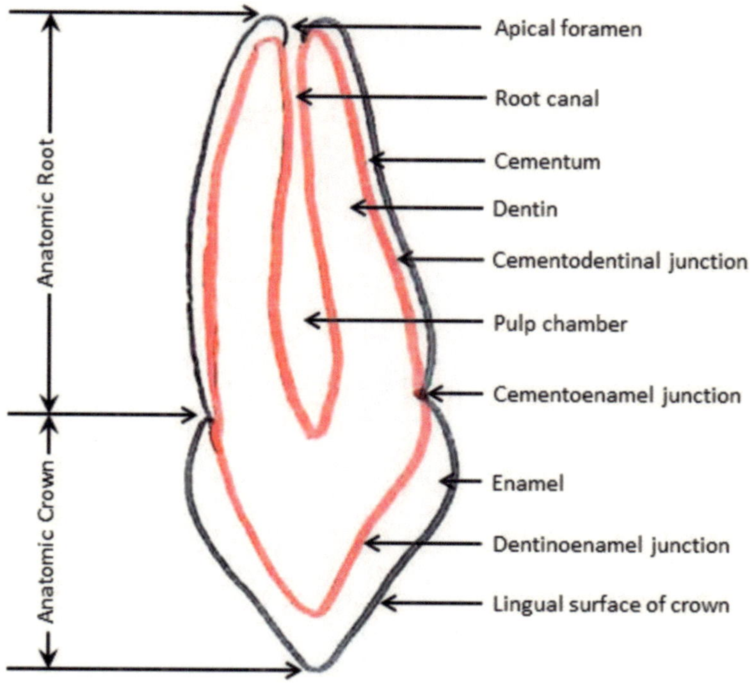

Figure 6.
Crown and root for permanent teeth.

called cementoenamel junction (CEJ) [1]. Please note that in **Figure 6**, the lingual surface of the crown is at the bottom of the diagram.

Human teeth have four types of tissues; the first three are enamel, dentin, and cementum, and these are referred to as hard tissues [1]. The fourth, pulp, is referred to as soft tissue [1]. In terms of the root, as shown in **Figure 6**, the pulp chamber consists of soft connective tissue that enervates and provides the blood supply to the tooth. The pulp chamber is surrounded by dentin, which is the inner portion of the tooth (surrounded by red in the diagram).

Dentin makes up the largest proportion of tissue in the tooth. In the root, the dentin is covered by a layer of cementum. At the top of the root is the apical foramen, where the nerves and blood supply can enter the pulp and transit to the pulp through the root canal. In terms of the crown, the dentin is surrounded by enamel, and where they meet is called the dentinoenamel junction [1].

As described earlier, the crown portion is covered by enamel, and the bulk of the crown is composed of dentin. The crown morphology varies among the dentition. The crowns of anterior teeth, such as central and lateral incisors, have cutting edges. Other teeth in the dentition have cusps to aid in chewing; canines have a single cusp, while premolars and molars have two or more cusps [1].

Regardless of type of tooth—molar, premolar, canine, or incisor—all adult teeth have features labeled with particular terminology. These features are illustrated in **Figure 7** using the example of a canine anterior tooth. Note in **Figure 7**, the apex of the root refers to the tip of the root, and the cusp refers to the opposite end of the tooth. The line between the apex of the root and the tip of the cusp is referred to as the root axis line. Per **Figure 7**, on the front view, the cusp can be said to start at where the slope starts; the distal slope and the mesial slope are labeled, and from here to the tip of the cusp is the cusp. The line that separates the crown from the root is called the cervical line, and the area where the crown meets the root is called the cervix [1].

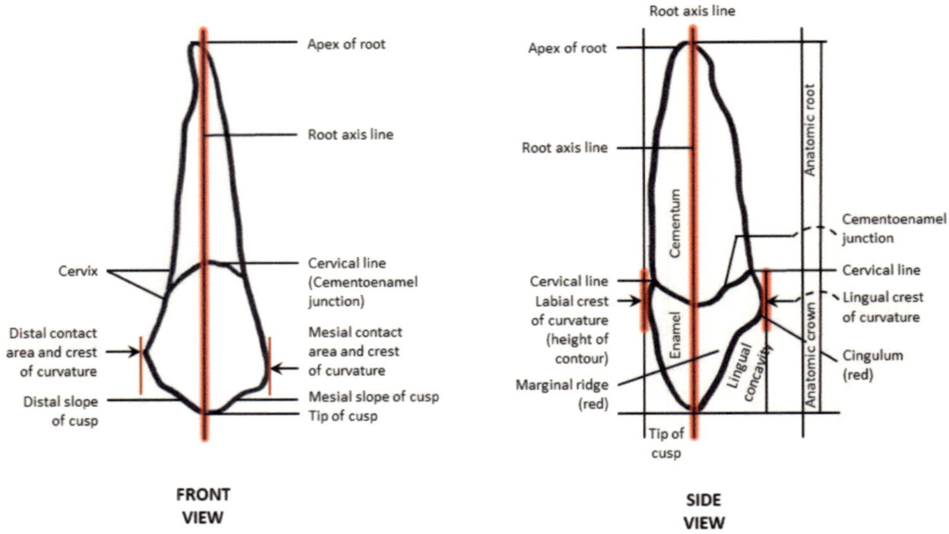

Figure 7.
Diagram of canine anterior tooth.

The curves in the crown are referred to as curvature. **Figure 7** shows the distal contact area and crest along with the mesial contact area and crest of the curvature from the front view, and the labial crest and lingual crest in the side view. Note in the side view that the lingual concavity, marginal ridge, and cingulum refer to the features behind the tooth.

Referring to **Figure 7**, please observe the sharp distal and mesial slopes of the cusp which give the canine tooth its cutting edge and make canine teeth optimized for tearing food [5]. The incisors share similar sharp edges, but are better at cutting food rather than tearing it [5]. Both the premolars and the molars have flatter surfaces; the distance between the tip of the cusp and the apex of the root are much shorter [5].

3. Stages of tooth formation

Tooth development goes through different stages: the bud stage, the cap stage, the bell stage, and finally, maturation. This section will explain the staging of tooth development so it is possible to understand both the embryological and the morphological aspects that take place along a continuum.

3.1 Bud stage

In the bud stage, the tooth bud forms, and the cells from the tooth bud come originally from the ectomesenchyme. The ectomesenchyme originates from the neural crest, which is a group of cells situated in the cranial region during the early development of the vertebrate. This ectomesenchyme layer takes the lead in the formation of the hard tissue in the body that includes bone and teeth. Ectomesenchymal cells congregate deep into the bud, forming an aggregation of cells, which is the initiation of the condensation of the ectomesenchyme [6].

One of the earliest signs in the formation of the tooth that can be seen microscopically is the dental lamina, situated next to the vestibular lamina, which begins to form the tooth bud (see **Figure 8**). The vestibular and dental lamina both originate from the buccopharyngeal membrane [1]. The vestibular lamina is responsible of the creation of the vestibular, which is the area between the junction

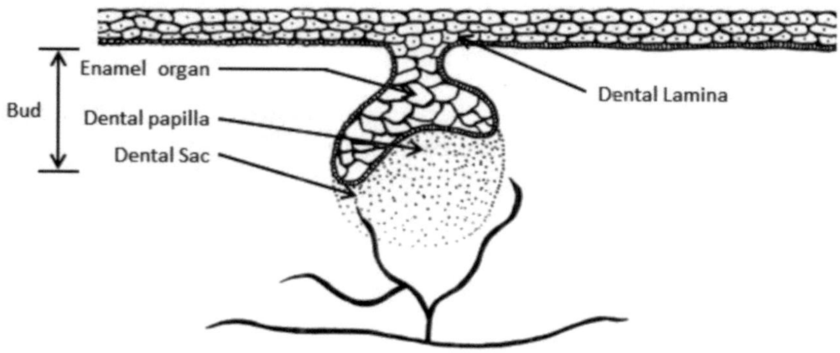

Figure 8.
Bud stage.

of the gingiva and the tissue of the cheek (not shown). It is usually formed after the formation of the dental lamina, around 37 days *in utero*.

The dental lamina is a bundle of epithelium tissue which appears as the earliest sign of tooth development, at 6 weeks *in utero*. When the dental lamina starts forming a tooth bud, it is called the bud stage (or initiation stage) (see **Figure 8**). The dental lamina connects the developing tooth bud to the epithelial layer of the mouth until full separation happens and the tooth forms [6].

As shown in **Figure 8**, first, the tooth bud appears with a random number of cells. Next, the epithelial cells proliferate into the ectomesenchyme of the jaw. This proliferation occurs when the fetus is about 8 weeks old.

From this proliferation, 10 round epithelial structures form. Each one of them will form its own bud, which will then develop into a tooth at the distal aspect of the dental lamina of each arch. This set of 10 teeth will represent the primary teeth of each dental arch. After this, each tooth bud becomes separated from the ectomesenchyme through the development of a basement membrane.

3.2 Cap stage

In the bud stage, the cells are randomly arranged, but once the cap stage is reached, the orderly arrangement of cells takes place (see **Figure 9**). A minor group of ectomesenchymal cells suppresses the production of extracellular substances, which leads to an aggregation of these cells within the dental follicle, forming the

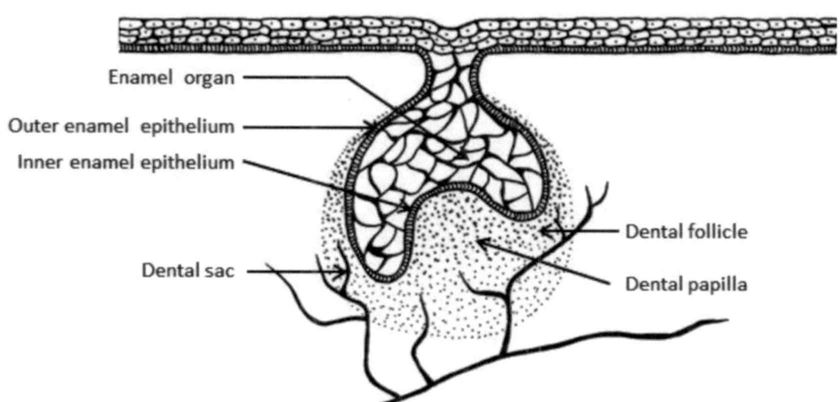

Figure 9.
Cap stage.

dental papilla. At this stage, the tooth bud grows around the dental papilla, forming the appearance of a cap, and becomes the enamel organ covering the dental papilla. Ectomesenchymal cells form the dental sac surrounding the enamel organ and limit the dental papilla. Eventually, the enamel organ will form enamel, the dental papilla will form dentin and pulp, and finally, the dental sac will form all the supporting structures of a tooth, and the periodontium [7].

Notice the Inner enamel epithelium (IEE) in **Figure 9**. During the cap stage, this undergoes rapid division called mitosis to increase cells that will later form the tooth pulp.

3.3 Bell stage

The bell stage is the third stage in the process of odontogenesis, where the enamel organ comes to resemble a bell shape (see **Figure 10**). At this stage, the interior of the enamel organ's cells is called stellate reticulum (SR), because of the star-shaped appearance of the cells. This is also the stage where histodifferentiation and morphodifferentiation take place, in which the different tissues of the tooth form and tooth shapes are established [8]. Notice in **Figure 10**, the SR of the enamel organ is bordered by a layer of ameloblasts, followed by a layer of odontoblasts; these are tissues where histodifferentiation and morphodifferentiation have taken place. Ameloblasts will evolve into enamel, and odontoblasts, which originate in the dental papilla, will later play a role in forming the organic matrix on which minerals will be deposited as part of tooth formation.

The bell stage is divided into two stages: the early bell stage and the late bell stage. They will be described here.

3.3.1 Early bell stage

The early bell stage is when morphodifferentiation and histodifferentiation take place, and the tooth crown assumes its final shape (see **Figure 11**). It has four different layers of epithelial cells. The outer enamel epithelium (OEE) is a layer of cuboidal cells that covers the enamel organ in a developing tooth. The IEE is a layer of columnar cells which covers the recess of the enamel organ in a developing tooth. The stratum intermedium (SI) is the layer of the cells between the IEE and the SR. As described before, the SR is a set of cells situated in the center of the enamel organ of a developing tooth that are shaped like a star. The rim of the enamel organ where the OEE and IEE link on each side is called the cervical loop (see **Figure 11**) [8].

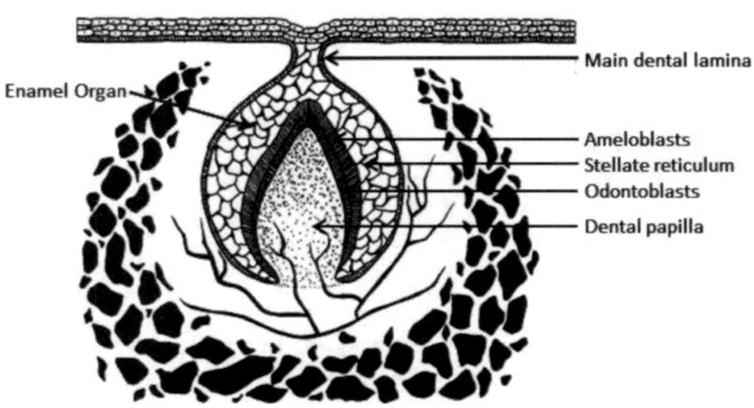

Figure 10.
Bell stage.

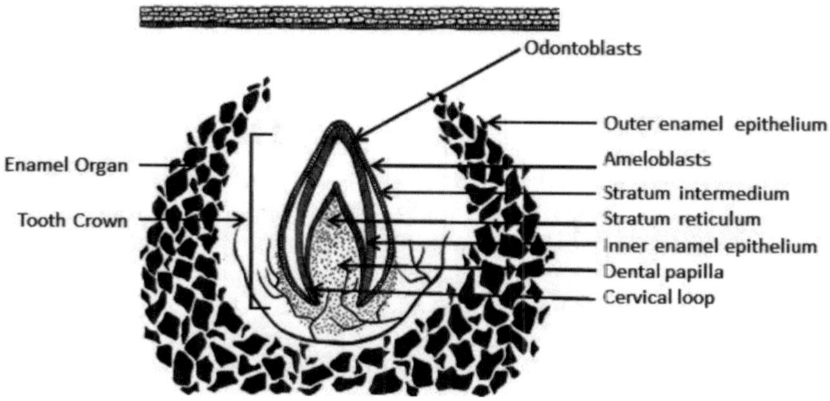

Figure 11.
Early bell stage.

The early bell stage represents sets of tissue that will evolve into the full tooth. The tissue layers that will develop, in order from innermost to outermost, will be composed of dentin, enamel (formed by IEE made of ameloblasts, as they move outward and upward), IEE, and SI. SI are stratified cells that support the synthetic activity of the IEE. Next, as shown in **Figure 11**, is the initial enamel organ, the center of which is made up of SR cells that serve to safeguard the enamel organ. there are all enclosed by the OEE layer [9].

Further events happen during the early bell stage. The dental lamina disintegrates, emancipating the developing tooth, which completely parts from the epithelium of the oral cavity. The developing tooth will remain separated from the epithelium until later, after the late bell stage, when the tooth will erupt into the mouth. During the early bell stage, the crown of the tooth takes shape, guided by the shape of the IEE.

3.3.2 Advanced bell stage

Throughout the advanced bell stage, hard tissues, including enamel and dentin, are developed. Some researchers call this phase the "crown stage." In the advanced bell stage, significant cellular changes occur, and the mitosis that went on during the cap stage is arrested. As shown in **Figure 12**, at this time, the initial mineralized

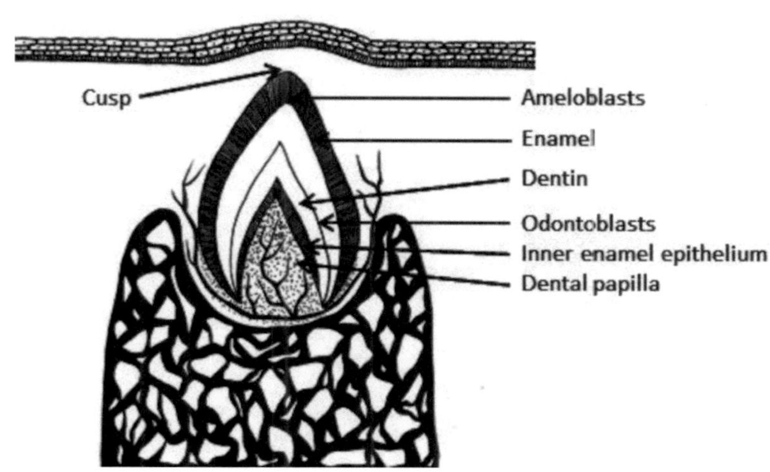

Figure 12.
Advanced bell stage.

hard tissues form into the dentin and the enamel. The IEE cells adjust in shape from cuboidal to columnar and evolve into preameloblasts simultaneously. The nuclei of these preameloblasts move outward, away from the dental papilla as they evolve, and their surface stretches [8].

The cells that form dentin originate in the dental papilla. They randomly grow in size and discern into odontoblasts (see **Figure 12**). Researchers believe that the odontoblasts would not form if it was not for the developments occurring in the IEE. The odontoblasts secrete a substance into their immediate surroundings during development that forms an organic matrix. This reaches the IEE, and the formation of odontoblasts continues from the tip of the cusp [10].

Dentin formation requires materials that are present in the organic matrix. As odontoblasts deposit minerals onto the organic matrix to create predentin, they move toward the center of the dental papilla. Dentin begins forming on the surface nearest to the outside of the tooth and continues inward. In contrast, the enamel grows outward.

Cytoplasmic extensions are left behind as the odontoblasts move inward. The resulting unique tubular microscopic appearance allows for the creation of dentin around these extensions. The cells of the IEE conceal an organic matrix against the dentin after dentin formation begins. This matrix directly mineralizes, and becomes the primary layer of the tooth's enamel. Ameloblasts proliferate to facilitate the final formation of the enamel layer.

3.3.3 Maturation stage

The maturation stage, also called "apposition," is considered by many as the final stage of tooth formation. However, others do not agree with this nomenclature, as it essentially refers to the final period after the tooth is fully formed.

In the maturation stage, both enamel and dentin increase in thickness, and cementum forms after eruption, and follows the development of the root (see **Figure 13**). This stage is extremely important for crown formation, as any disturbance at this stage will cause a major deformity in crown development. Potential

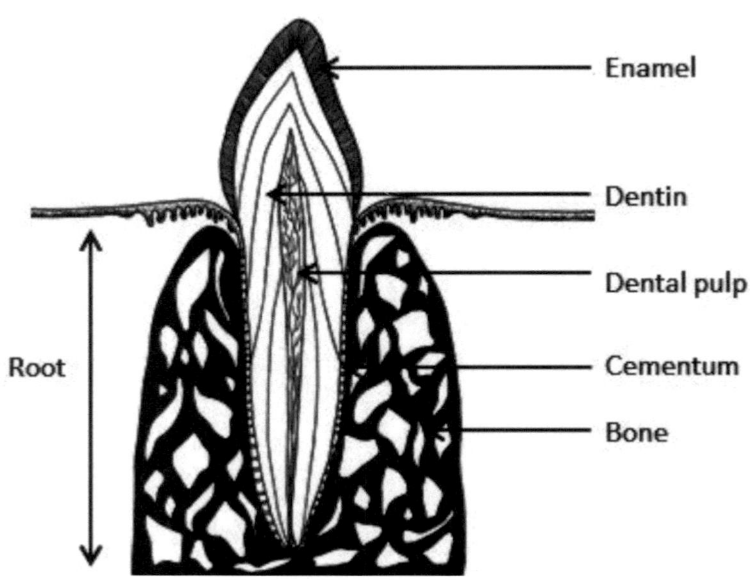

Figure 13.
Maturation stage.

deformities include enamel hypoplasia or hypocalcification, which can manifest clinically as white or yellowish spots on the crown. In addition, tooth development at this stage is very sensitive to any illness in the mother during pregnancy, which can impact primary teeth. Further, illness in the first year of the child's life can impact enamel formation in permanent teeth [11].

4. Tooth morphology hypotheses

Throughout the mouth, though all teeth develop through these stages, it is still not clear why teeth form various crown shapes—for instance, incisors vs. canines. There are two dominant hypotheses. The first is the "field model," which suggests that the elements for each type of tooth shape originate in the ectomesenchyme during tooth development. The elements for specific kinds of teeth, such as incisors, are localized in one area and dissipate quickly in different parts of the mouth. Therefore, for instance, the "incisor field" has factors that grow teeth into the incisor form, and this field is focused in the central incisor area but decreases rapidly in the canine area [1].

The second dominant hypothesis, the "clone model," suggests that the epithelium programs a set of ectomesenchymal cells to produce teeth of specific shapes. This set of cells, called a clone, persuades the dental lamina into tooth growth, producing a tooth bud to form. Development of the dental lamina persists in an area called the "progress zone." As soon as the progress zone travels a certain distance from the first tooth bud, this marks the beginning of the development of a second tooth bud [1, 12].

These two hypotheses are not automatically mutually exclusive, and widely accepted dental science does not see them as contradictory. It is assumed that both models explain tooth development at different times.

5. Conclusion

In conclusion, this chapter presented an overview of tooth morphology. First, nomenclature was defined and then tooth numbering systems were described. After this, the anatomy of the crown and root, as well as explanations of the tooth surfaces and ridges were presented. The next section focused on tooth development, starting with the bud stage. A description of the formation of the tooth continued through the section on the cap stage and the bell stage, and finally, the maturation stage was described. The chapter ended with a discussion of two tooth morphology hypotheses that are thought to help explain tooth development.

In order to grasp the morphology of the human tooth, it is necessary to understand the stages of tooth development. These stages give rise to the final morphology of a variety of human teeth with different surfaces and ridges, which are named using an entomologic system, and enumerated using numbering systems. This chapter provides a guide to the various stages of tooth development and the tissue composition of teeth at various stages of development, and provides insight into the vocabulary and numbering systems used to identify and describe human teeth

Acknowledgements

The authors would like to thank Dr. Hanan Abdulla Al Ghayhab for creating the illustrations for the stages of tooth formation. The authors would also like to thank Ms. Sarah Ibrahim ALHarthi and Ms. Sama Subhi ALHarthi for assisting with the other illustrations.

Conflict of interest

All of the authors declare that they have no conflict of interest with this publication.

Nomenclature

Advanced bell stage	last part of the bell stage, where hard tissues of the tooth are developed; also called the crown stage
Anterior teeth	teeth toward the front of the mouth, including central incisors, lateral incisors, and canines
Apex of the root	tip of the root
Apical foramen	the top of the root, where nerves and blood supply can enter the pulp and transit to the pulp through the root canal
Bell stage	the third stage of tooth formation, where the enamel organ comes to resemble a bell shape
Buccal surfaces	surfaces of posterior teeth facing the buccal mucosa
Bud stage	first stage of tooth development where the tooth bud forms
Canine teeth	one canine tooth is present next to each central incisor in the maxillary and mandibular
Cap stage	stage after bud stage, where orderly arrangement of cells takes place
Cementoenamel junction	where the crown of the tooth meets the root
Cementum	a layer of hard tissue covering dentin in the tooth
Central incisors	the two front teeth in the maxillary and mandibular
Cervical line	line that separates the crown from the root
Cervical loop	the rim of the enamel organ where the outer enamel epithelium and the inner enamel epithelium meet
Cervix	area where the crown meets the root
Clone model	hypothesis of tooth formation that suggests that the epithelium programs a set of ectomesenchymal cells to produce teeth of specific shapes
Crown	the portion of the tooth visible in the oral cavity
Curvature	curves in the crown
Cusp	tip of the tooth; canines have a single cusp, while premolars and molars have two or more cusps
Dental lamina	layer of cells next to the vestibular lamina that begin to form the tooth bud
Dental papilla	formed during the cap stage from an aggregation of cells within the dental follicle
Dental sac	group of ectomesenchymal cells that surround the enamel organ and limit the dental papilla during the cap stage
Dentin	a hard tissue that makes up the largest proportion of the tooth
Distal surface	the proximal surface of a tooth furthest from a vertical line drawn down the center of the face
Early bell stage	first part of the bell stage, where morphodifferentiation and histodifferentiation take place
Ectomesenchymal cells	cells from which tooth formation originates

Enamel	a hard tissue forming the outer layer of the tooth
Federation Dentaire Internationale (FDI) System	tooth numbering system that is easy to memorize and has been adopted by the International Standard Organization
Field model	hypothesis of tooth formation that suggests that the elements for each type of tooth shape originate in the ectomesenchyme during tooth development
Inner enamel epithelium (IEE)	a layer of columnar cells which covers the recess of the enamel organ in a developing tooth
Labial surfaces	surfaces of anterior teeth facing the lips
Lateral incisors	the teeth on either side of the central incisors in the maxillary and mandibular
Lower left quadrant	left portion of the mandibular
Lower right quadrant	right portion of the mandibular
Mandibular	lower jaw
Maturation stage	final stage of tooth formation; also called apposition
Maxillary	upper jaw
Mesial surface	the proximal surface of a tooth closest to a vertical line drawn down the center of the face
Molars	in the adult mouth, three molars follow the two premolars in the maxillary and the mandibular. For primary teeth, there are no premolars, and only two molars. The first molar will be exfoliated and replaced by the two premolars, and the second molar will be exfoliated and replaced by the three molars
Occlusal surfaces	surfaces of posterior teeth which occlude opposing posterior surfaces
Odontoblasts	cells that originate in the dental papilla that ultimately secrete a substance that forms an organic matrix
Outer enamel epithelium	layer of cuboidal cells covering the enamel organ in a developing tooth
Palatal surfaces	surfaces of the tooth facing the palate
Palate	upper portion of the mouth
Permanent teeth	teeth that replace primary teeth later on in childhood; also called succedaneous teeth
Posterior teeth	teeth toward the back of the mouth, including premolars and molars
Preameloblasts	during the advanced bell stage, inner enamel epithelium cells evolve into preameloblasts
Predentin	cells created from odontoblasts depositing minerals onto an organic matrix
Premolars	in the adult mouth, next to each canine tooth in the maxillary and mandibular are two premolars
Primary teeth	first set of teeth humans have in their lifetime; also called deciduous dentition
Proximal surface	a surface of a tooth that is facing an adjacent tooth
Pulp	soft tissue in the root of the tooth that enervates and provides blood supply to the tooth
Ridge	a raised area of a tooth
Root	the portion of the tooth between the cementoenamel junction and the apical foramen
Root axis line	line between the apex of the root and the tip of the cusp

Root canal	canal starting at the apical foramen leading to the pulp chamber that allows nerves and blood supply to enter the pulp
Stellate reticulum	interior of the enamel organ's cells
Stratum intermedium	layer of cells between the inner enamel epithelium and the stellate reticulum
Surface	a flat area of a tooth
Tooth bud	the first stage of tooth formation
Universal System	tooth numbering system adopted by the American Dental Association that lacks an anatomical reference
Upper left quadrant	left portion of the maxillary
Upper right quadrant	right portion of the maxillary
Vestibular lamina	layer of cells next to the dental lamina that begin to form the tooth bud
Zsigmondy-Palmer System	eight numerical quadrant system for tooth numbering used in the late 1800s

Author details

Abeer ALShami[1], Shatha ALHarthi[1]*, Munerah Binshabaib[1] and Monika Wahi[2]

1 Princess Nourah Bint Abdulrahman University, Riyadh, Saudi Arabia

2 Laboure College, Milton, Massachusetts, USA

*Address all correspondence to: shsalharthi@pnu.edu.sa

References

[1] Nelson SJ. Wheeler's Dental Anatomy, Physiology and Occlusion—E-Book. St. Louis, Mo: Elsevier Health Sciences; 2009. p. 401

[2] Koch G, Poulsen S, Espelid I, Haubek D. Pediatric Dentistry: A Clinical Approach. United Kingdom: John Wiley & Sons; 2017. p. 408

[3] Havale R, Sheetal BS, Patil R, Hemant Kumar R, Anegundi RT, Inushekar KR. Dental notation for primary teeth: A review and suggestion of a novel system. European Journal of Paediatric Dentistry. 2015;**16**(2):163-166

[4] Turp JC, Alt KW. Designating teeth: The advantages of the FDI's two-digit system. Quintessence International. 1995;**26**(7):501-504

[5] Dental Health Foundation. Tooth Types [Internet]. 2010. Dental Health Foundation. Available from: https://www.dentalhealth.ie/children/toothdevelopment/types/ [Accessed: 7 April 2019]

[6] Hovorakova M, Lesot H, Peterka M, Peterkova R. Early development of the human dentition revisited. Journal of Anatomy. 2018;**233**(2):135-145

[7] Sunderland EP, Smith CJ, Sunderland R. A histological study of the chronology of initial mineralization in the human deciduous dentition. Archives of Oral Biology. 1987;**32**(3):167-174

[8] Hovorakova M, Lesot H, Peterka M, Peterkova R. The developmental relationship between the deciduous dentition and the oral vestibule in human embryos. Anatomy and Embryology. 2005;**209**(4):303-313

[9] Fuller JL, Denehy GE, Schulein TM. Concise Dental Anatomy and Morphology. University of Iowa College of Dentistry; 2001. p. 218

[10] Peterkova R, Hovorakova M, Peterka M, Lesot H. Three-dimensional analysis of the early development of the dentition. Australian Dental Journal. 2014;**59**(Suppl 1):55-80

[11] Robinson C. Enamel maturation: A brief background with implications for some enamel dysplasias. Frontiers in Physiology. 2014. p. 388. Available from: https://www.ncbi.nlm.nih.gov/pmc/articles/PMC4189374/ [Accessed: 13 May 2019]

[12] Balic A. Concise review: Cellular and molecular mechanisms regulation of tooth initiation. Stem Cells. Jan 2018;**37**(1):26-32. DOI: 10.1002/stem.2917. Epub 20 Nov 2018

Chapter 6

External and Internal Anatomy of Maxillary Permanent First Molars

Abdulbaset A. Mufadhal, Mohammed A. Aldawla and Ahmed A. Madfa

Abstract

Adequate knowledge of the tooth morphology is of paramount importance for clinicians worked in the different branches of dentistry in order to maintain good oral health. Unfortunately, tooth morphology shows a high level of complexity and variability. These anatomical variations have been reported to be related to many factors including age, gender and ethnicity. The permanent first molars are the largest teeth in the maxilla which play an important role in mastication. Because of their early eruption, they are more vulnerable to caries and subsequent pulp and periapical pathoses. This chapter will summarize the internal and external morphologic features of these teeth with the reported variations in relation to age, gender and population in order to provide clinicians with the morphological knowledge necessary for performing successful dental treatments.

Keywords: morphology, maxillary, first molar, variations

1. External anatomy

1.1 Crown morphology

In the maxillary arch, the permanent first molar is the largest tooth. The anatomical crown of this tooth is broader buccolingually than mesiodistally (usually by 1 mm). This, however, may be changed from one individual to another. Even though, the crown is slightly shorter than premolars, it is wider both mesiodistally and buccolingually, giving the occlusal table its generous surface area that helps in food grinding [1].

This tooth has five cusps, four of which are well-developed to perform the intended function. These include the mesiobuccal, the mesiolingual, the distobuccal, and the distolingual cusps. The fifth one has yet been considered as a supplemental cusp of little physiological importance [1]. This little cusp have several names including accessory cusp, supplemental cusp, mesiolingual elevation, fifth lobe, Carabelli's tubercle, etc. [2] and can take various shapes ranging from a well-developed cusp to an interconnecting depressions, grooves, or pits on the mesial half of the palatal surface. The presence of this cusp or a developmental groove at its normal site is used to distinguish the maxillary first molar from other teeth [1]. In addition, it has been considered as a representative trait in anthropological and forensic studies for identifying different racial populations [1, 3]. High prevalence of Carabelli trait was reported in North West Europe origin Americans [4] whereas

Eskimo of unmixed descent had no Carabelli trait at all [5]. Russians [6], Brazilians [7], Malaysians [8] and Saudis [9] show moderate Carabelli trait prevalence.

1.2 Root morphology

Among the maxillary teeth, the permanent first molar has the strongest anchorage in the maxillary arch due to their well-developed widely separated roots [1]. Typically, this tooth has three roots, the mesiobuccal, distobuccal, and palatal [10]. These roots diverge in a manner parallel to the direction of the maximum force that could be applied diagonally against the crown in a buccolingual direction [1]. The palatal root is conical and smoothly rounded in shape. The mesiobuccal root is broader buccolingually with subsequent increased resistance to rotational forces. The distobuccal root is the smallest one with smooth rounded cross section. Normally, the palatal root is the longest one, and the other two roots have approximately similar lengths [1]. It has been reported that the average lengths of the mesiobuccal, distobuccal and palatal roots are 12.9 mm (8.5–18.8 mm); 12.2 mm (8.9–15.5 mm) and 13.7 mm (10.6–17.5 mm) respectively [11]. Generally, the average length of roots is approximately twice that of the crown [1].

Although anatomical variations have been reported in the literature however, the development of these teeth barely deviates from the typical morphology [1]. Several studies conducted in different populations (Korean, Thai, Chinese, polish, Russian, Burmese, and Kuwait populations) have reported that all or nearly all maxillary first molars presented with three separated roots [12–18]. It has also been reported that the prevalence of maxillary firs molars with two roots, four roots and single root are very low, (1.8%), (0.3%) and (0.2%) respectively [11]. However, Alrahabi and Sohail Zafar [19] used the CBCT technique to study the morphology of maxillary molars in a Saudi population and reported 94% of teeth with three separated roots, while the reminder 6% have four separated roots.

1.3 Root trunk and furcations

Normally, roots of the molars develop as one common root at the crown base before dividing into three roots (for the maxillary molars) or two roots (for the mandibular molars). This common root base is known as root trunk [1]. It extends from the cervical line to the entrance of the furcation [20]. In maxillary molars, the root trunk divides into three widely separated roots with three furcations, one buccally and two proximally. The access to these furcations is usually located in the coronal thirds of the roots. The buccal furcation entrance is approximately located at the center mesiodistally, while the entrances of the mesiopalatine and distopalatine furcations are slightly palatal to the center buccopalataly [21].

From a periodontal perspective, furcations of the maxillary first molars are more commonly involved than those of the mandibular first molars [22]. Additionally, the buccal furcations of the maxillary first molars are the most frequently affected, followed by the mesiopalatal and distopalatal furcations [23]. However, fortunately, the buccal furcation is the most accessible one for both patients and clinicians. The access to the periodontal lesion in proximal furcations represents a challenge for maintaining good oral hygiene and performing an optimal periodontal treatment [21].

It is generally accepted that root trunk length play an important role in the susceptibility of maxillary molars to periodontal disease [24]. Several studies evaluated the length of the root trunks in maxillary first molars [20, 25–30]. There was a general agreement in the majority of these studies that the mean trunk length in the buccal aspect is shorter than those in the mesial and distal ones [20, 25, 27, 29]. However, the mean length of the mesial and distal root trunks varies among different studies. Some authors found that the mean mesial root trunk is greater than the distal one [20, 27] whereas others reported that the distal root trunk was the longest one [28, 30]. Moreover, equal length of the mesial and distal root trunks has also been reported [26]. Although teeth with short root trunk are more susceptible for periodontal lesion on the furcation, however these teeth have a favorable prognosis after periodontal therapy since less attachment loss has occurred [31].

In maxillary first molars, a deep groove is frequently found on the buccal aspect of the root trunk which extends from the furcation to end as a shallow concavity at the cemento-enamel junction (CEJ) [1]. Jackson Lu [32] founded that about 94% of the evaluated furcations have a developmental depression of different depth on the root trunks of molars. These concavities may complicate the coronal adaptation of the membrane along the trunk surface during the guided tissue regeneration procedure. Furthermore, Kerns et al. [26] reported that the mean distances from the CEJ to these developmental grooves ranged between 1.35 mm and 1.65 in the maxillary first molars. Therefore, they stated that guided tissue regenerative therapy for short trunk molars could be compromised particularly if developmental root trunk grooves are present.

1.4 Root fusion

Root fusion is thought to be caused either by cementum deposition over time or due to inability of Hertwig epithelial sheath to form or fuse at the furcation area [33]. This is based on the fact that the three roots are initially developed as a single root projecting from the crown base then divided into three roots by the growth and fusion of the Hertwig root sheath. Frequently, root fusion in the mandibular molars takes the form of a C-shaped root, while maxillary molars may show different fusion patterns, such as partial or complete fusion of two or more roots [34]. According to Zhang et al. [34], there are six different patterns of root fusion in maxillary molars including Type 1 (MBR fused with DBR), Type 2 (MBR fused with PR), Type 3 (DBR fused with PR), Type 4 (MBR fused with DBR, PR fused MBR, or DBR), Type 5 (PR fused with MBR and DBR) and Type 6 (PR, MBR, and DBR fused to a cone-shaped root).

Generally, root fusion is less prevalent in maxillary first molars. The proportion of fused roots in maxillary second molars is about four folds greater than that in maxillary first molars [35]. Concluded from several cone beam computed tomographic studies, the averages of different types of root fusion in maxillary first molars are Types I (1.13%), type III (1.1%), type II (0.23%), type IV (0.2%), type V (0.2%) and type VI (0.1%) [11].

Although it is a rare variation, several studies have reported different proportions of root fusion in the maxillary first molars in different populations [10, 12, 36, 37]. Using cone-beam computed tomography (CBCT), Kim et al. [12] identified 0.73% of the first molars in a Korean population show fused roots. Neelakantan et al. [36] reported that root fusion present in 2.2% of the first maxillary molars in an Indian population. By using clearing techniques, Rwenyonyi et al. [37] found fused roots in 4.1% of the same teeth in Uganda. However, Al Shalabi et al. [38] reported that 11% of the maxillary first molars teeth of Irish population have fused roots. These variations could be in part due to that there has been no widely accepted definition of the fused root [12, 34]. Some authors have considered roots as fused if fusion extended along the entire root length. Others have categorized teeth in the fused group if one third or less of the roots were fused and subsequently ended up with higher prevalence. Therefore, the defining criteria of fused roots have to be clarified in to justify whether these differences in prevalence were true variations [12].

Root fusion has a strong clinical impact in periodontics and oral surgery and to a less extent in endodontics [35]. However, taking in consideration that a high proportion of fused roots also have their main root canals merging, it is obvious that root fusion represent challenges not only to root canal preparation but also to endodontic microsurgery [11, 35]. For example, merging canals can create angles which increase the stress on endodontic instruments. Moreover, roots with multiple canals show more isthmi and more complicated apical anatomy which may negatively influence the approach of the endodontic microsurgery [35].

1.5 Direction of apical root curvature

Knowledge of the apical root curvature is also an important factor that should be assessed properly before root canal treatment as well as prior to tooth extraction. Such knowledge enables the clinicians to perform a safe and efficient dental treatment through the selection of suitable instruments and approaches. According to Versiani et al. [11], the direction of the apical curvature for the three roots of the maxillary first molar has been reported. 78% of the mesiobuccal roots had distal apical curvature while 21% were straight and the remaining 1% showed s-shaped root. Although majority of the distobuccal roots were straight (54%), mesial curved, distal curved and s-shaped distobuccal roots have also been reported (19, 17 and 10% respectively). The palatal root showed buccal apical curvature in 55% of teeth while it was straight in 40.7%. In 3.2 and 1.1% of teeth, the palatal root showed mesial and distal curvature respectively. It is worth mentioning that root curvatures in the buccolingual direction are frequently underestimated and undiscovered clinically through the conventional projections of the two-dimensional intra-oral radiography. Therefore, different angled projections are necessary to identify the presence and direction of root curvature.

2. Internal anatomy

In 1907, Fischer [39] showed, for the first time, the anatomical complexity of the apical root canal by injecting the teeth with a collodion solution. Due to this unpredictability and complexity of the canal morphology, he came up with the widely used description "root canal System". Therefore, the thought of a single uniform root canal with a single centered apical foramen is a misconception [40]. Generally, pulp cavity consists of the pulp chamber that is situated within the anatomical crown and the root canal system that is located inside the anatomical root [41]. Other anatomical features of the pulp space include pulp horns, canal orifices, furcation, lateral and accessory canals, inter-canal anastomosis, and apical foramina [41].

2.1 Pulp chamber morphology

Generally, the shape of the pulp chamber follows the shape of the tooth crown. Therefore, the pulp chamber of maxillary first molar is rather rectangular from the mesial aspect and squared from the buccal aspect of the tooth [1]. Theses shapes are usually constricted at the floor of the pulp chamber [21]. This tooth has a relatively large pulp chamber with four prominent projections (horns) under the well-developed four cusps [1]. However, the size of the pulp chamber is reduced with age either physiologically by the continued formation of secondary dentine or pathologically through the formation of reparative or tertiary dentine as a consequent of pulp irritation or dental trauma [42]. Moreover, the formation of the secondary dentin is not uniformly distributed. Greater amount of secondary dentine production takes place at the roof and floor of the pulp chamber when compared with the other walls [43]. Therefore, a flattened, disc-like pulp chamber is frequently seen in old aged patients which may complicate the access cavity preparation and canals identification during root canal treatment [41]. In such situation, the pulp chamber roof is very close to the floor which decreases the clinician's tactile perception and may result in perforation during access cavity preparation [44, 45].

It is clear that knowledge of the average dimensions and general location of the pulp chamber in molars may decrease the occurrence of chamber perforations during the access preparation. Unfortunately, few studies have been conducted to correlate external anatomical landmarks with the floor and roof of the chamber [46]. Sterrett et al. [47] measured the distance from the pulp chamber floor to the furcation of the maxillary and mandibular molars. They found that this distance range from 2.7 to 3 mm in maxillary and mandibular molars. In their study, Majzoub and Kon [48] reported that the average distance from the chamber floor to the furcation was not more than 3 mm in 86% of the measured maxillary molars. Several distances from multiple anatomical landmarks have been measured in the maxillary molars by Deutsch and Musikant [46]. The mean distance from the chamber floor to the furcation was 3.05 mm, from the chamber roof to furcation was 4.91 mm, from the tip of the buccal cusp to the furcation was 11.15 mm, from the buccal cusp tip to the chamber floor was 8.08 mm and from the buccal cusp tip to the chamber roof was 6.24 mm. They also found that the roof pulp chamber was located at the same level of the cementoenamel junction (CEJ) in 98% of the maxillary molars. Townsend et al. [49] conducted similar study on the maxillary first molars of an Indian population and found comparable results as follows: the distance from chamber floor to the furcation = 2.7 ± 0.63; distance from the chamber roof to the furcation = 5.34 ± 0.9; distance from the palatal cusp tip to the furcation = 11.58 ± 1.01; distance from the tip of the palatal cusp to the chamber floor = 8.86 ± 0.68; distance from the tip of the palatal cusp to the chamber roof = 6.2 ± 0.66. Similarly, the roof of the pulp chamber was found at the level of the CEJ in 96% of the measured teeth.

2.2 Canal orifices locations

The canal orifices of the maxillary first molars form a triangular shape in the floor of the pulp chamber; the base of the triangle connects the mesiobuccal and the palatal canals while the orifice of the distobuccal canal represents the apex of the triangle. The orifice of the palatal canal is located at the center lingually. The orifice of the mesiobuccal canal is located at the acute corner of the pulp chamber while the distobuccal canal is located somewhat distal and palatal to the mesiobuccal canal, close to the obtuse corner of the pulp chamber. If it is present, the second mesiobuccal canal (MB2) will be positioned palatal to the mesiobuccal canal and at or slightly mesial to the imaginary line connecting the mesiobuccal and the palatal canals [1].

This knowledge has a direct clinical influence on the form and extent of the endodontic access cavity. Conventionally, a triangular shaped access cavity was prepared during root canal treatment of these teeth. However, this seems to be inconsistent with the fact that maxillary first molars frequently have an extra-canal (MB2) in the mesiobuccal root which is difficult to locate and prepare [50, 51]. The presence of MB2 has to be expected by the clinician until the clinical and radiographic assessment show the opposite [50]. In order to locate the extra-canals, it has been proposed that the outline form of the access cavity should be guided by the morphology of the pulp chamber floor [52]. Therefore, several authors have advised to re-assess the shape and design of the endodontic access cavity for maxillary molar teeth [53–55]. To locate MB2 in maxillary molars, the shape of the access opening should be first modified from the conventional triangular outline to the rhomboidal shape [56]. Besides the access cavity modification, different angled radiographs, NaOCl bubble test, surgical loupe and operating microscope represent other clinical facilities for locating extra-canals [51, 52].

2.3 Root canal morphology

Root canal is the radicular portion of the pulp space. It starts as a funnel shaped orifice on the floor of the pulp chamber at or somewhat apical to cervical line, and ends as one or multiple apical foramina at or lateral (0–3 mm) to the center of the anatomical apex of the root [21, 57, 58].

The root canal morphology of the maxillary first molar is one of the most complex root canal anatomies in human dentition [11]. Generally, the most frequent pattern of the maxillary permanent first molar in the literature has three roots and four canals with a high incidence of a second canal in the mesiobuccal root (MB2) [10, 11]. This is consistent with the broad buccolingual dimension of the mesiobuccal root and with the root depressions on its proximal surfaces [1].

The horizontal shape of the root canals varies along its length. From the canal orifice to the midroot, the mesiobuccal canal is oval or flat oval in cross section and then tapers to terminate as a round canal with very small diameter. Frequently, the palatal canal and distobuccal canal are oval or round in shape and taper gradually to the apex [1, 11].

2.3.1 Accessory and lateral canals

Any branch of the pulp cavity, other than the main canals, that communicates with the periodontium is called an accessory canal. Additionally, any accessory canal extending horizontally from the cervical or middle third of the main canal is called a lateral canal [59]. These canals are thought to be formed during the calcification due to the entrapment of blood vessels from the periodontium into the Hertwig's root sheath [60]. Studying root canal anatomy of the human permanent teeth, Vertucci [57] reported that accessory canals were more commonly located in the apical third of the root (73.5%), followed by the middle third (11.4%) and the coronal third (6.3%). In the maxillary permanent first molars, he found that accessory canals are more prevalent in the mesiobuccal and palatal roots (51% and 48% respectively) than those in the distobuccal root (36%). In multi-rooted teeth, accessory canals can also be located in the trifurcation or bifurcation, and are called furcation canals [61]. They are forms as a consequence of blood vessels entrapment during the fusion of the root diaphragm [60]. The incidence of such canals in the maxillary first molars is 18% [11, 57]. Accessory canals represent an additional pathway for the transmission of irritants mainly from the pulp space to the periodontium, resulting in primary endodontic lesions [41].

2.3.2 Isthmi

An isthmus is a thin transverse anastomosis that connects two roots canals [62]. It can be found in any root with multiple canals [41]. This intercanal connection serves as a bacterial reservoir which is difficult to be cleaned mechanically even with the most sophisticated engine driven endodontic instruments. It has been reported that 52% of the mesiobuccal roots of the maxillary first molar show transverse anastomosis (10% coronally, 75% at midroot and 15% apically) [11, 41]. Weller et al. [63] reported that most of the anastomosis in the mesiobuccal root of the maxillary first molars was found at 3–5 mm short of the apex. The presence of such anastomosis may jeopardize the outcome of the surgical endodontic treatment [64, 65]. Therefore, Cambruzzi and Marshall [62] emphasized that these anastomosis should be cleaned, prepared and filled during endodontic surgery. They also suggested the use of methylene blue stain to facilitate the identification of an isthmus occurrence in the resected root surface.

2.3.3 Apical anatomy

In a large proportion of maxillary first molars, the apical foramina of the three root canals are located lateral to the corresponding root tip (82% of the palatal roots, 81% of the distobuccal roots and 76% of the mesiobuccal roots) [11]. On average, majority of the MB2 canals (61.6%) merge with the mesiobuccal canals at the midroot or apical region and share the same foramen while minority of them (38.4%) end in a separated foramen [10].

The presence of more than one apical foramen is not uncommon. Morfis et al. [66] used a scanning electron microscope to study the apical anatomy of 213 permanent teeth. They found that the presence of more than one apical foramen was observed in all roots except for the distal root of mandibular molars and the palatal root of the maxillary molars. They also reported that the mesiobuccal root of the maxillary molars showed a high prevalence of multiple apical foramina (41.7%).

Marroquín et al. [67] studied the apical anatomy of the maxillary and mandibular molars in an Egyptian population using stereomicroscope. They found that most of the roots (70%) have oval apical constrictions. The average of the narrow and wide diameters of the apical constriction in maxillary molars was 0.18–0.25 mm in the mesiobuccal and distobuccal root, and 0.22–0.29 mm in the palatal root. They also found a high frequency (71%) of two main foramina in the mesiobuccal root of the maxillary first molars. Additionally, the accessory foramina were found in about 33% of these roots.

Moreover, apical ramifications have been reported to be found in 32–86% of maxillary first molar teeth [11]. All these anatomical irregularities show the complex nature of the root canal system in maxillary first molars which invariably complicates the root canal treatment procedures.

2.3.4 Root canal curvature

Preoperative recognition of the root canal curvature is of paramount importance during the root canal treatment. This is considered as an important factor in determining the level of difficulty, and the probability of procedural errors during root canal treatment [68]. This will invariably guide the clinician to select the most appropriate technique and instruments to effectively prepare the root canal system. Root canal curvature could be a gradual smooth curve of the whole canal or a sharp bent in the apical part of the canal [41]. Versiani et al. [11] have reported the range of curvature degree for each root canal of the maxillary first molars in the clinical view (MB1 0–42°; MB2 23–49°; DB, 0–48°; P, 0–47°) as well as proximal views (MB1, 0–54°; MB2, 0–36°; DB, 0–41°; P, 0–38°). Several methods [69–71] have been proposed to assess the root canal curvature, by measuring the angle of the curvature and/or the radius of the curvature. Radiographically, Schäfer et al. [72] evaluated the degree of curvature of more than 1160 root canals in all human teeth from the clinical (0–75°) and proximal views (0–69°). They reported that the most severe curvature was found in the clinical projection of the mesiobuccal root canals of maxillary permanent molars and in the mesial root canals of the mandibular permanent molars. According to Vertucci [41], almost all root canals in human are curved apically, especially in the buccolingual direction. Therefore, in order to recognize the presence, severity, and direction of the root canal curvature, it is necessary to evaluate the tooth radiographically from different angled projections.

2.4 Variations in the root canal anatomy

2.4.1 Variations in the occurrence of MB2 in maxillary first molars

The internal anatomy of the mesiobuccal root is the main focus of many morphological studies as the incidence of more than one canal is highly variable [41, 73]. In addition to the variations due to the age [55, 74] and gender [74, 75], several studies in various populations revealed that, the anatomy of root canal system has ethnic features [13, 76–78]. Therefore, many researchers had studied the internal root anatomy of the maxillary first molar, mesiobuccal root in particular, in different racial populations and subpopulations using different techniques [12–15, 19, 38, 52, 57, 78–82].

A wide range of ethnic variations has been inferred from several studies conducted to evaluate the root and canal anatomy of mesiobuccal root of maxillary first molar in various populations. For example, a high prevalence of the MB2 has been reported in Japanese (88.2%) [52], Iranian (86.6%) [78], Ireland (78%) [38], Australian (73.6%) [83], Caucasian (71%) [84] and Saudi (70.6%) [19] populations. However, a lower prevalence has been reported in Korean (63.59%) [12], Thailand (63.3%) [13], Russian (59.8%) [17], Polish (59.5%) [15], Greek (53.2%) [85] and Pakistani (48%) [81] populations. According to two different studies, the lowest reported incidence of MB2 was in Brazil (42.63%) [80] and (25%) [86]. As a result of such ethnic variations, the evaluation of root canal anatomy for all populations and ethnic groups is indispensable [36, 87].

Regarding the variation with age, many studies concluded that the prevalence of MB2 decreases by aging, due to dentine apposition which subsequently results in narrowing and obliteration of the canal [55, 88, 89]. For example, Razumova et al. [17] evaluated the presence of MB2 canal in different age groups; young (20–44 years), middle-aged (45–60 years) and elderly (>60 years). They observed that the presence of MB2 was higher in young group with 48.8% than that in middle with 33.2% and elderly group with 18%. Similar results were obtained in a study by Zheng et al. [14] in which they observed a higher prevalence of MB2 among patients between 20 and 30 years of age. However, these findings are in contrast with those of Ratanajirasut et al. [13] and Katarzyna and Pawlicka [15] who did not find correlation between age and the prevalence of MB2 in the maxillary first molars. Unexpectedly, in a study conducted on a Chilean population, a higher occurrence of the MB2 canal in the maxillary first and second molars in older patients was observed [90]. These differences could be related to the sample size and the anatomical variations among populations. However, MB2 could exist in any age group, and the clinician should be aware of finding and treating it [17].

Few studies have reported gender differences in the morphology of the root canal system [91]. Sert and Bayirli [75] studied the root canal morphology of 2800 extracted teeth (1400 teeth from each gender) from Turkish individuals by using decalcification and clearing method. For each gender, they included 100 teeth of each type of the permanent dentition, except the third molars, in their sample. Even though only 100 teeth of each tooth type for each gender were evaluated, a significant morphological difference has been noted between males and females. Regarding the mesiobuccal root, type I Vertucci canal configuration was found in only 3% of males compared to 10% of females. Therefore, they suggested that morphological variations due to gender and ethnic background should be considered during the preoperative evaluation for the root canal therapy. Similarly, Kim et al.

[12] reported higher numbers of additional canals in males' mesiobuccal root of maxillary first molars. However, there are conflicting results with respect to gender and the number of canals [55, 75, 89, 92].

In addition to the previously mentioned variation factors, differences in reported results may also be influenced by the design of the study (clinical versus laboratory) [93]. Some authors conducted studies to compare the results of in vivo versus in vitro techniques. Seidberg et al. [94] found MB2 canal in 33.3% of 201 first maxillary molars in their clinical in vivo study compared to 62% in their in vitro sectioning evaluation of 100 of the same tooth type. These results were comparable to another study conducted by Pomeranz and Fishelberg [95]. They reported that MB2 canal was found in 31% of 100 teeth examined in vivo. This percentage increased to 69% when the same number of teeth was evaluated in their in vitro study. The more common use of SOM or loupes in recent clinical studies has resulted in an increased prevalence of the clinical detection of the MB2 canal [73, 96]. The effect of magnification on the incidence of MB2 was assessed in a clinical study by Buhrley et al. [96]. They reported that MB2 canal was located in 71.1% of the maxillary first molars treated with the aid of surgical operating microscope (SOM). When the dental loupe was used, this percentage was reduced to 62.5%. In the non-magnification group, the percentage was decreased dramatically to only 17.2% of the teeth. Sempira and Hartwell [73] concluded that the incidence of MB2 increased significantly when the SOM is used during the root canal therapy.

In conclusion, the wide variation in the reported prevalence of MB2 canal is significantly affected by the method of evaluation being used. As a result, any attempt to compare MB2 prevalence of different populations should take in consideration the similarity of the evaluation methods. For example, considering only CBCT in vivo studies, MB2 prevalence vary from 86% in Iran [78] to 30.9% in China [97], with in-between proportions in other countries such as Portugal (71%) [84], Korea (63.6%) [12], and Brazil (44.4%) [80]. Another issue is that all these studies were conducted by different research teams which can lead to variations in the CBCT assessment among different observers. This in turn affects the validity of any attempt of direct comparison.

To overcome these drawbacks, recent global in vivo study [98] has been conducted to evaluate the prevalence of the MB2 canal in the maxillary first molars in 21 different geographic regions around the world using CBCT method. The special issue in this study is that twenty-one observers from different countries have been uniformly pre-calibrated to reduce the inter-observers variability. They found that MB2 prevalence ranged widely from 48.0 to 97.6% among the studied countries, with a global MB2 proportion of 73.8%. However, the authors also clarified some drawbacks of their study. Bearing in mind the effect of age and gender on the MB2 prevalence, it seems to be difficult to compare the different regions in this study due to the high variations in their mean age and gender proportions. In addition, although serious attempts were performed to pre-calibrate the observers, assessment differences may still present due to the differences in personal experience and beliefs. They suggested that these limitations can be overcome by gathering CBCT databases of patients having the same age and enrolling both genders equally in the all different regions. Then, all these databases have to be assessed by a single qualified observer [98].

2.4.2 Bilateral existence of MB2 in maxillary first molars

Several studies have investigated the simultaneous presence of MB2 root canal in the contra-lateral maxillary first molars among different populations. High proportions of bilateral occurrence of MB2 canal in maxillary first molars have been reported in selected Korean [12], Malaysians [99], and Chinese [100] populations (82.9; 82.36;

and 74% respectively). Clinically, previous knowledge about the presence of MB2 in one maxillary first molar should make the clinician aware about the increased likelihood of MB2 occurrence in the contra-lateral molar of the same patient.

2.4.3 Variations in the number of distobuccal and palatal root canals

According to Cleghorn et al. review [10], single canal (98.3%) with a single apical foramen (98%) is the most frequent canal pattern in the distobuccal root. In a similar manner, the majority of the palatal roots have a single canal and a single foramen (99 and 98.8% respectively). Although anatomical variations for these root canals have been reported, they are significantly rare. Several studies addressed this issue in different populations. Alrahabi and Sohail Zafar [19] conducted a study on a Saudi population and found that the distobuccal and the palatal root had one root canal in 100% of cases. In Razumova et al. [17] study on a Russians population, the distobuccal root contained single canal in most of cases and two canals in 0.5%. Similar results were obtained by Ratanajirasut et al. [13] (Thai population), Zheng et al. [14] (Chinese), Neelakantan et al. [36] (Indians), and Kim et al. [12] (Koreans), in which second distobuccal was found in 1, 1.2, 2.2, and 1.25% of cases, respectively.

2.5 Anatomical anomalies

Generally, the most frequent pattern of the maxillary permanent first molar in the literature has three roots and four canals with a high incidence of a second canal in the mesiobuccal root (MB2), [10, 11]. Although anatomical anomalies have been reported in the literature however, they are barely mentioned in studies [10]. Maxillary first molar with four roots [101], five roots [101], two roots [102], single conical root [103, 104] and single O-shaped root [105] have been reported. Additionally, it has been inferred from several CBCT studies that the incidence of C-shaped root canals in maxillary first molars ranges from 0.3% to 1.1% with an average equal to 0.83% [11]. Other anatomical anomalies such as maxillary first molars with One canal [103], five canals [106], six canals [107], seven canals [108], eight canals [109], and hypertaurodontism [110] are extremely rare and have been documented as case reports.

Enamel pearls and trunk developmental grooves are most prevalent in the maxillary molars [1]. These anatomical anomalies are considered as local cofactors that increase the risk of periodontal disease development [111].

3. Clinical remarks

Maxillary first molars present the greatest clinical challenge for endodontic treatment. This is because the complexity of the root canal system surpasses that of all other teeth within the human dentition [11]. It is generally accepted that the mesiobuccal root of these teeth has a second canal in majority of cases. Although this canal is usually difficult to be negotiated, it must be expected to be there until clinical and radiographic examinations prove its absence [50]. Clinically, the location of this canal varies to a large extent, but it is frequently positioned mesial to or along the imaginary line connecting the mesiobuccal and palatal canals, within average area of 2 mm mesially and 3.5 mm palatally from the orifice of the MB1 canal [112]. Radiographically, it is mandatory to take and carefully evaluate two or more different angled radiographs which would provide much required information about the morphology of the root canal system [41, 113].

According to Görduysus et al. [112], 16% of MB2 canals cannot be negotiated down beyond the orifice. This could be due to several reasons such as the presence of a dentine ledge which covers the orifice, its mesiobuccal inclined entrance on the chamber floor, its route coronally which frequently shows single or multiple sharp curves and its tendency to be more calcified especially in old aged individuals [11, 41]. Therefore, Vertucci [41] suggested that countersinking or troughing of the developmental groove, which is located palatal to the MB1 canal, by using ultrasonic tips would eliminate most of these obstacles. During this procedure, the groove should be deepened apically (0.5–3 mm) and widened mesially. This may require a slight modification in the access outline to extend more mesially. Due to the presence of a concavity on the distal surface of this root, troughing should be prepared with cautions to avoid perforation into the furcation.

Despite their frequency of occurrence, high variations in the number of canals for maxillary first molars have been reported in the literature. Accordingly, the mesiobuccal and the palatal roots may have one, two, or three canals, whereas the distobuccal root may contain one or two canals [11]. In order to locate these additional canals properly, several diagnostic aids should be taken in consideration. These include examination of the chamber floor by using a sharp endodontic explorer, using methylene blue to stain the orifices, visual inspection of the bleeding points, performing the 'champagne bubble' test using sodium hypochlorite and magnification of the pulp floor using dental loupe or surgical operating microscope [41, 51, 52]. Surgical operating microscope (SOM) significantly enhances the visibility and lightening of minute details. Using SOM, clinician is able to remove obstacles and calcifications selectively in a precise manner that would minimize the procedural errors [41].

Although the palatal root usually has a large and easily accessible canal on the pulpal floor, it requires skillful cleaning and shaping procedure. This root canal often curves buccally in its apical part. Since it is difficult to be recognized with the two dimensional intra-oral radiograph, this may results in under-estimation of the working length with subsequent short preparation and obturation of this canal [21].

Author details

Abdulbaset A. Mufadhal[1*], Mohammed A. Aldawla[1] and Ahmed A. Madfa[1,2]

1 Department of Conservative Dentistry, Faculty of Dentistry, Sana'a University, Sana'a, Yemen

2 Department of Conservative Dentistry, Faculty of Dentistry, Thamar University, Dhamar, Yemen

*Address all correspondence to: dr.obad99@gmail.com

References

[1] Nelson S, Ash M. Wheeler' s Dental Anatomy, Physiology, and Occlusion. St. Louis, Missouri: Saunders Elsevier; 2010

[2] Kirthiga M et al. Ethnic Association of Cusp of Carabelli trait and shoveling trait in an Indian population. Journal of Clinical and Diagnostic Research: JCDR. 2016;**10**(3):ZC78

[3] Mavrodisz K et al. Prevalence of accessory tooth cusps in a contemporary and ancestral Hungarian population. The European Journal of Orthodontics. 2007;**29**(2):166-169

[4] Meredith HV, Hixon EH. Frequency, size, and bilateralism of Carabelli's tubercle. Journal of Dental Research. 1954;**33**(3):435-440

[5] Pedersen PO. Dental Investigations of Greenland Eskimos [Summary]. In: Proceedings of the Royal Society of Medicine. 1947;**40**(12):726-732

[6] Carbonell VM. The tubercle of Carabelli in the Kish dentition, Mesopotamia, 3000 BC. Journal of Dental Research. 1960;**39**(1):124-128

[7] Ferreira MA et al. Presence and morphology of the molar tubercle according to dentition, hemi-arch and sex. International Journal of Morphology. 2010;**28**(1):121-125

[8] Rusmah M. The cusp of Carabelli in Malaysians. Odonto-stomatologie Tropicale = Tropical Dental Journal. 1992;**15**(1):13-15

[9] Syed S et al. The prevalence of fifth cusp (Cusp of Carabelli) in the upper molars in Saudi Arabian school students. International Journal of Morphology. 2012;**30**(2):757-760

[10] Cleghorn BM, Christie WH, Dong CC. Root and root canal morphology of the human permanent maxillary first molar: A literature review. Journal of Endodontia. 2006;**32**(9):813-821

[11] Versiani MA, Basrani B, Sousa-Neto MD. The Root Canal Anatomy in Permanent Dentition. Springer, Cham; 2018

[12] Kim Y, Lee SJ, Woo J. Morphology of maxillary first and second molars analyzed by cone-beam computed tomography in a korean population: Variations in the number of roots and canals and the incidence of fusion. Journal of Endodontia. 2012;**38**(8):1063-1068

[13] Ratanajirasut R, Panichuttra A, Panmekiate S. A cone-beam computed tomographic study of root and canal morphology of maxillary first and second permanent molars in a Thai population. Journal of Endodontia. 2018;**44**(1):56-61

[14] Zheng QH et al. A cone-beam computed tomography study of maxillary first permanent molar root and canal morphology in a Chinese population. Journal of Endodontia. 2010;**36**(9):1480-1484

[15] Katarzyna O, Pawlicka H. The morphology of maxillary first and second molars analyzed by cone-beam computed tomography in a Polish population. BMC Medical Imaging. 2017;**17**(1):68

[16] Ng YL et al. Root and canal morphology of Burmese maxillary molars. International Endodontic Journal. 2001;**34**(8):620-630

[17] Razumova S et al. Evaluation of anatomy and root canal morphology of the maxillary first molar using the cone-beam computed tomography among residents of the Moscow region.

Contemporary Clinical Dentistry. 2018;**9**(Suppl 1):S133-S136

[18] Pattanshetti N, Gaidhane M, Al Kandari AM. Root and canal morphology of the mesiobuccal and distal roots of permanent first molars in a Kuwait population—A clinical study. International Endodontic Journal. 2008;**41**(9):755-762

[19] Alrahabi M, Sohail Zafar M. Evaluation of root canal morphology of maxillary molars using cone beam computed tomography. Pakistan Journal of Medical Sciences. 2015;**31**(2):426-430

[20] Dababneh R et al. Root trunk: Types and dimension and their influence on the diagnosis and treatment of periodontally involved first molars. Journal of the Royal Medical Services. 2011;**18**(1):45

[21] Scheid RC. Woelfel's Dental Anatomy. Philadelphia: Lippincott, Williams & Wilkins; 2012

[22] Cattabriga M, Pedrazzoli V, Wilson TG Jr. The conservative approach in the treatment of furcation lesions. Periodontology 2000. 2000;**22**(1):133-153

[23] Sánchez-Pérez A, Moya-Villaescusa MJ. Periodontal disease affecting tooth furcations. A review of the treatments available. Medicina Oral Patologia Oral y Cirugia Bucal. 2009;**14**(10):554-557

[24] Desanctis M, Murphy KG. The role of resective periodontal surgery in the treatment of furcation defects. Periodontology 2000. 2000;**22**:154-168

[25] Plagmann HC, Holtorf S, Kocher T. A study on the imaging of complex furcation forms in upper and lower molars. Journal of Clinical Periodontology. 2000;**27**(12):926-931

[26] Kesas DG et al. Root trunk dimensions of 5 different tooth types. International Journal of Periodontics & Restorative Dentistry. 1999;**19**(1):82-91

[27] Porciúncula HF, Zuza EP, Mendes A. Root trunk height as a risk factor for periodontal furcation involvement in maxillary first molars: An in vitro study. Journal of the International Academy of Periodontology. 2007;**9**(3):89-95

[28] Roussa E. Anatomic characteristics of the furcation and root surfaces of molar teeth and their significance in the clinical management of marginal periodontitis. Clinical Anatomy: The Official Journal of the American Association of Clinical Anatomists and the British Association of Clinical Anatomists. 1998;**11**(3):177-186

[29] Rosenberg M. Furcation Involvement: Periodontic, Endodontic and Restorative Interrelationships. Periodontal and Prosthetic Management for Advanced Cases. Chicago: Quintessence; 1988. p. 247

[30] Gher MW Jr, Dunlap RW. Linear variation of the root surface area of the maxillary first molar. Journal of Periodontology. 1985;**56**(1):39-43

[31] McClain PK, Schallhorn RG. Focus on furcation defects–guided tissue regeneration in combination with bone grafting. Periodontology 2000. 2000;**22**(1):190-212

[32] Jackson Lu H-K. Topographical characteristics of root trunk length related to guided tissue regeneration. Journal of Periodontology. 1992;**63**(3):215-219

[33] Al-Fouzan KS. C-shaped root canals in mandibular second molars in a Saudi Arabian population. International Endodontic Journal. 2002;**35**(6):499-504

[34] Zhang Q et al. Root and root canal morphology in maxillary second molar

with fused root from a native Chinese population. Journal of Endodontics. 2014;**40**(6):871-875

[35] Martins JN et al. Prevalence of root fusions and main root canal merging in human upper and lower molars: A cone-beam computed tomography in vivo study. Journal of Endodontics. 2016;**42**(6):900-908

[36] Neelakantan P et al. Cone-beam computed tomography study of root and canal morphology of maxillary first and second molars in an Indian population. Journal of Endodontia. 2010;**36**(10):1622-1627

[37] Rwenyonyi CM et al. Root and canal morphology of maxillary first and second permanent molar teeth in a Ugandan population. International Endodontic Journal. 2007;**40**(9):679-683

[38] Al Shalabi RM et al. Root canal anatomy of maxillary first and second permanent molars. International Endodontic Journal. 2000;**33**(5):405-414

[39] Fischer G. Über die feinere Anatomie der Wurzelkanäle menschlicher Zähne. Dtsch Monatsschr Zahnheilk. 1907;**25**:544-552

[40] Hargreaves KM. Cohen's Pathways of the Pulp. St. Louis, Mosby: Elsevier; 2011

[41] Vertucci FJ. Root canal morphology and its relationship to endodontic procedures. Endodontic Topics. 2005;**10**(1):3-29

[42] Carrotte P. Endodontics: Part 4 Morphology of the root canal system. British Dental Journal. 2004;**197**:379

[43] Kronfeld R. Dental Histology and Comparative Dental Anatomy. Philadelphia: Lea & Febiger; 1937

[44] Alhadainy HA. Root perforations: A review of literature. Oral Surgery, Oral Medicine, Oral Pathology. 1994;**78**(3):368-374

[45] Goon WW, Lundergan WP. Redemption of a perforated furcation with a multidisciplinary treatment approach. Journal of Endodontics. 1995;**21**(11):576-579

[46] Deutsch AS, Musikant BL. Morphological measurements of anatomic landmarks in human maxillary and mandibular molar pulp chambers. Journal of Endodontics. 2004;**30**(6):388-390

[47] Sterrett JD, Pelletier H, Russell CM. Tooth thickness at the furcation entrance of lower molars. Journal of Clinical Periodontology. 1996;**23**(7):621-627

[48] Majzoub Z, Kon S. Tooth morphology following root resection procedures in maxillary first molars. Journal of Periodontology. 1992;**63**(4):290-296

[49] Townsend G et al. How studies of twins can inform our understanding of dental morphology. Frontiers of Oral Biology. 2009;**13**:136-141

[50] Ting P, Nga L. Clinical detection of the minor mesiobuccal canal of maxillary first molars. International Endodontic Journal. 1992;**25**(6):304-306

[51] Stropko JJ. Canal morphology of maxillary molars: Clinical observations of canal configurations. Journal of Endodontics. 1999;**25**(6):446-450

[52] Imura N et al. Two canals in mesiobuccal roots of maxillary molars. International Endodontic Journal. 1998;**31**(6):410-414

[53] Kulid JC, Peters DD. Incidence and configuration of canal systems in the mesiobuccal root of maxillary first and

second molars. Journal of Endodontics. 1990;**16**(7):311-317

[54] Hartwell G, Bellizzi R. Clinical investigation of in vivo endodontically treated mandibular and maxillary molars. Journal of Endodontics. 1982;**8**(12):555-557

[55] Neaverth EJ, Kotler LM, Kaltenbach RF. Clinical investigation (in vivo) of endodontically treated maxillary first molars. Journal of Endodontics. 1987;**13**(10):506-512

[56] Kaptan F, Kayahan B, Bayırlı G. Anatomy of the pulp chamber floor of the permanent maxillary and mandibular molars. Balkan Journal of Stomatology. 2008;**12**(1):18-19

[57] Vertucci FJ. Root canal anatomy of the human permanent teeth. Oral Surgery, Oral Medicine, and Oral Pathology. 1984;**58**(5):589-599

[58] Gutierrez JH, Aguayo P. Apical foraminal openings in human teeth. Number and location. Oral Surgery, Oral Medicine, Oral Pathology, Oral Radiology, and Endodontics. 1995;**79**(6):769-777

[59] Endodontists, A.A.o., Glossary of Endodontic Terms. Chicago: American Association of Endodontists; 2003

[60] Cutright DE, Bhaskar SN. Pulpal vasculature as demonstrated by a new method. Oral Surgery, Oral Medicine, Oral Pathology. 1969;**27**(5):678-683

[61] Vertucci F, Seelig A, Gillis R. Root canal morphology of the human maxillary second premolar. Oral Surgery, Oral Medicine, and Oral Pathology. 1974;**38**(3):456-464

[62] Cambruzzi J, Marshall F. Molar endodontic surgery. Journal (Canadian Dental Association). 1983;**49**(1):61

[63] Weller RN, Niemczyk SP, Kim S. Incidence and position of the canal isthmus. Part 1. Mesiobuccal root of the maxillary first molar. Journal of Endodontics. 1995;**21**(7):380-383

[64] Rubinstein RA, Kim S. Short-term observation of the results of endodontic surgery with the use of a surgical operation microscope and Super-EBA as root-end filling material. Journal of Endodontics. 1999;**25**(1):43-48

[65] Rubinstein RA, Kim S. Long-term follow-up of cases considered healed one year after apical microsurgery. Journal of Endodontics. 2002;**28**(5):378-383

[66] Morfis A et al. Study of the apices of human permanent teeth with the use of a scanning electron microscope. Oral Surgery, Oral Medicine, Oral Pathology. 1994;**77**(2):172-176

[67] Marroquín BB, El-Sayed MA, Willershausen-Zönnchen B. Morphology of the physiological foramen: I. Maxillary and mandibular molars. Journal of Endodontics. 2004;**30**(5):321-328

[68] Faraj S, Boutsioukis C. Observer variation in the assessment of root canal curvature. International Endodontic Journal. 2017;**50**(2):167-176

[69] Schneider SW. A comparison of canal preparations in straight and curved root canals. Oral Surgery, Oral Medicine, Oral Pathology. 1971;**32**(2):271-275

[70] Weine F. Endodontic Therapy. 3rd ed. St. Louis: CV Mosby Co; 1982. pp. 283-286

[71] Pruett JP, Clement DJ, Carnes DL. Cyclic fatigue testing of nickel-titanium endodontic instruments. Journal of Endodontics. 1997;**23**(2):77-85

[72] Schäfer E et al. Roentgenographic investigation of frequency and degree of

canal curvatures in human permanent teeth. Journal of Endodontics. 2002;**28**(3):211-216

[73] Sempira HN, Hartwell GR. Frequency of second mesiobuccal canals in maxillary molars as determined by use of an operating microscope: A clinical study. Journal of Endodontia. 2000;**26**(11):673-674

[74] Weine FS. Endodontic Therapy. 6th ed. India: Mosby Publications; 2004

[75] Sert S, Bayirli GS. Evaluation of the root canal configurations of the mandibular and maxillary permanent teeth by gender in the Turkish population. Journal of Endodontia. 2004;**30**(6):391-398

[76] Weine FS et al. Canal configuration of the mesiobuccal root of the maxillary first molar of a Japanese sub-population. International Endodontic Journal. 1999;**32**(2):79-87

[77] Caliskan MK et al. Root canal morphology of human permanent teeth in a Turkish population. Journal of Endodontia. 1995;**21**(4):200-204

[78] Naseri M et al. Survey of anatomy and root canal morphology of maxillary first molars regarding age and gender in an Iranian population using cone-beam computed tomography. Iranian Endodontic Journal. 2016;**11**(4):298-303

[79] Ghoncheh Z, Zade BM, Kharazifard MJ. Root morphology of the maxillary first and second molars in an Iranian population using cone beam computed tomography. Journal of Dentistry (Tehran, Iran). 2017;**14**(3):115-122

[80] Silva EJ et al. Evaluation of root canal configuration of maxillary molars in a Brazilian population using cone-beam computed tomographic imaging: An in vivo study. Journal of Endodontia. 2014;**40**(2):173-176

[81] Wasti F, Shearer AC, Wilson NH. Root canal systems of the mandibular and maxillary first permanent molar teeth of south Asian Pakistanis. International Endodontic Journal. 2001;**34**(4):263-266

[82] Weine FS et al. Canal configuration in the mesiobuccal root of the maxillary first molar and its endodontic significance. Oral Surgery, Oral Medicine, and Oral Pathology. 1969;**28**(3):419-425

[83] Thomas RP, Moule AJ, Bryant R. Root canal morphology of maxillary permanent first molar teeth at various ages. International Endodontic Journal. 1993;**26**(5):257-267

[84] Martins JNR et al. Root and root canal morphology of the permanent dentition in a Caucasian population: A cone-beam computed tomography study. International Endodontic Journal. 2017;**50**(11):1013-1026

[85] Nikoloudaki GE, Kontogiannis TG, Kerezoudis NP. Evaluation of the root and canal morphology of maxillary permanent molars and the incidence of the second mesiobuccal root canal in Greek population using cone-beam computed tomography. The Open Dentistry Journal. 2015;**9**:267-272

[86] Pecora JD et al. Morphologic study of the maxillary molars. Part II: Internal anatomy. Brazilian Dental Journal. 1992;**3**(1):53-57

[87] Sperber GH. The phylogeny and odontogeny of dental morphology. From Apes to Angels. 1990:215-219

[88] Gilles J, Reader A. An SEM investigation of the mesiolingual canal in human maxillary first and second molars. Oral Surgery, Oral Medicine, and Oral Pathology. 1990;**70**(5):638-643

[89] Fogel HM, Peikoff MD, Christie WH. Canal configuration in the mesiobuccal root of the maxillary

first molar: A clinical study. Journal of Endodontia. 1994;**20**(3):135-137

[90] Abarca J et al. Assessment of mesial root morphology and frequency of MB2 canals in maxillary molars using cone beam computed tomography. International Journal of Morphology. 2015;**33**(4):1333-1337

[91] Caputo BV et al. Evaluation of the root canal morphology of molars by using cone-beam computed tomography in a Brazilian population: Part I. Journal of Endodontics. 2016;**42**(11):1604-1607

[92] Çalişkan MK et al. Root canal morphology of human permanent teeth in a Turkish population. Journal of Endodontics. 1995;**21**(4):200-204

[93] Alavi A et al. Root and canal morphology of Thai maxillary molars. International Endodontic Journal. 2002;**35**(5):478-485

[94] Seidberg BH et al. Frequency of two mesiobuccal root canals in maxillary permanent first molars. Journal of the American Dental Association (1939). 1973;**87**(4):852-856

[95] Pomeranz HH, Fishelberg G. The secondary mesiobuccal canal of maxillary molars. The Journal of the American Dental Association. 1974;**88**(1):119-124

[96] Buhrley LJ et al. Effect of magnification on locating the MB2 canal in maxillary molars. Journal of Endodontics. 2002;**28**(4):324-327

[97] Jing Y et al. Cone-beam computed tomography was used for study of root and canal morphology of maxillary first and second molars. Beijing da xue xue bao. Yi xue ban = Journal of Peking University. Health Sciences. 2014;**46**(6):958-962

[98] Martins JN et al. Worldwide analyses of maxillary first molar second mesiobuccal prevalence: A multicenter cone-beam computed tomographic study. Journal of Endodontics. 2018;**44**(11):1641-1649.e1

[99] Al-Kadhim AH et al. Morphology of maxillary first molars analyzed by cone-beam computed tomography among Malaysian: Variations in the number of roots and canals and the incidence of fusion. International Medical Journal Malaysia. 2017;**16**(2):33-39

[100] Wang H et al. Evaluation of root and canal morphology of maxillary molars in a Southern Chinese subpopulation: A cone-beam computed tomographic study. International Journal of Clinical and Experimental Medicine. 2017;**10**(4):7030-7039

[101] Barbizam JVB, Ribeiro RG, Tanomaru Filho M. Unusual anatomy of permanent maxillary molars. Journal of Endodontics. 2004;**30**(9):668-671

[102] Fava LRG. Root canal treatment in an unusual maxillary first molar: A case report. International Endodontic Journal. 2001;**34**(8):649-653

[103] Gopikrishna V, Bhargavi N, Kandaswamy D. Endodontic management of a maxillary first molar with a single root and a single canal diagnosed with the aid of spiral CT: A case report. Journal of Endodontics. 2006;**32**(7):687-691

[104] Saxena A et al. A rare case of maxillary first molar with single root and single canal diagnosed using spiral computed tomographic scan. Journal of Indian Society of Pedodontics and Preventive Dentistry. 2014;**32**(3):242-245

[105] Shin Y, Kim Y, Roh B-D. Maxillary first molar with an O-shaped root morphology: Report of a case. International Journal of Oral Science. 2013;**5**:242

[106] Beatty RG. A five-canal maxillary first molar. Journal of Endodontics. 1984;**10**(4):156-157

[107] Albuquerque DV et al. Endodontic management of maxillary permanent first molar with 6 root canals: 3 case reports. Oral Surgery, Oral Medicine, Oral Pathology, Oral Radiology, and Endodontology. 2010;**110**(4):e79-e83

[108] Kottoor J et al. Maxillary first molar with seven root canals diagnosed with cone-beam computed tomography scanning: A case report. Journal of Endodontics. 2010;**36**(5):915-921

[109] Kottoor J, Velmurugan N, Surendran S. Endodontic management of a maxillary first molar with eight root canal systems evaluated using cone-beam computed tomography scanning: A case report. Journal of Endodontics. 2011;**37**(5):715-719

[110] Sert S, Bayırlı G. Taurodontism in six molars: A case report. Journal of Endodontics. 2004;**30**(8):601-602

[111] Blieden TM. Tooth-related issues. Annals of Periodontology. 1999;**4**(1):91-96

[112] Görduysus MÖ, Görduysus M, Friedman S. Operating microscope improves negotiation of second mesiobuccal canals in maxillary molars. Journal of Endodontics. 2001;**27**(11):683-686

[113] Martínez-Lozano MÁ, Forner-Navarro L, Sánchez-Cortés JL. Analysis of radiologic factors in determining premolar root canal systems. Oral Surgery, Oral Medicine, Oral Pathology, Oral Radiology, and Endodontology. 1999;**88**(6):719-722

Chapter 7

External and Internal Root Canal Anatomy of the First and Second Permanent Maxillary Molars

Said Dhaimy, Lamyae Bedida, Hafsa El Merini and Imane Benkiran

Abstract

A successful endodontic treatment depends on a comprehensive knowledge of the morphology of canal and its variations, an appropriate access cavity, cleaning and shaping, and adequate root canal filling. Lack of knowledge in this regard and missing a root canal are among the most common causes of failure of root canal treatments. Most previous studies on maxillary molars have reported that they usually have three roots and four canals since an extra canal is often found in the mesiobuccal root. Other anatomical variations, such as an extra C-shaped canal, have also been reported in distobuccal and palatal roots. Thus, because of having a more complex anatomy compared to other teeth, maxillary molars have the highest rate of endodontic failure. Several studies have assessed the morphology of root canal anatomy in different populations using different techniques such as sectioning, root canal clearing, association of a dental operating microscope and ultrasonic tips, periapical radiography, and computed tomography scanning. Recently, CBCT was suggested to three-dimensionally explore the root canal details before an endodontic treatment. The purpose of this chapter was to highlight the importance of having a thorough knowledge about the root canal morphology of the permanent first and second maxillary molar.

Keywords: permanent maxillary first molars, permanent maxillary second molars, root canal complex, internal morphology, anatomic variation

1. Introduction

The root canal configuration is complex and has many variations depending on the group of teeth. Understanding and mastering this internal anatomy is essential for the planning and executing endodontic therapies [1].

In order to explore root canal anatomy for better understanding, several benchmarks were chosen in combination with appropriate information from the literature, encompassing: general description of teeth, overall length and root's length, chronology of root formation [2–8], the degree of canals curvature [9–11], the number of roots [12], root's curvature and fusion [13], number and configuration of canals [12], diameter of the canal at 1, 2, and 5 mm from the apex [1, 14], apical foramen position, accessory canals, and lateral and apical ramifications [12].

The divergence of results reported in several studies may be due to the type of the study (clinical/laboratory study); however, different methods have been used in these studies.

Studies done in the laboratory to describe the internal anatomy include various types of methods:

- Decalcification with injection of India's ink [12, 15, 16]
- Injection of sodium fluorescein and microscopy [17]
- In vitro radio-opaque gel infusion and radiography [18]
- In vitro endodontic with radiography and instruments [19] or only with instruments [20]
- In vitro macroscopic examination [13]
- Cone beam computed tomography (CBCT) [21–25, 26]
- Micro-computed tomography [10, 26–29]
- Sectioning and microscopy [11, 14, 18]

While clinical methods include:

- Clinical evaluation during endodontic treatment using enlargement or operating microscope [30]
- In vivo treatment of the root canal and radiography [31]

2. The method of internal anatomy analysis

2.1 Conventional radiography

The retro-alveolar image shows the totality of each X-rayed tooth up to the apex, and provides information on canal anatomy as well as on the integrity of the periodontium [32].

Some studies combined the radiographic technique and radio-opaque sodium iothalamate gel infused in the root canal system [18]. In another use of radiography, Kulild and Peters [19] assessed the internal anatomy of 83 maxillary molars by taking radiography of instruments into the canals (**Figure 1(a)**).

In a retrospective study of 520 completed endodontic treatments of maxillary second molar, radiographs reviewed were useful to detect the anatomical root and canal variations [31].

Unfortunately, the maxillary molar area is often a difficult area to obtain a good radiographic quality because of the superimposition of the maxillary process of the zygomatic bone [34].

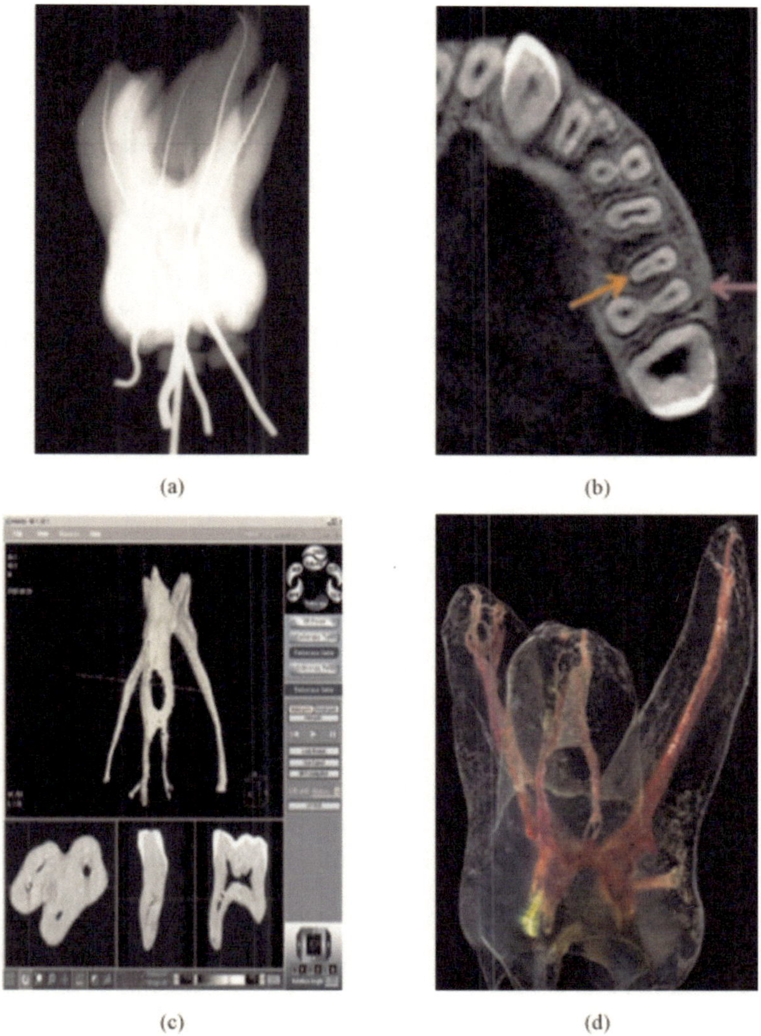

Figure 1.
Methods of study of internal anatomy. (a) Conventional radiography with instruments showing a maxillary first molar with five roots [33]. (b) Cross section, from a CBCT imaging, representing the second mesiobuccal canal of a maxillary first molar [26]. (c) The 3D root canal system of each maxillary first molar was reconstructed with Micro-CT and mathematical modeling [10]. (d) Diaphanization technique showing the complexity of the internal morphology of a maxillary molar [15].

2.2 Cone beam computed tomography (CBCT)

Several studies compared the use of cone beam computed tomography (CBCT) imaging to study root and canal anatomy with some laboratory methods such as histological sectioning and clearing technique and, more recently with the gold standard nondestructive high-resolution micro-computed tomography (Micro-CT) [26].

In order to identify the root canal system, CBCT was used next to charged coupled device (CCD) and photostimulable phosphor (PSP) [22]. For CCD and PSP, the endodontist evaluators correctly identified the number of root canal systems 78 and 80% of the time, respectively, when compared with CBCT 100%.

Numerous in vivo studies used CBCT to highlight the second mesiobuccal canal, with prevalence of 42.63 [21] and 70.5% [25] for the first maxillary molar, and between 34.32 [21] and 41.6% [25] for the second maxillary molar (**Figure 1(b)**).

2.3 Micro-computed tomography (Micro-CT)

X-ray micro-computed tomography has also been denominated as micro-computed tomography, microcomputer tomography, high-resolution X-ray tomography, X-ray microtomography, Micro-CT, and similar terminologies. Nowadays, despite the impossibility of employing micro-CT for in vivo human imaging, it has been considered the most important and accurate research tool for the study of fine details of root canal anatomy [26].

In Markvart et al.'s [28] article, he investigated the Micro-CT and segmentation precision of the surface models of molars for the detection of small volumes, such as the reduced pulp cavity, formation of mineral deposits, detection of narrow root canals, and to improve the clinical and morphological understanding of the number of root canals and their configuration. Other study was done by Peters et al. [29] on 12 maxillary molars; Micro-CT was used to detailing root canal geometry.

Bjørndal et al. [35] correlated the shape of the root canals to the corresponding root surface of five maxillary molars. While in 2006, Lee et al. [10] measured the three-dimensional (3D) canal curvature in maxillary first molars using Micro-CT and mathematical modeling (**Figure 1(c)**).

2.4 Diaphanization

Diaphanization is a histological term that refers to the whole body, organ, or structure transparency [15].

Dental diaphanization has been frequently used to observe several anatomical features of the root canal system, including the presence and the type of root canal, number of roots, fusion, lateral canals, transverse anastomoses, position of apical foramen, and apical deltas [12], additional canals such as MB2 in mesiobuccal roots of maxillary molars [16] (**Figure 1(d)**).

To prove the effectiveness of diaphanization technique in the identification of root canal morphology, many authors compared between diaphanization and other techniques. Baratto Filho et al. [36] showed that the incidence of 4 roots in 140 maxillary first molars was high in vivo assessment (67.14%).

3. Permanent maxillary first molar

3.1 The anatomical particularities of the maxillary first molar

3.1.1 General

The maxillary first molars are the first permanent molars to erupt and sometimes referred to as 6-year molar; they erupt distal to the deciduous dentition and they are considered succedaneous, as they do not replace any deciduous teeth; they contact the maxillary second premolar on the mesial and the maxillary second molar on the distal, the maxillary first molars occlude with the mandibular first and second molars; and they are considered the cornerstones in the development of occlusion because of their eruption pattern and location in the arch [37].

Numbering system	Right	Left
Universal	3	14
Palmer	6┘	└6
International	16	26

3.1.2 Development

- Initial calcification: at birth
- Enamel completed: 3–4 years
- Eruption is between: 6–7 years
- Root completed: 9–10 years

3.1.3 Dimensions

See **Table 1**.

3.1.3.1 Crown dimensions

The mesiodistal crown dimension is greater than the cervico-occlusal crown dimension [2, 5, 6]; the average difference is as great as 3.3 mm and as small as 2.5 mm [2, 5] (**Figure 2(a)**).

The buccolingual crown dimension is greater than the cervico-occlusal crown dimension [2, 5, 6], the average difference is as great as 4.1 mm and as small as 3 mm [6] (**Figure 2(b)**).

Overall length	22.0 mm
Crown length	8 mm
Crown width	10.8 mm
Crown buccolingual	11.6 mm
Root length	12.7 mm (DB)
	12.9 mm (MB)
	14.0 mm (P)

Table 1.
Average dimensions (mm) of the maxillary first molar [37].

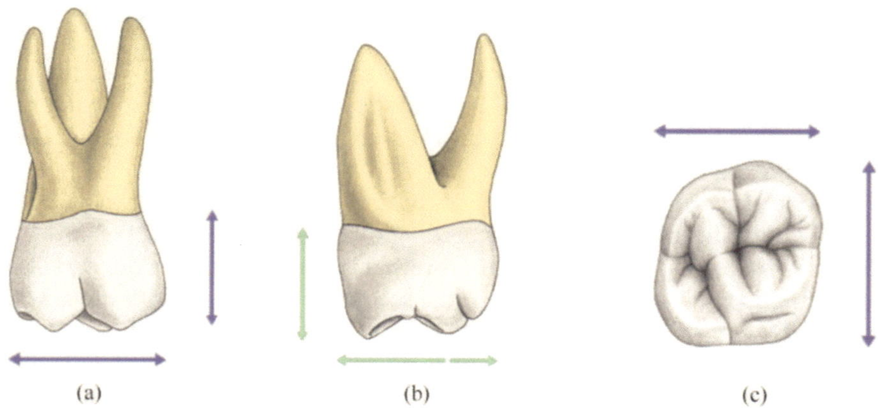

Figure 2.
The crown dimensions (reprinted from 3D tooth atlas version 9) [37]. (a) Crown buccal dimension, (b) crown mesial dimension, and (c) crown occlusal dimension.

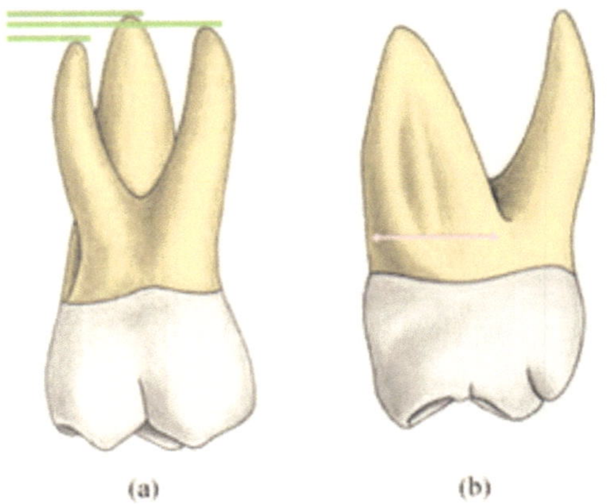

Figure 3.
Roots dimensions (reprinted from 3D tooth atlas version 9) [37]. (a) Root length and (b) mesial root dimension.

The buccolingual crown dimension is greater than the mesiodistal dimension [2, 5, 6]. Diamond [6] indicates that the two dimensions are the same. The inequity of the two measurements appears slight from an occlusal view [2] (**Figure 2(c)**).

3.1.3.2 Roots dimensions

The three roots are nearly the same length (within 1.5 mm), but the palatal root is the largest [3]: the mesiobuccal root is slightly longer than the distobuccal root [3]; the two buccal roots are approximately the same length [2]; and the distobuccal root is the shortest root [3] (**Figure 3(a)**).

The buccolingual dimension of the mesiobuccal root at its base equals two-third of the buccolingual dimension of the root trunk [3] (**Figure 3(b)**).

3.2 External root canal anatomy of maxillary first molars

3.2.1 Number of roots

The maxillary first molar root anatomy is predominantly a three-rooted form, as shown in these anatomic studies [12, 13, 18] of this tooth (**Figure 4(a)**).

The single root or conical form of root anatomy in the first maxillary molar is very rarely reported [12, 13] (**Figure 4b**).

The two-rooted form is rarely reported, and may be due to fusion of the distobuccal root to palatal root (5%) [13], fusion of the mesiobuccal root and the palatal root (0%) [13], or fusion of the distobuccal root to the mesiobuccal root (6%) [12] (**Figure 4(c)**).

Over 95% of maxillary first molars had three roots and 3.8% had two roots in four studies that included 416 teeth, according to a literature review [40].

The four-rooted anatomy in its various forms is also very rare in the maxillary first molar and is more likely to occur in the second or third maxillary molars (**Figure 4(d)**).

Review data from two studies that included 2480 teeth show that the maxillary first molars had an incidence of C-shaped canals of 0.12% indicating that this type of anomaly is a rare occurrence in the maxillary first molar [40].

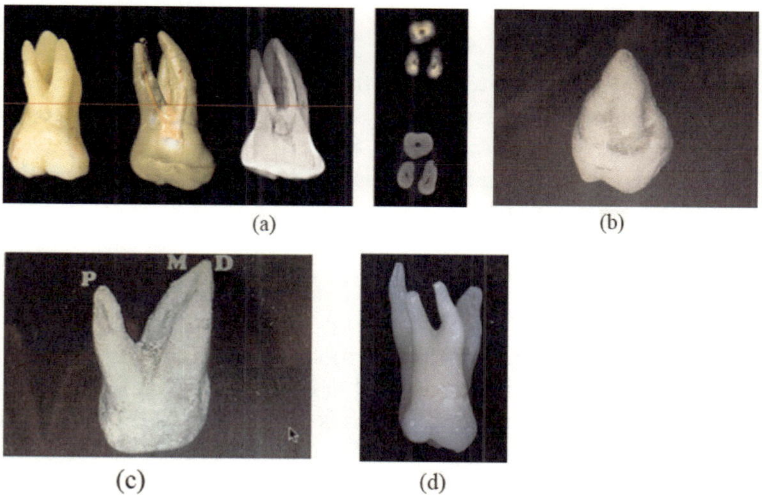

Figure 4.
Variation of root number in maxillary first molar. (a) Buccal view of maxillary right first molar (reprinted from 3D tooth atlas version 9) [37]. (b) First maxillary molar with single root [38]. (c) Fusion of mesiobuccal and distobuccal roots [38]. (d) Maxillary right molar with bifurcated with double palatal root [39].

3.2.2 Shape of roots

3.2.2.1 Buccal aspect

The roots are described as all being roughly ovoid in cross-sectional form at the mid-root area [4] (**Figure 5(a)**).

The buccal furcation is often near the junction of the cervical and middle thirds of the root [3]; the buccal bifurcation is located about 4 mm apical to the cervical line [2] (**Figure 5(b)**).

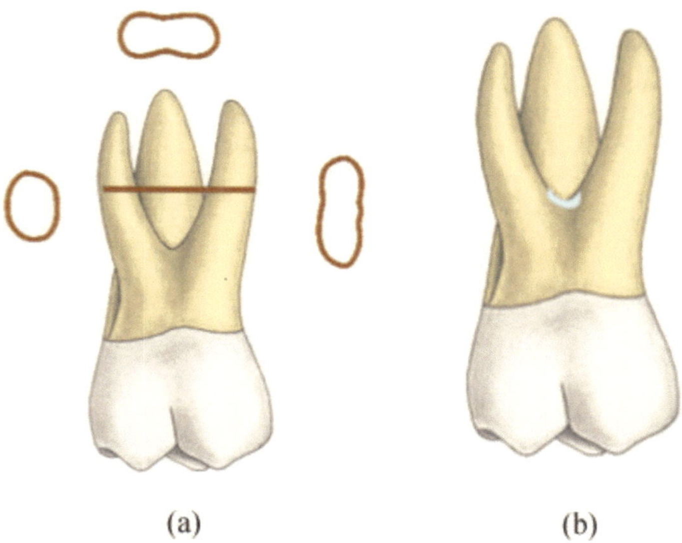

Figure 5.
Buccal aspect of maxillary first molar roots (reprinted from 3D tooth atlas version 9) [37]. (a) Cross-sectional root form and (b) buccal bifurcation.

3.2.2.2 Mesial aspect

The mesial bifurcation is located closer to the cervical line than the buccal bifurcation [2]. There is a smooth concavity extending occlusally and lingually from the furcation almost to the cervical line [2] (**Figure 6(a)**).

The lingual root is the largest; it diverges boldly to the lingual [7], and it is bent like a banana [2, 3]. **Figure 6(b, c)**.

3.2.2.3 Distal aspect

The distal bifurcation is located 5 mm or more apical to the cervical line, thereby being the most apically located furcation [2] (**Figure 7(a)**).

The buccal surface of the distobuccal root is not located as far buccally as the mesiobuccal root; the distal surface on the distobuccal root has no longitudinal depressions [3].

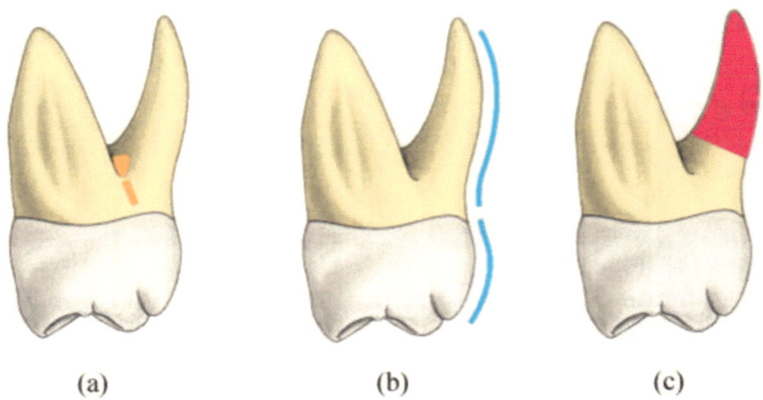

Figure 6.
Mesial aspect of maxillary first molar roots (reprinted from 3D tooth atlas version 9) [37]. (a) Mesial furcation, (b) lingual outline form, and (c) palatal root form.

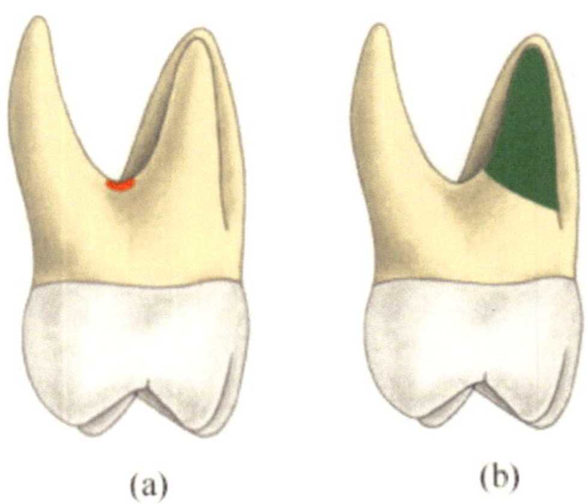

Figure 7.
Distal aspect of maxillary first molar roots (reprinted from 3D tooth atlas version 9) [37]. (a) Distal bifurcation and (b) distobuccal root.

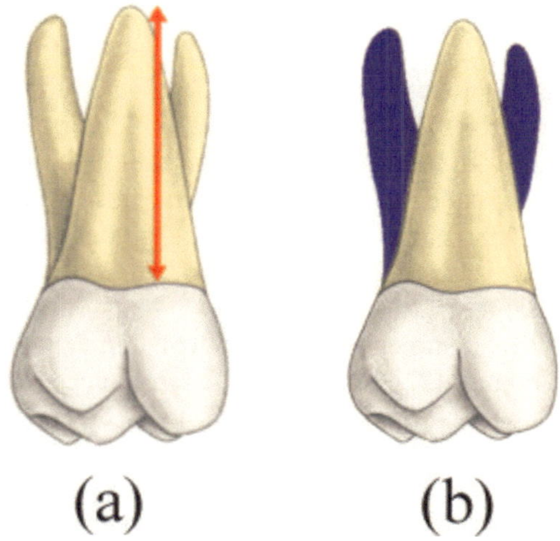

Figure 8.
Palatal aspect of maxillary first molar roots (reprinted from 3D tooth atlas version 9) [37]. (a) Palatal root length and (b) buccal roots visibility.

The distobuccal root is the smallest, shortest, and weakest root and it is a little larger buccolingually than the mesiodistally [4] (**Figure 7(b)**).

3.2.2.4 Lingual aspect

The lingual root of the maxillary first molar has an average length of 13–13.7 mm, depending on the authors [2, 3] (**Figure 8(a)**). It is the third longest root in the maxilla after the canine and the second premolar [3].

The lingual root is the longest, largest, and strongest of the three first molar roots [4].

The lingual root is conical and has a bluntly rounded apex [2]. The buccal roots are visible from a lingual view due to their wide mesiodistal spread [3] (**Figure 8(b)**).

3.3 Internal root canal anatomy of maxillary first molars

3.3.1 Pulp chamber and canal entries

3.3.1.1 Morphology of pulp chamber

The bulk of the pulp chamber is contained within the root trunk, with only the pulp horns extending more coronally. Similar to the outer tooth contour, the pulp chamber is broader buccolingually than mesiodistally. The pulp chamber might undergo calcific metamorphosis, which will reduce its volume considerably [37].

A total of 134 maxillary first molars were studied by Acosta Vigouroux and Trugeda Bosaans [20]; the floor of the pulp chamber was found exactly in the center of the tooth; the most frequent shapes corresponded to trapezoids, rectangles, and inverted trapezoids [20] (**Figure 9**).

The transverse cross-sectional shape of the pulp chamber was trapezoidal in 94 teeth (81.0%); triangular-shaped pulp chambers were found in 13 teeth (11.2%). The shape of the pulp chamber was elliptical in 9 teeth (7.8%) as claimed by Thomas et al. [18].

3.3.1.2 Description and location of canal entries

As stated in Acosta Vigouroux and Trugeda Bosaans' study [20], the largest funnel-shaped entry was that of the lingual canal, which was circular in 45.70% of the cases, and elliptical in 54.30%. The opening to the distobuccal canal was elliptical with a larger buccolingual diameter in 95% of the cases and circular in 5%, the mesiobuccal canal opens at a narrow groove leaning slightly toward the distal aspect and noticeably toward the lingual, which has its origin in the mesiobuccal angle of the floor of the pulp chamber [20].

The average horizontal distance between the MB1 and the MB2 is 1.21 ± 0.5 mm according to Spagnuolo et al. [27], and 1.55 ± 0.56 mm according to Peeters et al. [42] (**Figure 10**).

Spagnuolo et al. [27] also depict a vertical distance between MB1 and MB2 of 1.68 ± 0.83 mm.

The access cavity has a rhomboid shape, due to the presence of four canals with the corners corresponding to the four orifices, as described in "Cohen's Pathways of the Pulp" [41]; the access cavity should not extend into the mesial marginal ridge. From the distal side, the preparation can invade the mesial portion of the oblique ridge; the buccal wall should be parallel to a line connecting the mesiobuccal and distobuccal orifices (**Figure 11**).

In a recent study done by Rover et al. [43] on 30 maxillary first molars, they assess the influence of contracted endodontic cavities (CECs) on root canal detection. The traditional endodontic cavities (TECs) were used as a reference for comparison. The results show that it was possible to locate more root canals in the TEC group in stages 1 and 2 than the CEC group.

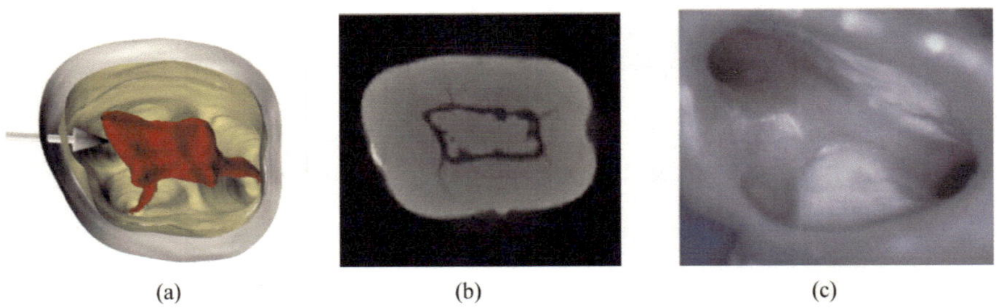

Figure 9.
The morphology of pulp chamber. (a/b) trapezoid form of the pulp chamber (reprinted from 3D tooth atlas version 9) [37]. (c) pulp chamber shape of maxillary first molar with three canals [41].

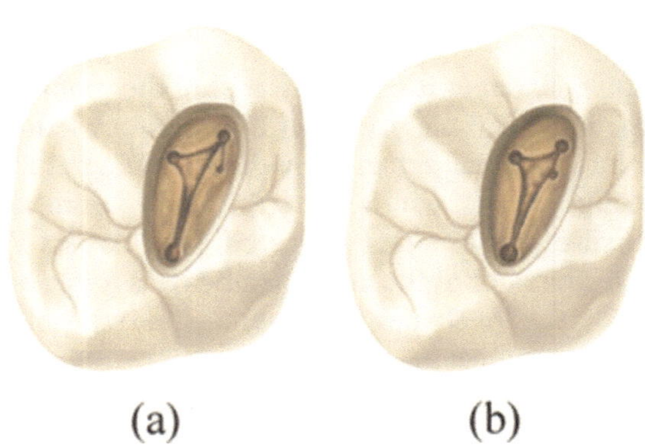

Figure 10.
The two locations of the second mesiobuccal (MB-2) canal orifices in a maxillary first molar : (a) first location, (b) second location [41].

3.3.2 Morphology of the canals

3.3.2.1 Mesiobuccal canal

According to a book chapter "Ingle's Endodontics" [39], a meta-analysis has done by Cleghorn and Goodacre contained the most data of the mesiobuccal canal morphology, a total of 8515 teeth from 37 studies (**Figure 12(a)**).

The incidence of two canals in the mesiobuccal root was 57.1%, and of one canal was 42.9% in a weighted average of all reported studies. The incidence of two canals in the mesiobuccal root was higher in laboratory studies (61.1%) compared to clinical studies (54.7%).

The mesiobuccal canal has a similar volume (2.76 mm^3), and considerably larger surface area (up to 24 square mm^2) compared to the distobuccal one; canal lengths are similar and can reach up to 24 mm [29] (**Figure 12(b)**).

On 100 maxillary first molar studied by Karaman et al. [11]; the degree of primary curvature in type II, MB (25.63 ± 7.43°) and ML (34.74 ± 8.99°), and in type III, MB (27.33 ± 9.70°) and (ML 36.98 ± 9.41°) in clinical view was not significantly different.

As Vertucci claimed that the median canal diameter at 1, 2, and 5 mm from the apex for **MB1** was 0.19, 0.37, 0.46 mm, respectively, buccally and lingually, and

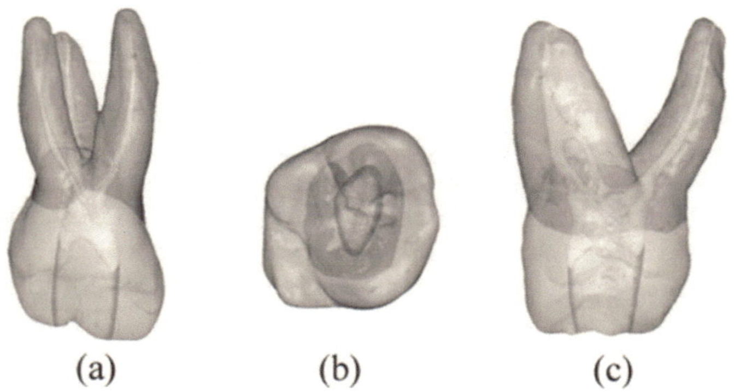

Figure 11.
The shape of the access cavity of maxillary first molars from different views [41]. (a) Buccal view, (b) occlusal view, and (c) mesial view.

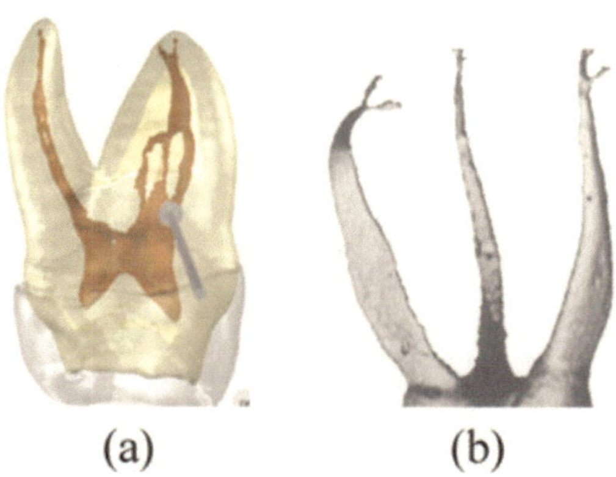

Figure 12.
Three-dimensional configuration of internal anatomy of maxillary first molar. (a) Mesiobuccal canal (reprinted from 3D tooth atlas version 9) [37]. (b) Micro-CT data showing the detailed anatomy of root canal system [29].

0.13, 0.27, 0.32 mm mesially and distally; for **MB2,** the median canal diameter was: 0.19, 0.31, 0.38 mm, respectively, buccally and lingually, 0.16, 0.16, 0.16 mm mesially and distally [1].

3.3.2.2 Distobuccal canal

According to "Ingle's Endodontics" meta-analysis [39]: 15 studies consisting of 2606 teeth, results show that the distobuccal root had only one canal in 98.3% of teeth studied, two canals were found in 1.7% (**Figure 13**).

It is the smallest of the canals present in terms of volume, length, and surface area with around 2.25 mm^3, 24 mm, and 18.75 mm^2, respectively [29].

The distobuccal canal has a clear curvature of $0.29 \pm 0.13\ mm^{-1}$. However, it is generally less curve that the mesiobuccal root canals [29].

The median canal diameter at 1, 2, and 5 mm from the apex for the distobuccal canal was: 0.22, 0.33, and 0.49 mm, respectively, buccally and lingually, and 0.17, 0.25, 0.31 mm mesially and distally [1].

3.3.2.3 Palatal canal

In a literature review [40] already mentioned included 14 in vivo and in vitro studies based on 2576 maxillary first molars; 99.0% and 98.8% of the palatal roots contained one canal and a single foramen respectively, while the remaining of 1.0% contained 2 canals (**Figure 14**).

Clinical cases reporting the existence of two canals within a palatal root are not uncommon [44], or two distinct palatal roots [45].

The palatal canal is the largest of the root canals present in maxillary molars, with regards to both length and volume; canal length may be up to 25 mm or more, the volume varies $6.96 \pm 1.81\ mm^3$, and area up to 30.43 mm^2 [29].

The median canal diameter at 1, 2, and 5 mm from the apex for the palatal canal was: 0.29, 0.40, and 0.55 mm, respectively, buccally and lingually, and 0.33, 0.40, 0.74 mm mesially and distally [1].

The palatal canal is unique, wide, and rectilinear except for a slight curvature in order of 0.23–0.12 mm^{-1} [29].

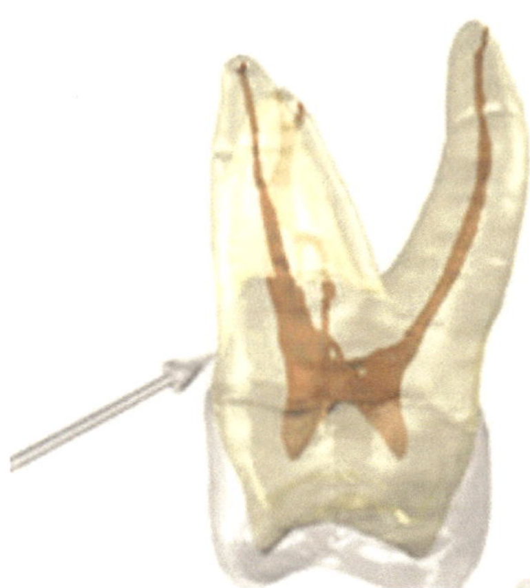

Figure 13.
Distobuccal canal system of maxillary first molar (reprinted from 3D tooth atlas version 9) [37].

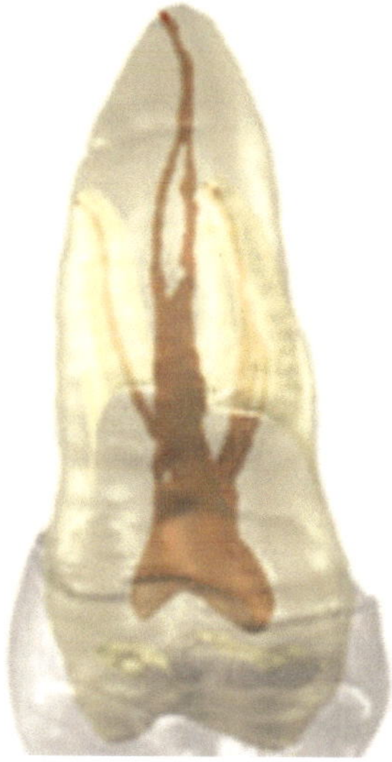

Figure 14.
Palatal canal system of maxillary first molar (reprinted from 3D tooth atlas version 9) [37].

The apical foramen is in the center of the apex in 18.0% of cases, and lateral in 82.0% of cases on the palatal root of the first maxillary molar [1].

4. Permanent maxillary second molar

4.1 The anatomical particularities of the maxillary second molar

4.1.1 General

The maxillary second molars are the seventh teeth from the midline, because they erupt at about age 12, they are occasionally referred to as 12-year molars [37].

They contact the maxillary first molar on the mesial and the maxillary third molar on the distal, and they occlude with the mandibular second and third molar [37].

Numbering system	Right	Left
Universal	2	15
Palmer	7⏌	⎿7
International	17	27

4.1.2 Development

- Initial calcification: 2.5–3 years
- Enamel completed: 7–8 years
- Eruption is between: 12–13 years
- Root completed: 14–16 years

4.1.3 Dimensions

See **Table 2.**

4.1.3.1 Crown dimensions

The mesiodistal crown dimension is greater than the occlusocervical crown dimension [2, 3]. The average difference is as great as 2.2 mm [3] (**Figure 15(a)**).

The buccolingual crown dimension is greater than the occlusocervical crown dimension [2, 3]. The average difference is as great as 4.3 mm [7] (**Figure 15(b)**).

The buccolingual crown is greater than the mesiodistal crown dimension [2, 3]. The average distance is as great as 2.3 mm [7] and as small as 1 mm [6] (**Figure 15(c)**).

The distal half of the crown has a smaller occlusocervical dimension than the mesial half [3] (**Figure 15(d)**).

4.1.3.2 Root's dimensions

The buccal roots are about the same length [2], and the palatal root is the longest root [2, 3] (**Figure 16(a)**).

The mesiobuccal root is wider buccolingually than the distobuccal root [3] (**Figure 16(b)**).

The distobuccal root is shorter and exhibits less buccolingual dimension than the mesiobuccal root [3] (**Figure 16(c)**).

4.2 External root canal anatomy of maxillary second molars

4.2.1 Number of roots

As stated in "Ingle's Endodontics" [39], a majority of maxillary second molars in three anatomical studies were found to be three-rooted 88.6% (n = 1272); this result is lower than that found in the maxillary first molar, while the incidence of root fusion was 25.8% (n = 1960) as claimed in seven studies (**Figure 17**), and C-shaped canals with (4.9%) when compared to the maxillary first molar.

Other studies show different numbers. Indeed, the periodontologists Ross and Evanchik [46] observed 657 maxillary molars in 170 patients in their dental offices

Overall length	21.4 mm
Crown length	7.7 mm
Crown width	9.7 mm
Crown buccolingual	11.4 mm
Root length	12.5 mm (DB)
	13.1 mm (MB)
	13.7 mm (P)

Table 2.
Average dimensions (mm) of the maxillary second molar [37].

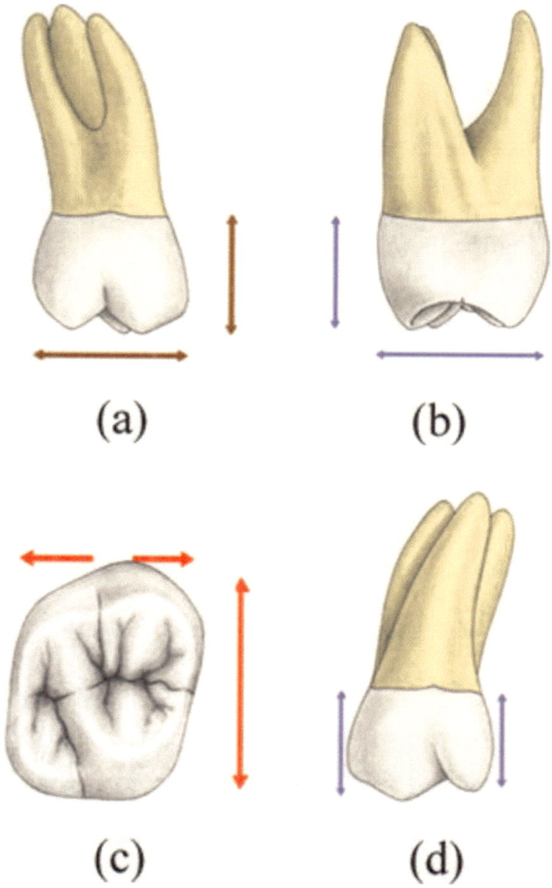

Figure 15.
The crown dimensions (reprinted from 3D tooth atlas version 9) [37]. (a) Crown buccal dimension, (b) crown mesial dimension, (c) crown occlusal dimension, and (d) occlusocervical crown dimension.

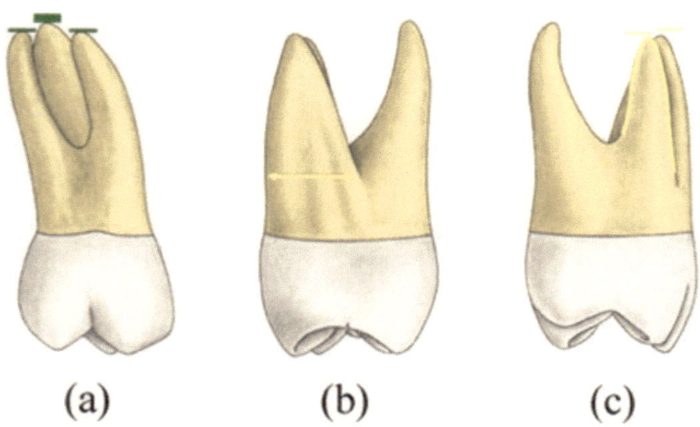

Figure 16.
Roots dimensions (reprinted from 3D tooth atlas version 9) [37]. (a) Root length, (b) mesial root dimension, and (c) distobuccal root dimension.

and concluded that the root fusion in the maxillary second molars percentage is up to 52.9% (n = 157) versus 47.1% (n = 140) without root fusion.

4.2.2 Shape of roots

4.2.2.1 Buccal aspect

The buccal roots are nearly parallel [2, 3]. The roots are relatively straight, and the second molar roots are relatively close together [3] (**Figure 18(a)**).

The roots have a distal inclination [2, 3] (**Figure 18(b)**). The root trunk is relatively long [3] (**Figure 18(c)**).

4.2.2.2 Mesial aspect

The lingual root is relatively straight [3] (**Figure 19(a)**).

The mesiobuccal root has a similar morphology of the maxillary first molar, but the furrow that runs through its mesial face is less marked, or nonexistent [8] (**Figure 19(b)**).

4.2.2.3 Distal aspect

The lingual root apex is frequently aligned with the distolingual cusp tip [2] (**Figure 20(a)**).

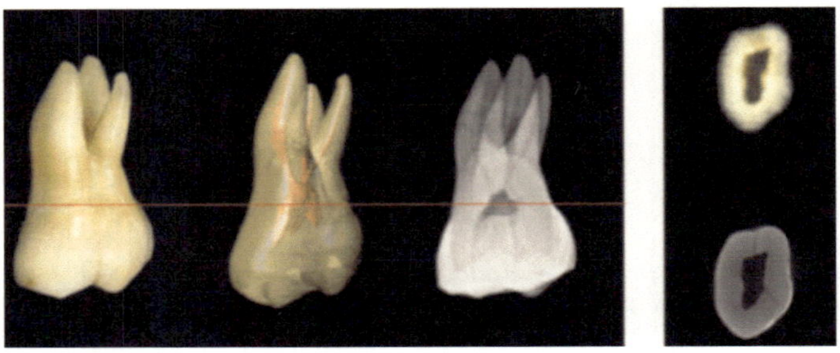

Figure 17.
Buccal view of maxillary right second molar with three roots (reprinted from 3D tooth atlas version 9) [37].

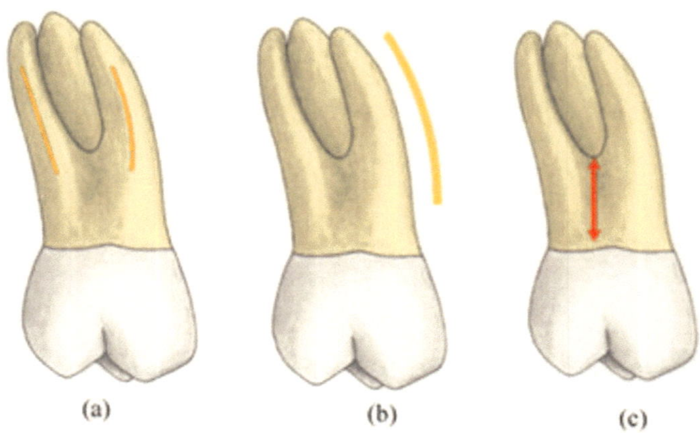

Figure 18.
Buccal aspect of maxillary second molar roots (reprinted from 3D tooth atlas version 9) [37]. (a) Root form/proximity, (b) root curvature, and (c) root trunk.

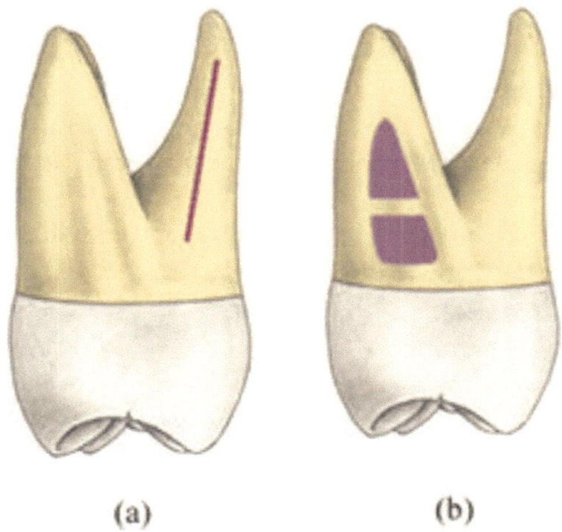

Figure 19.
Mesial aspect of maxillary second molar roots (reprinted from 3D tooth atlas version 9) [37]. (a) Lingual root form and (b) mesiobuccal root surface form.

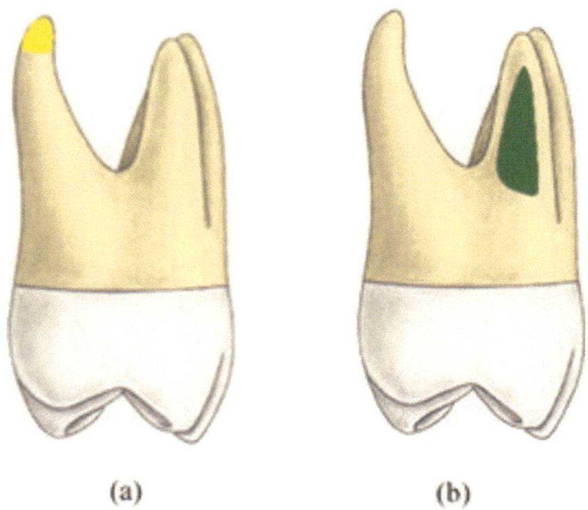

Figure 20.
Distal aspect of maxillary second molar roots (reprinted from 3D tooth atlas version 9) [37]. (a) Lingual root apex location and (b) distobuccal root surface/form.

The distobuccal root of the second maxillary molar differs morphologically. The background the mesiobuccal root on a distal view is visible [8] (**Figure 20(b)**).

4.2.2.4 Lingual aspect

The lingual root is not curved when seen from the lingual view, but it does taper apically to a blunt or rounded apex. The buccal roots are spread out far enough that they are usually visible behind the lingual root from this view (**Figure 21(a)**).

The apex of the lingual root is in line with the distolingual cusp tip instead of the lingual groove, as was found on the first molar [2].

The palatal root curves distally [5] (**Figure 21(b)**).

4.3 Internal root canal anatomy of maxillary second molars

4.3.1 Pulp chamber and canal entries

4.3.1.1 Morphology of pulp chamber

The general outline of the pulp chamber in second maxillary molars resembles first molars; four pulp horns of various sizes are present corresponding to the arrangement of the cusps [37].

The floor of the pulp chamber is markedly convex, which gives the canal orifices a slight funnel shape [41].

In Karaman et al.'s [11] research, among 100 maxillary second molars, the shape of the pulp chamber can be trapezoidal about 74% (n = 74), triangular about 21% (n = 21), or elliptical about 5% (n = 5) (**Figure 22**).

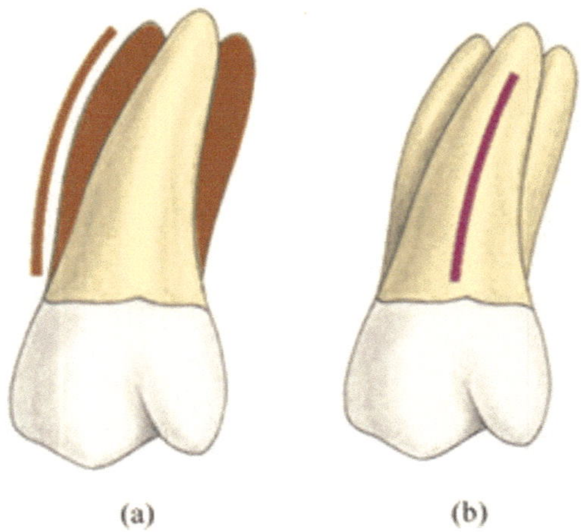

Figure 21.
Palatal aspect of maxillary second molar roots (reprinted from 3D tooth atlas version 9) [37]. (a) Buccal roots visibility and (b) lingual root curvature.

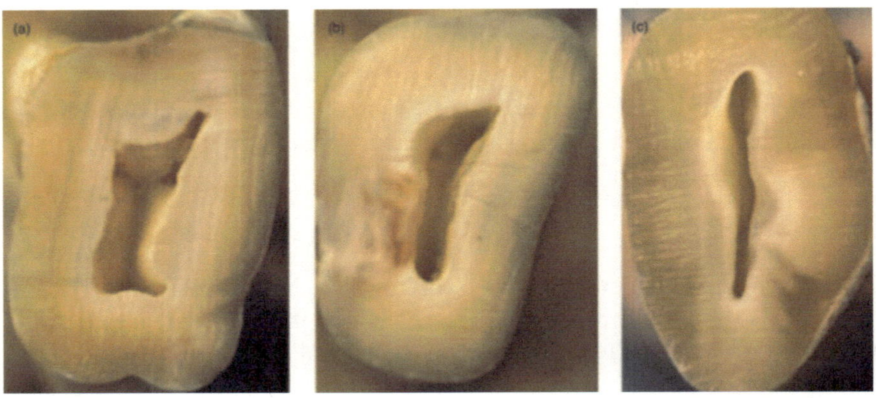

Figure 22.
Photograph of three second maxillary molars with pulp chambers [11]: trapezoidal (a), triangular (b), and elliptical (c).

When four canals are present, the access cavity preparation of the maxillary second molar has a rhomboid shape, if only three canals are present, the access cavity is a rounded triangle, the mesial marginal ridge need not be invaded with the base to the buccal; if only two canals are present, the access outline form is oval and widest in the buccolingual dimension [41] (**Figure 23**).

4.3.1.2 Description and location of canal entries

The canals' orifices in the maxillary second molars are closer mesially to each other than they are in maxillary first molar [41].

The three main orifices (MB, DB, and P) usually form a flat triangle and sometimes almost a straight line [41] (**Figure 24**).

The mesiobuccal canal orifice is located more to the buccal and mesial than in the first molar; the distobuccal orifice approaches the midpoint between mesiobuccal and palatal orifices; and the palatal orifice usually is located at the most palatal aspect of the root [41].

The distance between orifices in pulp chamber floor was claimed as: 3.09 ± 0.22 mm in type II (n = 20), and 3.89 ± 0.23 mm in type III (n = 8) according to Karaman et al. [11].

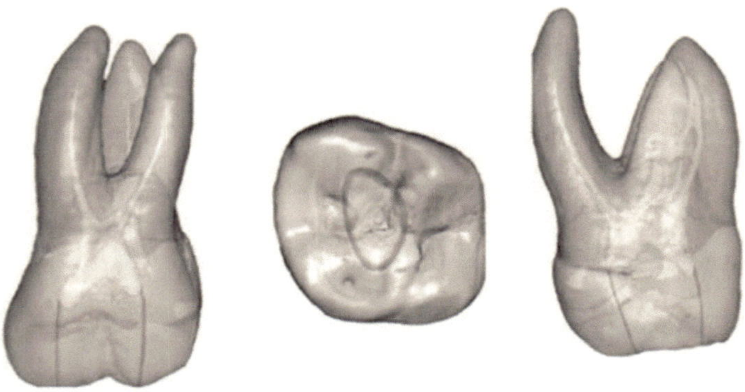

(a) (b) (c)

Figure 23.
The shape of the access cavity of maxillary second molars from different views [41]: (a) buccal view, (b) occlusal view, and (c) mesial view.

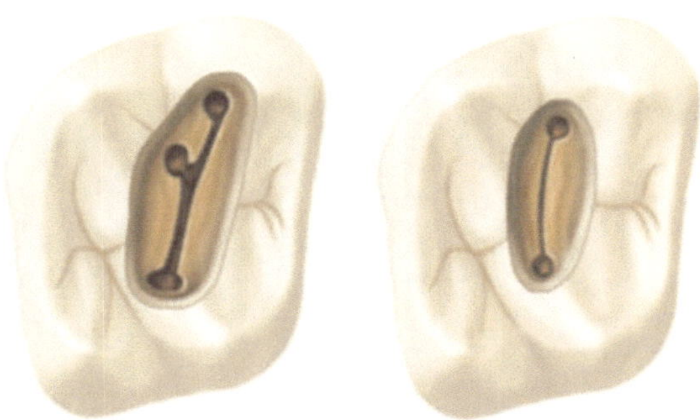

(a) (b)

Figure 24.
Canal entries [41]. (a) Three canal orifices in a maxillary second molar. (b) Two canal orifices in a maxillary second molar.

4.3.2 Morphology of the canals

4.3.2.1 Mesiobuccal canal

As mentioned in the fifth chapter of "Cohen's Pathways of the Pulp" [41]. Seventeen anatomical studies found a wide range of canal incidence in the mesiobuccal root; we calculated the average of one canal's incidence, the results

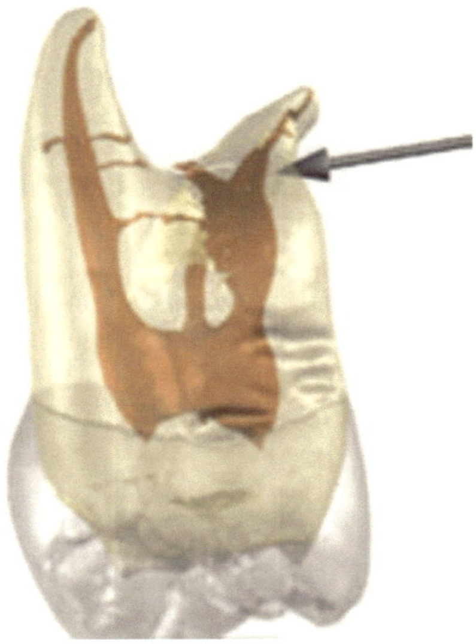

Figure 25.
Mesiobuccal canal system of maxillary second molar (reprinted from 3D tooth atlas version 9) [37].

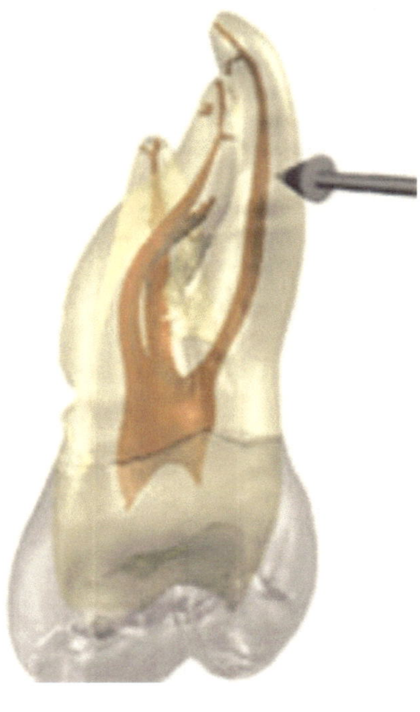

Figure 26.
Distobuccal canal system of maxillary second molar (reprinted from 3D tooth atlas version 9) [37].

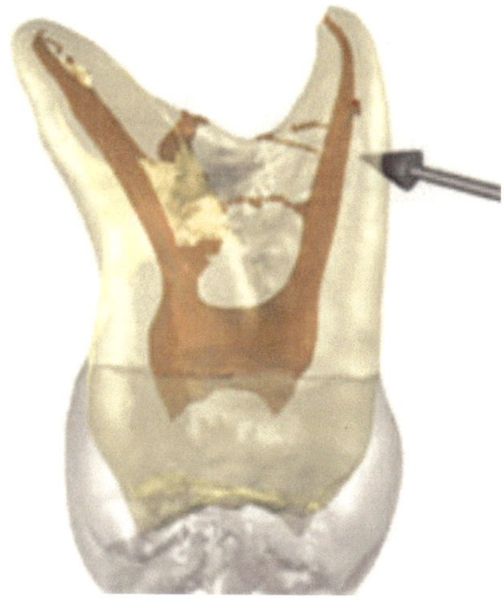

Figure 27.
Palatal canal system of maxillary second molar (reprinted from 3D tooth atlas version 9) [37].

were 69.3%, of two canals was 29%, while the incidence of three and four canals was, respectively, 2.6 and 1% in two studies (**Figure 25**).

There was a single apical foramen found in the mesiobuccal root over 68% in 1352 maxillary second molars studied [39].

The mean degrees of primary canal curvature that obtained for type II and type III configurations in maxillary second molar in clinical view were, respectively, ($26.13 \pm 9.18°$) and ($18.97 \pm 4.71°$) [11].

4.3.2.2 Distobuccal canal

These canals can be quite small and smaller at the mid-root and exit the pulp in a relatively straight line, occasionally there may be acute apical curves in mesial as well as distal directions [37] (**Figure 26**).

The distobuccal roots exhibited a single canal over 99% of the time in 10 reported anatomical studies, according to Cleghorn and Goodacre [39].

Otherwise stated in a book chapter: “Tooth Morphology, Isolation, and Access” [41] reporting seven anatomical studies, one single canal was found in the rate of 100%.

4.3.2.3 Palatal canal

In maxillary second molars, palatal canals are mostly straight with an apical curve to the buccal, apical to this marker is a deposition of secondary dentin along the palatal surface of the palatal canal [37] (**Figure 27**).

The internal canal morphology of the palatal root of the maxillary second molar was assessed in seven studies, showing the incidence of one canal over 99% [41]. While one study found that two palatal roots and two palatal canals occur in 1.47% of these teeth [31].

Neelakantan et al. [23] used CBCT to analyze 191 extracted maxillary second molars from an Indian population; the incidence of a single canal in a palatal root was 87.8%, and the presence of two or more canals was approximately 5.3%.

5. Conclusion

The roots' variation and the canal system's morphology knowledge constitute for each tooth a daily mission to the dental surgeon, in order to minimize the potential risks that lead to a failure of the therapy, especially in the endodontic.

An accurate diagnosis and a successful therapy could be resulted by highlighting the entire roots and canals network of molars in particular.

The preoperative radiography is the first complementary test to the diagnosis; although the results of the retro-alveolar radiography in ortho-centered incidence are important, they are not as significant as those of the meso-centric in terms of their impact, which appeared to display three roots of maxillary molars distinctly.

The cone beam computed tomography technology offers a high accuracy, when the data collected by the clinic and conventional radiography are not sufficiently contributory to the diagnosis. Unfortunately, the micro-computed tomography is not applicable in vivo human imaging; however, it forms a detailed means to evaluate the root canal anatomy quantitatively and qualitatively.

Respecting the maxillary molars' axis, the endodontic access cavity in a trapezoidal shape allows: a direct access, and a possible discovery of an additional canal. This incidence appears to be increasing with the use of the surgical operating microscope during the access opening procedure, while a lower magnification of Galilean loupes are limited.

Furthermore, the canal entries could be located by using micro-openers, ultrasound inserts, round burs, or fine taper files. The use of dyes, with or without transillumination, could also be useful.

The working length must ideally be determined through an apex locator, and validated by retro-alveolar radiography. Cleaning and shaping with the k-files remains a prerequisite for Ni-Ti instrumentation.

The techniques that are used to fill a canal network of maxillary molars act according to the principle of vertical warm compaction or thermo-mechanical condensation with Gutta condenser.

Abbreviation

CBCT	cone beam computed tomography
Micro-CT	micro-computed tomography
CCD	charged coupled device
PSP	photostimulable phosphor

Author details

Said Dhaimy*, Lamyae Bedida, Hafsa El Merini and Imane Benkiran
Department of Restorative Dentistry and Endodontics, Faculty of Dental Medicine, University Hassan II, Casablanca, Morocco

*Address all correspondence to: saiddhaimy@gmail.com

References

[1] Vertucci FJ. Root canal morphology and its relationship to endodontic procedures. Endodontic Topics. 2005; **10**(1):3-29

[2] Nelson SJ. Wheeler's Dental Anatomy, Physiology, and Occlusion. 10th ed. St. Louis, Missouri: Elsevier Saunders; 2015

[3] Scheid RC, Woelfel JB. Woelfel's Dental Anatomy. 8th ed. Philadelphia: Wolters Kluwer/Lippincott Williams & Wilkins Health; 2012

[4] Fuller JL, Denehy GE, Schulein TM. Concise Dental Anatomy and Morphology. Iowa City, Iowa: University of Iowa; 2001

[5] Jordan R, Abrams L, Kraus B. Kraus' Dental Anatomy and Occlusion. 2nd ed. St. Louis: Mosby Year Book, Inc; 1992

[6] Diamond M. Dental Anatomy. 2nd ed. Revised and Enlarged. New York: Macmillan; 1929

[7] Black GV (Greene V. Descriptive Anatomy of the Human Teeth. Philadelphia : Wilmington Dental Manufacturing Company; 1890

[8] Tallec P. Anatomie Dentaire : Cours de Morphologie et Technologie Appliquées à l'art Dentaire. Nouvelle éd. Aix-en-Provence: École de Prothèse Dentaire, IFOSUPD; 1983. 352 p

[9] Bone J, Moule AJ. The nature of curvature of palatal canals in maxillary molar teeth. International Endodontic Journal. 1986;**19**(4):178-186

[10] Lee J-K, Ha B-H, Choi J-H, Heo S-M, Perinpanayagam H. Quantitative three-dimensional analysis of root canal curvature in maxillary first molars using micro-computed tomography. Journal of Endodontia. 2006;**32**(10):941-945

[11] Karaman GT, Onay EO, Ungor M, Colak M. Evaluating the potential key factors in assessing the morphology of mesiobuccal canal in maxillary first and second molars. Australian Endodontic Journal: The Journal of the Australian Society of Endodontology Inc. 2011; **37**(3):134-140

[12] Shalabi RMA, Omer J Glennon OE, Jennings M, Claffey NM. Root canal anatomy of maxillary first and second permanent molars: Rewarming of cooled teeth. International Endodontic Journal. 2000;**33**(5):405-414

[13] Pécora JD, Woelfel JB, Sousa Neto MD. Morphologic study of the maxillary molars. 1. External anatomy. Brazilian Dental Journal. 1991;**2**(1):45-50

[14] Gani O, Visvisian C. Apical canal diameter in the first upper molar at various ages. Journal of Endodontia. 1999;**25**(10):689-691

[15] Barrington C, Balandrano F. Diaphanization techniques in the study of root canal anatomy. In: Versiani MA, Basrani B, Sousa-Neto MD, editors. The Root Canal Anatomy in Permanent Dentition. Cham: Springer International Publishing; 2019:57-88

[16] Pécora JD, Woelfel JB, Sousa Neto MD, Issa EP. Morphologic study of the maxillary molars. Part II: Internal anatomy. Brazilian Dental Journal. 1992; **3**(1):53-57

[17] Pais A, Deo A, Martin A, Cunha R, Fontana C, Bueno C. Sodium fluorescein and cobalt blue filter coupled to a dental operating microscope to optimise root canal location in maxillary first molars. ENDO. 2014;**8**(3):193-198

[18] Thomas RP, Moule AJ, Bryant R. Root canal morphology of maxillary permanent first molar teeth at various

ages. International Endodontic Journal. 1993;**26**(5):257-267

[19] Kulild JC, Peters DD. Incidence and configuration of canal systems in the mesiobuccal root of maxillary first and second molars. Journal of Endodontia. 1990;**16**(7):311-317

[20] Acosta Vigouroux SA, Trugeda Bosaans SA. Anatomy of the pulp chamber floor of the permanent maxillary first molar. Journal of Endodontia. 1978;**4**(7):214-219

[21] Silva EJNL, Nejaim Y, Silva AIV, Haiter-Neto F, Zaia AA, Cohenca N. Evaluation of root canal configuration of maxillary molars in a Brazilian population using cone-beam computed tomographic imaging: An in vivo study. Journal of Endodontia. 2014;**40**(2): 173-176

[22] Matherne RP, Angelopoulos C, Kulild JC, Tira D. Use of cone-beam computed tomography to identify root canal systems in vitro. Journal of Endodontia. 2008;**34**(1):87-89

[23] Neelakantan P, Subbarao C, Ahuja R, Subbarao CV, Gutmann JL. Cone-beam computed tomography study of root and canal morphology of maxillary first and second molars in an Indian population. Journal of Endodontia. 2010;**36**(10):1622-1627

[24] Guo J, Vahidnia A, Sedghizadeh P, Enciso R. Evaluation of root and canal morphology of maxillary permanent first molars in a North American population by cone-beam computed tomography. Journal of Endodontia. 2014;**40**(5):635-639

[25] Lee J-H, Kim K-D, Lee J-K, et al. Mesiobuccal root canal anatomy of Korean maxillary first and second molars by cone-beam computed tomography. Oral Surgery, Oral Medicine, Oral Pathology, Oral Radiology, and Endodontics. 2011; **111**(6):785-791

[26] Martins JNR, Versiani MA. CBCT and micro-CT on the study of root canal anatomy. In: Versiani MA, Basrani B, Sousa-Neto MD, editors. The Root Canal Anatomy in Permanent Dentition. Cham: Springer International Publishing; 2019:89-180

[27] Spagnuolo G, Ametrano G, D'Antò V, et al. Microcomputed tomography analysis of mesiobuccal orifices and major apical foramen in first maxillary molars. The Open Dentistry Journal. 2012;**6**:118-125

[28] Markvart M, Bjørndal L, Darvann TA, Larsen P, Dalstra M, Kreiborg S. Three-dimensional analysis of the pulp cavity on surface models of molar teeth, using X-ray micro-computed tomography. Acta Odontologica Scandinavica. 2012;**70**(2):133-139

[29] Peters OA, Laib A, Rüegsegger P, Barbakow F. Three-dimensional analysis of root canal geometry by high-resolution computed tomography. Journal of Dental Research. 2000;**79**(6): 1405-1409

[30] Stropko JJ. Canal morphology of maxillary molars: Clinical observations of canal configurations. Journal of Endodontia. 1999;**25**(6):446-450

[31] Peikoff MD, Christie WH, Fogel HM. The maxillary second molar: Variations in the number of roots and canals. International Endodontic Journal. 1996;**29**(6):365-369

[32] Saint-Pierre F, Fanelli G, Mokhbi J, Lombry Y, Pocholle P, Tuil L. Traitement Endodontique-Rapport d'évaluation; 2008. Available from: https://www.has-sante.fr/portail/upload/docs/application/pdf/2009-01/rapport_traitement_endodontique.pdf

[33] Barbizam JVB, Ribeiro RG, Tanomaru Filho M. Unusual anatomy of permanent maxillary molars. Journal of Endodontia. 2004;**30**(9):668-671

[34] Slowey RR. Radiographic aids in the detection of extra root canals. Oral Surgery, Oral Medicine, and Oral Pathology. 1974;**37**(5):762-772

[35] Bjørndal L, Carlsen O, Thuesen G, Darvann T, Kreiborg S. External and internal macromorphology in 3D-reconstructed maxillary molars using computerized X-ray microtomography. International Endodontic Journal. 1999; **32**(1):3-9

[36] Baratto Filho F, Zaitter S, Haragushiku GA, de Campos EA, Abuabara A, Correr GM. Analysis of the internal anatomy of maxillary first molars by using different methods. Journal of Endodontia. 2009;**35**(3): 337-342

[37] Montgomery K, Herbranson E. Dental anatomy & 3D tooth atlas version 9.0. 3D Tooth Atlas 9 | eHuman. Illinois: Quintessence; 2018. Available from: https://ehuman.com/product/3d-tooth-atlas-9/

[38] Yang Z-P, Yang S-F, Lee G. The root and root canal anatomy of maxillary molars in a Chinese population. Dental Traumatology. 1988;**4**(5):215-218

[39] Ingle JI, Bakland LK, Baumgartner JC. Ingle's Endodontics. Hamilton, ON: BC Decker; 2008

[40] Cleghorn BM, Christie WH, Dong CCS. Root and root canal morphology of the human permanent maxillary first molar: A literature review. Journal of Endodontia. 2006;**32**(9):813-821

[41] Cohen S. In: Hargreaves KM, Berman LH, Rotstein I, editors. Cohen's Pathways of the Pulp. 11th ed. St. Louis, Missouri: Elsevier; 2016

[42] Peeters HH, Suardita K, Setijanto D. Prevalence of a second canal in the mesiobuccal root of permanent maxillary first molars from an Indonesian population. Journal of Oral Science. 2011;**53**(4):489-494

[43] Rover G, Belladonna FG, Bortoluzzi EA, De-Deus G, Silva EJNL, Teixeira CS. Influence of access cavity design on root canal detection, instrumentation efficacy, and fracture resistance assessed in maxillary molars. Journal of Endodontia. 2017;**43**(10):1657-1662

[44] Hartwell G, Bellizzi R. Clinical investigation of in vivo endodontically treated mandibular and maxillary molars. Journal of Endodontia. 1982; **8**(12):555-557

[45] Baratto-Filho F, Fariniuk LF, Ferreira EL, Pecora JD, Cruz-Filho AM, Sousa-Neto MD. Clinical and macroscopic study of maxillary molars with two palatal roots. International Endodontic Journal. 2002;**35**(9):796-801

[46] Ross IF, Evanchik PA. Root fusion in molars: Incidence and sex linkage. Journal of Periodontology. 1981;**52**(11): 663-667

Chapter 8

Morphology of Root Canal System of Maxillary and Mandibular Molars

Svetlana Razumova, Anzhela Brago, Haydar Barakat and Ammar Howijieh

Abstract

The root canal system is complicated and has many anatomical variations among different populations. It is so important to understand the morphology of root canal system before any endodontic procedure, since the lack of knowledge of root canal system could lead to missing the additional root canals which causes failure of endodontic treatment. The study of root canal anatomy was carried out by many researchers and among different populations using various techniques. The presence of additional root canals was most commonly observed in molars. The aim of this chapter is to provide an overview of the morphology of root canal system of maxillary and mandibular molars and its variation among populations.

Keywords: root canal, configuration, number of root canals, number of roots

1. Introduction

The success of endodontic treatment depends on the precise knowledge of root and root canal anatomy and morphology, which is an important challenge due to the complexity of the root canal system and the anatomical variations [1, 2]. This knowledge helps the clinicians in endodontic treatment planning and decreases the percent of endodontic failure. The root canal contains the dental pulp, which occupies the internal cavity of the tooth [3].

Root canal system varies among the teeth, especially in molar teeth. Recent studies have demonstrated that root canal system is very complex due to splitting and union of canals during their way to the apex [4, 5]. The root canal starts from the orifice in the pulp chamber and ends apically with an open orifice into the periodontium. The root canals present different configurations between the teeth and among different populations [6]. Many techniques have been used to study the root canal system from clearing and radiographs to microcomputed tomography and cone-beam computed tomography scanning, which has the advantage of the high-quality three-dimensional slices [2, 5, 7].

2. The classification of root canal system

The root canal system has been classified by different authors to set terms for communication, diagnosis, and treatment planning. The ideal classification of root canal system is to define a number of roots, number of canals in each root, and the canal configurations [8]. Different configurations of root canals have been identified in numerous studies. Weine et al. [9] in 1969 were the first who studied the root canal configuration of maxillary second molars and defined four types as follows (**Figure 1**):

- Type I (1-1): single canal runs from the orifice to the apex.
- Type II (2-1): two canals start from the pulp chamber and join in one closer to the apex.
- Type III (2-2): two canals run separately from the orifice to the apex.
- Type IV (1-2): one canal starts from the pulp chamber floor and divides into two canals when coming closer to the apex.

In 1984, Vertucci [10] presented another classification for root canal configurations in maxillary first molars, and it has been commonly used in different studies. The classification was as follows (**Figure 2**):

- Type 1 (1-1): single canal runs from the orifice to the apex.
- Type II (2-1): two canals begin from the pulp chamber and join in one at the apex.
- Type III (1-2-1): one canal runs from the pulp chamber, splits into two canals during its way, and then unites into one canal at the apex.
- Type IV (2-2): two canals run separately from the orifice to the apex.
- Type V (1-2): one canal runs from the pulp chamber and splits into two canals when coming closer to the apex.
- Type VI (2-1-2): two canals run from the pulp chamber; during its way they unite into one canal and then again split into two canals at the apex.
- Type VII (1-2-1-2): one canal starts from the pulp chamber, then divides into two canals, again unites into one canal, and finally at the apex divides into two canals.
- Type VIII (3-3): three canals run from the orifice to the apex.

In the last decade, some authors studied the root canal configurations all over the world and added new types to Vertucci's classification, which demonstrates the complexity of root canal system. Kartal and Yanıkoğlu [12] identified two root canal configurations in mandibular anterior teeth: type (1-2-1-3) and type (2-3-1). In 2001 Gulabivala et al. [13] added seven new configurations to Vertucci's classification: type (3-1), type (3-2), type (2-3), type (2-1-2-1), type (4-2), type (4-4), and type (5-4) (**Figure 3**).

Also, in 2004, Sert and Bayirli [14] added 15 configurations (**Figure 4**), which have been observed in maxillary and mandibular teeth in Turkey. They were classified in the following order: type IX (1-3), type X (1-2-3-2), type XI (1-2-3-4), type XII (2-3-1), type XIII (1-2-1-3), type XIV (4-2), type XV (3-2), type XVI (2-3), type XVII (1-3-1), type XVIII (3-1), type XIX (2-1-2-1), type XX (4), type XXI (4-1), type XXII (5-4), and type XXIII (3-4).

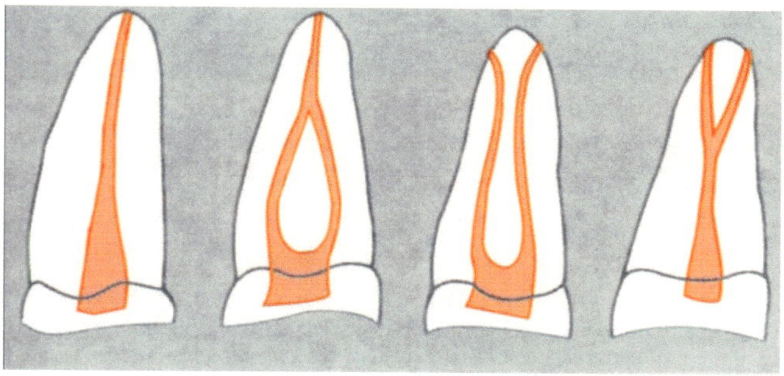

Figure 1.
Weine's classification of root canal configuration.

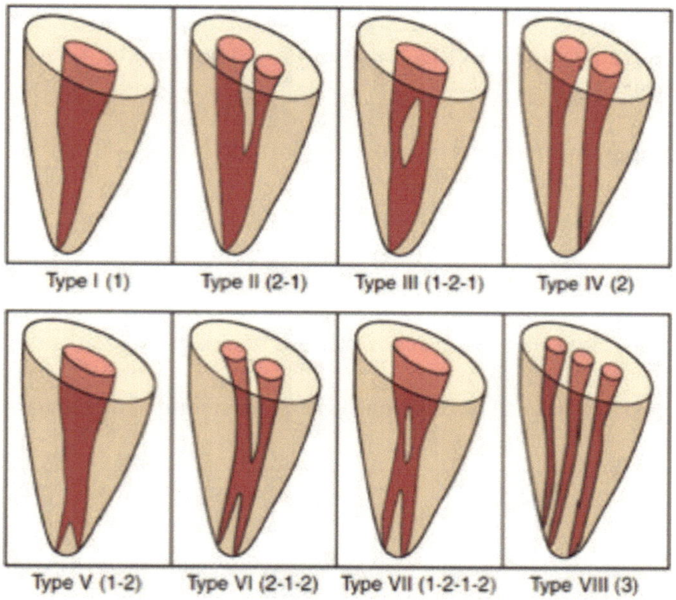

Figure 2.
Vertucci's classification of root canal configuration [11].

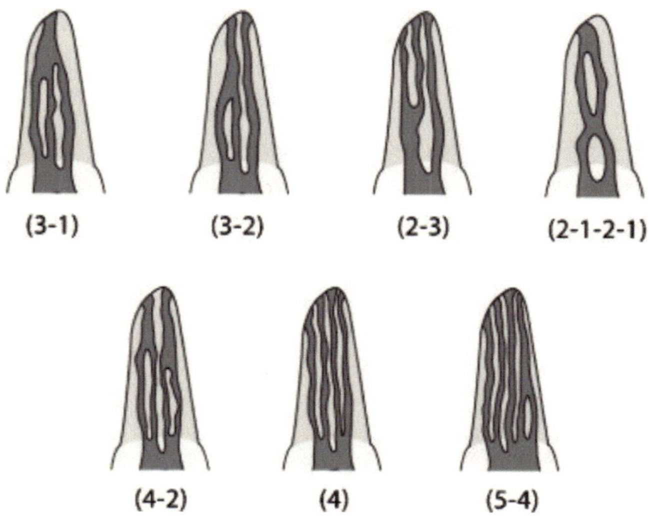

Figure 3.
Gulabivala's classification of root canal configurations.

Peiris et al. in 2008 observed two additional root canal configurations (1-2-3) and (3-1-2) in their study (**Figure 5A**) on mandibular first molar of a Sri Lankan population [15]. In 2008, Al-Qudah added four new types for root canal configurations of mandibular molars in Jordan population [16]: type XX (2-3-1), type XXI (2-3-2), type XXII (3-2-1), and type XXIII (3-2-3) (**Figure 5B**).

In addition to describing root canal system, many authors studied the root canal shape and the presence of isthmus (which is a narrow ribbon-shaped communication between two root canals that contain pulp tissue). The isthmus was found in 15% in maxillary anterior teeth, for maxillary premolars—it was identified in 16% at a 1-mm level of the apex and in 52% at a 6-mm level of the apex. The prevalence of the isthmus was high in mesiobuccal root of maxillary first molars (about 30–50%) in the apical third of the root. For mandibular first molars, 80% of mesial roots have connection in the middle and apical third of the root. Root canal shape varies between round, oval, and C-shaped. Kim et al. [17] classified root canal shape and the presence of connections between canals into five types (**Figure 6**):

- Type I: incomplete isthmus between two canals
- Type II: two canals with a definite connection between them
- Type III: very short complete isthmus between two canals
- Type IV: a complete or incomplete isthmus between three or more canals
- Type V: two or three canals without visible connection between them.

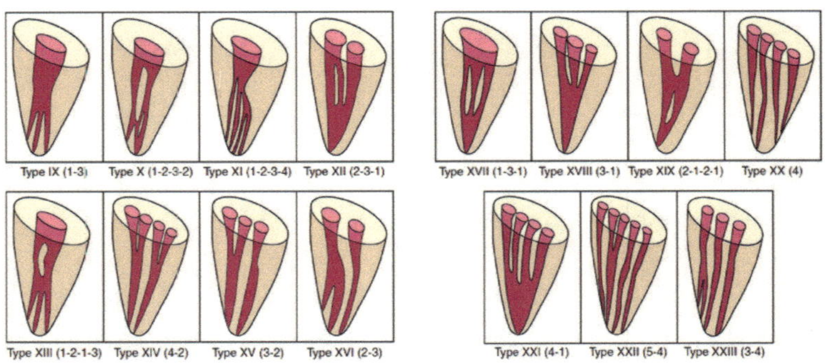

Figure 4.
Sert and Bayirli classification of root canal configurations [11].

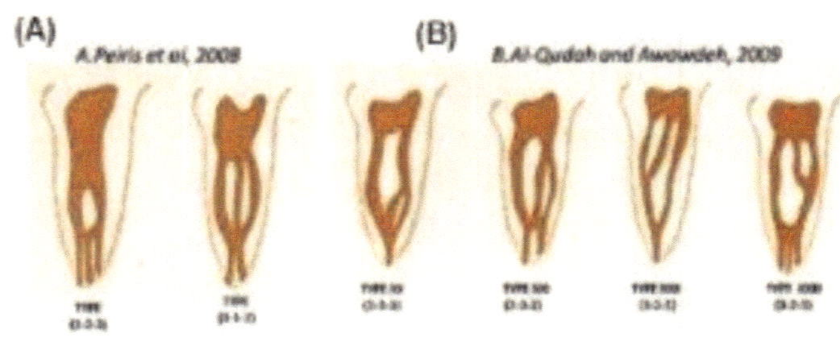

Figure 5.
Root canal configurations according to (A) Beiris and (B) Al-Qudah [8].

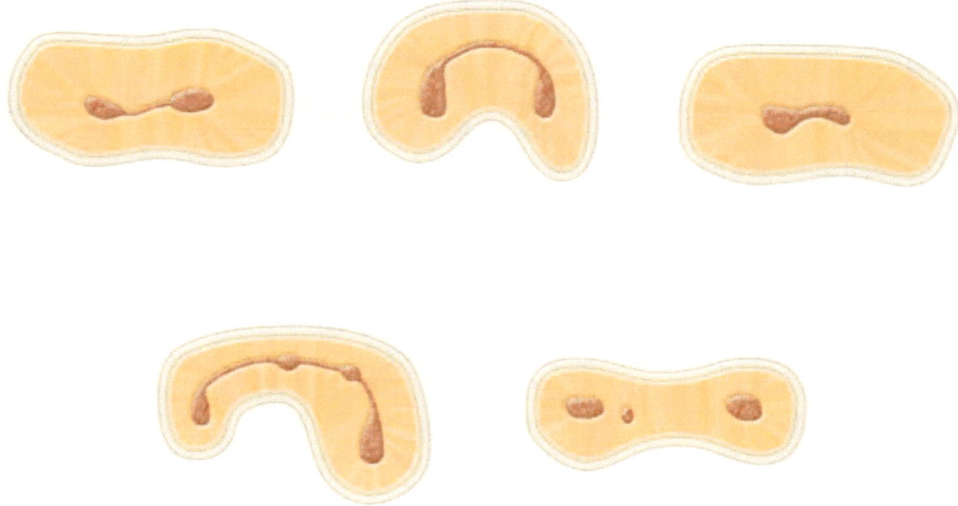

Figure 6.
Kim's classification of root canal shape [17].

In 2018, a review was conducted to study classification of root canal configuration to find a simple, reliable, accurate, and easy nomenclature system to identify the root canal depending on the tooth type, the number of roots, the course of the canal in each root, and the number of foramens [8].

3. Root canal morphology of maxillary molars

3.1 Maxillary first molar

The maxillary first molar is the earliest permanent tooth that appears in the oral cavity and that makes it vulnerable to caries and furthers to the need of endodontic treatment. It has three roots [mesiobuccal (MB), distobuccal (DB), and palatal (P)] with four canals. Despite this, in some populations these variations were observed: one, two, or four roots in the maxillary first molar [18–20]. Root fusion of this tooth was observed in about 0.9–3% [20–23]. The root canal system of the maxillary first molar is complex and has many variations among races; due to that it has the highest rate of endodontic failure. The palatal root is the longest and has the largest diameter; in most cases, it contains one round canal from the orifice of the pulp chamber to the apex. The presence of two or three canals in this root has been reported; in some population as in India, two canals were found in 5% [24]. The distobuccal root is conical and has one canal in most cases. The presence of the second distobuccal canal (DB2) has been documented in some studies, and its prevalence ranged from 0.5 to 9.5% (**Figure 7**) [25, 26]. The most common root canal morphology of the palatal and distobuccal roots is type I (1-1) (**Table 1**). The mesiobuccal root contains two canals (MB1, MB2) with a ribbon form type I by Kim et al. in most cases (**Figure 8**). The MB2 is one of the mysteries in endodontics; its orifice is located mesially or in the pulpal groove between the main mesiobuccal canal and palatal canal, 3.5 mm palatally and 2 mm mesially from the main mesiobuccal canal [27]. The prevalence of MB2 ranged from 48 to 88%, for example, in Russia MB2 was found in 59.8% [25], in Poland 59.5% [28], in Japan 88.2% [29], and in Portugal 71% [30]. The root canal system of the mesiobuccal root has significant variations among populations. The most common canal configuration is type I (1-1) followed by type II (2-1) and then type IV (2-2) by Vertucci [20, 24, 25, 30–37]. Many recent studies have been conducted to analyze the morphology of root canal configuration of three rooted maxillary first molars among different populations as shown in **Table 1**. The most common root canal configuration of one and four rooted maxillary first molars is type 1 (one canal) [31].

3.2 Maxillary second molar

The maxillary second molar is smaller and shorter than the first molar. It has three separated roots in the most common form (MB, DP, and P). Available studies show this tooth can have from one to five roots [37, 38]. Moreover, fusion of roots of maxillary second molars is observed from 5.90 to 42.25% [39]. The fusion of palatal root with mesiobuccal root is the most prevalent form followed by fusion of buccal roots, and the least spread form is the fusion of the three roots (**Figure 9**) (Video 1)

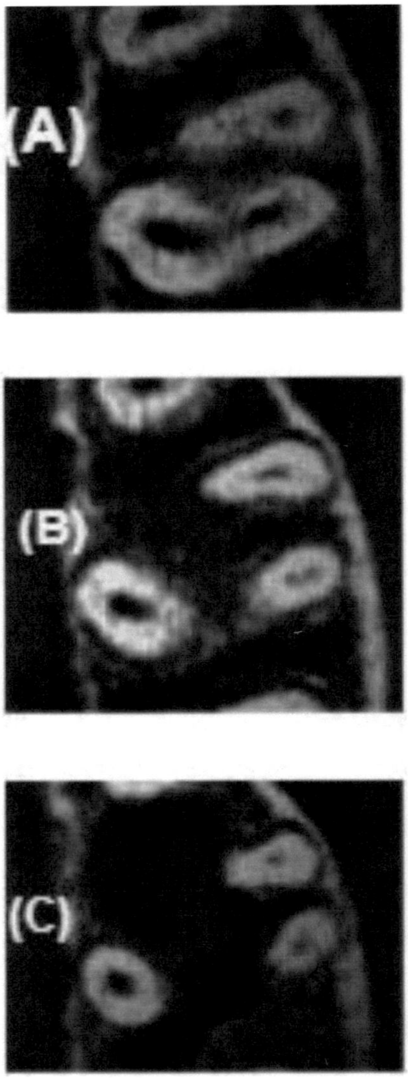

Figure 7.
A case of five canals in maxillary first molar. (A and B) Coronal and middle third: MB1, MB2, DB1, DB2, P. (C) Apical third: MB1 + MB2 + DP + P.

Author(s)	Country (year)	Root	Type (1-1)	Type (2-1)	Type (1-2-1)	Type (2-2)	Type (1-2)	Type (2-1-2)	Type (1-2-1-2)	Type (3-3)	Type (3-1-2)	type (1-3)	Type (3-2)	Type (2-3)	Type (2-1-2-1)
Neelakantan et al. [31]	India	MB	51.8	5.5	–	38.6	–	–	–	–	–	–	–	1	–
		DB	90.4	2.7	1.8	1.8	–	–	–	–	–	–	–	–	–
		P	88.1	1.8	–	4	1.4	–	–	–	–	–	–	–	–
Singh and Pawar [24]	South India (2015)	MB	69	24	–	4	2	–	–	1	–	–	–	–	–
		DB	100	–	–	–	–	–	–	–	–	–	–	–	–
		P	100	–	–	–	–	–	–	–	–	–	–	–	–
Alrahabi and Sohail Zafar [19]	Saudi Arabia (2015)	MB	29.4	47	11.8	11.8	–	–	–	–	–	–	–	–	–
		DB	100	–	–	–	–	–	–	–	–	–	–	–	–
		P	100	–	–	–	–	–	–	–	–	–	–	–	–
Martins et al. [30]	Portugal (2017)	MB	29	44.1	1	16.4	2	5.7	0.2	–	0.4	–	–	–	1.2
		DB	98	1.4	0.2	–	0.2	0.2	–	–	–	–	0.4	–	–
		P	98.2	0.4	1.4	–	–	–	–	–	–	–	–	–	–
Tian et al. [20]	China (2016)	MB	42.2	15.2	2.1	36.2	2	0.6	0.07	0.13			1.4		
		DB	98.2	0.3	0.6	0.3	0.5	–	–	–	–	–	–	–	–
		P	99.3	0.3	0.3	–	0.1	–	–	–	–	–	–	–	–
Ghobashy et al. [32]	Egypt (2017)	MB	25.4	45.6	0.99	27.2	0.5	–	–	–	–	–	–	–	–
		DB	100	–	–	–	–	–	–	–	–	–	–	–	–
		P	100	–	–	–	–	–	–	–	–	–	–	–	–
Pérez-Heredia et al. [33]	Spain (2017)	MB	13.8	56.5	–	23.2	–	4.3	–	–	–	–	0.7	–	1.4
		DB	97.1	1.4	–	–	1.4	–	–	–	–	–	–	–	–
		P	100	–	–	–	–	–	–	–	–	–	–	–	–

Author(s)	Country (year)	Root	Type (1-1)	Type (2-1)	Type (1-2-1)	Type (2-2)	Type (1-2)	Type (2-1-2)	Type (1-2-1-2)	Type (3-3)	Type (3-1-2)	type (1-3)	Type (3-2)	Type (2-3)	Type (2-1-2-1)
Ratanajirasut et al. [34]	Thailand (2018)	MB	36.4	28.8	2.7	25.3	5.3	1.1	–	–	–	–	–	–	–
		DB	99	–	–	0.2	0.8	–	–	–	–	–	–	–	–
		P	99.8	0.2	–	–	–	–	–	–	–	–	–	–	–
Rezaeian et al. [35]	Iran (2018)	MB	38.7	16.2		13.7	8.7	7.5	1.2	–	–	5	3.7	2.5	2.5
		DB	98.7	–	–	–	1.2	–	–	–	–	–	–	–	–
		P	100	–	–	–	–	–	–	–	–	–	–	–	–
Razumova et al. [25]	Russia (2018)	MB	40.2	22.4		37.3	–	–	–	–	–	–	–	–	–
		DB	99.5	0.5	–	–	–	–	–	–	–	–	–	–	–
		P	100	–	–	–	–	–	–	–	–	–	–	–	–

Table 1.
Root canal configurations of maxillary first molar in different populations.

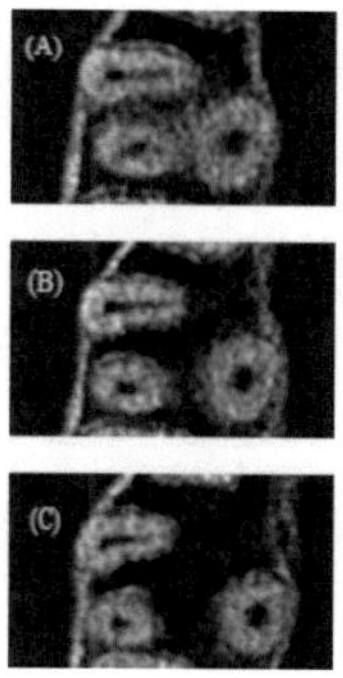

Figure 8.
A case of four canals in maxillary first molar. (A–C) Coronal, middle and apical third: MB1, MB2, DB, P.

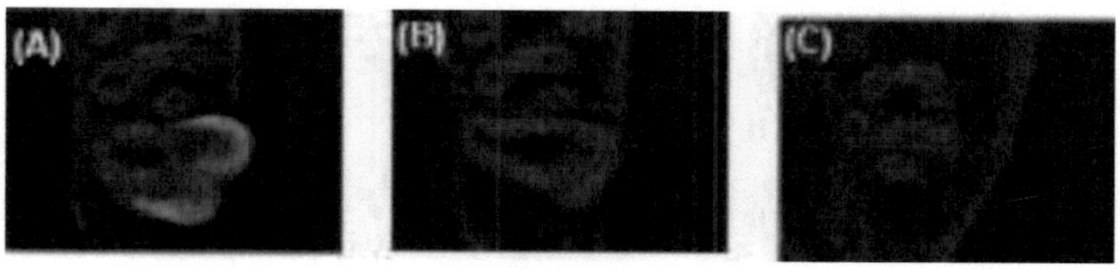

Figure 9.
A case of root fusion (MB + P) of maxillary second molar (A) coronal third of root canals, (B) middle third of root canal, (C) apical third of root canals.

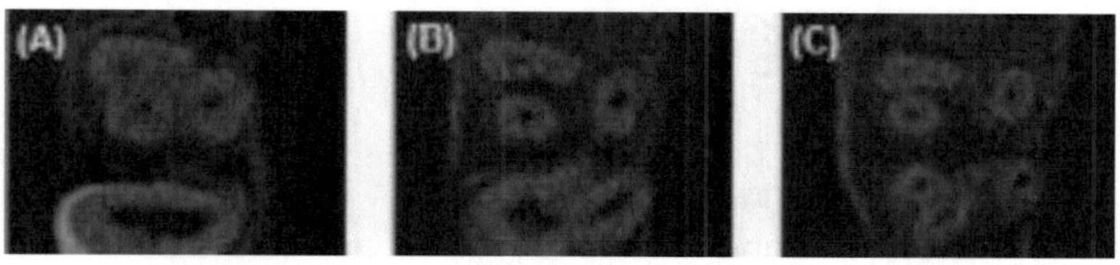

Figure 10.
A case of four canals in the coronal, middle and apical third of the maxillary second molar (A) coronal third of root canals, (B) middle third of root canal, (C) apical third of root canals.

[39]. Root canal morphology of this tooth varies among population and races. The most common root canal morphology of three-rooted second molar is four canals (MB1, MB2, DB, and P) (**Figure 10**). The incidence of MB2 ranged from 11.53 to 93.7% [40], in Russia—51.5%[41], and in Portugal—44% [30]. MB2 is located mostly 1 mm from the orifice of the mesiobuccal canal [39]. Root canal configuration of MB is so complex; type I (1-1) is common in MB root, followed by type II (2-1). Other types of root canal configurations were observed in some population like India, Portugal, and China [20, 30, 31]. Clinicians should pay attention to the presence of MB2 during endodontic treatment to avoid failure. The shape of the root canal in MB root could be ribbon-shaped when two canals exist or oval when just one canal (**Figure 11**).

For DB and P roots, they have one canal in most cases. Two canals in DB root were observed in some studies, and the prevalence of DB2 ranges from 0.6 to 4% [40]. Its orifice is located near the DB1. The most common root canal configuration in these roots is type 1 (1-1) (**Table 2**). The root canal shape of these roots is mostly round.

For one-, two-, and four-rooted maxillary second molars, type 1 (1-1) is mostly common [31]. **Table 2** presents the root canal configurations of three-rooted maxillary second molars in recent studies in different countries [20, 30–35, 42–44].

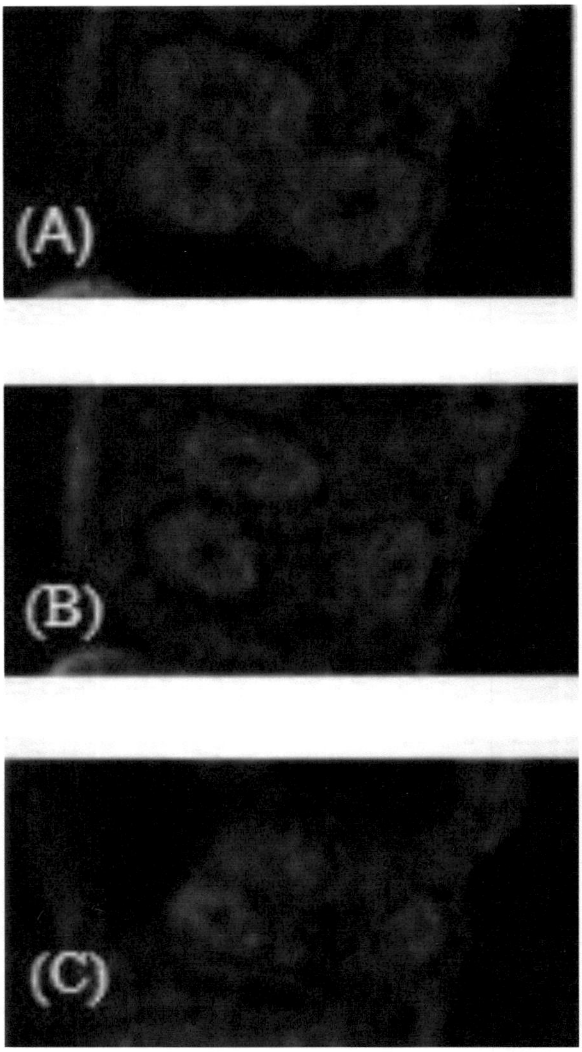

Figure 11.
Three canals of maxillary second molar. The shape of MB canal is oval while the shape of DB is round (A) coronal third of root canals, (B) middle third of root canal, (C) apical third of root canals.

3.3 Maxillary third molar

It is also known as wisdom tooth and generally erupts between the ages of 17 and 25 years old. The anatomy of the maxillary third molar is unpredictable and varies among populations, even in individuals in same populations [45–47]. A few studies were conducted to analyze the anatomy and root canal morphology of this tooth. It may have from one to five roots. Root fusion is common in this tooth, whereas Alavi et al. reported root fusion from 2 to 26.5% in Thai population [45]. Ahmad et al. found root fusion in 70% in Jordan population [46]. The fusion of three roots was the most common form. Regarding the number of root canals, it varies per root and generally ranges from one to six canals (**Figure 12**) [47]. **Table 3** shows the number of roots and root canals of maxillary third molar among different populations [41, 42, 45–51]. The most common root canal configuration for maxillary third molar is type I (1-1) followed by type II (2-1) (**Table 4**) [42, 47, 50, 51]. The incidence of C-shaped canals in this tooth was reported in two studies: in the USA (2.2%) [45] and in China (8.5%) [51]. The shape of the root canal in the coronal, middle, and

Author(s)	Country (year)	Root	Type (1-1)	Type (2-1)	Type (1-2-1)	Type (2-2)	Type (1-2)	Type (2-1-2)	Type (1-2-1-2)	Type (3-3)	Type (2-1-3)	type (3-1)	Type (3-2-1)	Type (2-1-2-1)
Weng et al. [41]	China (2009)	MB	82	8	–	6	4	–	–	–	–	–	–	–
		DB	92	2	–	–	6	–	–	–	–	–	–	–
		P	94	–	6	–	–	–	–	–	–	–	–	–
Neelakantan et al. [31]	India	MB	62	6.3		24.4	–	–	–	–	–	–	–	0.5
		DB	84.9	1.5	2.4	4.4	–	–	–	–	–	–	–	–
		P	87.8	–	–	3.4	0.9	–	–	0.5	–	0.5	–	–
Martins et al. [30]	Portugal (2017)	MB	56.2	27.1	0.7	7.6	3.4	4.2	0.2	–	–	–	0.2	0.4
		DB	100	–	–	–	–	–	–	–	–	–	–	–
		P	98.8	0.4	0.7	–	–	–	–	–	–	–	–	–
Tian et al. [20]	China (2016)	MB	70.3	12.9	5.3	6.8	3	0.4	0.3	0.1		0.9		
		DB	99.5	0.2	–	0.1	0.2	–	–	–	–	–	–	–
		P	99.7	0.2	0.1	–	–	–	–	–	–	–	–	–
Kalender et al. [42]	Turkey (2016)	MB	76.1	20.8	–	2.8	–	–	–	0.3	–	–	–	–
		DB	100	–	–	–	–	–	–	–	–	–	–	–
		P	100	–	–	–	–	–	–	–	–	–	–	–
Ghobashy et al. [32]	Egypt (2017)	MB	42.06	47.1	–	8.03	1.87	0.93	–	–	–	–	–	–
		DB	100	–	–	–	–	–	–	–	–	–	–	–
		P	100	–	–	–	–	–	–	–	–	–	–	–
Pérez-Heredia et al. [33]	Spain (2017)	MB	52.7	33	–	9.8	–	2.7	–	0.9	0.9	–	–	–
		DB	100	–	–	–	–	–	–	–	–	–	–	–
		P	100	–	–	–	–	–	–	–	–	–	–	–

Author(s)	Country (year)	Root	Type (1-1)	Type (2-1)	Type (1-2-1)	Type (2-2)	Type (1-2)	Type (2-1-2)	Type (1-2-1-2)	Type (3-3)	Type (2-1-3)	type (3-1)	Type (3-2-1)	Type (2-1-2-1)
Ratanajirasut et al. [34]	Thailand (2018)	MB	70.6	14.6	2.3	7.5	3.5	1.5	–	–	–	–	–	–
		DB	100	–	–	–	–	–	–	–	–	–	–	–
		P	99.7	0.3	–	–	–	–	–	–	–	–	–	–
Naseri et al. [43]	Iran (2018)	MB	23.5	18.5	3.2	11.5	7.6	26.8	–	–	–	–	–	–
		DB	94.3	–	0.6	–	3.8	1.3	–	–	–	–	–	–
		P	93.6	–	0.6	–	4.5	1.3	–	–	–	–	–	–

Table 2.
Root canal configurations of maxillary second molars in different populations.

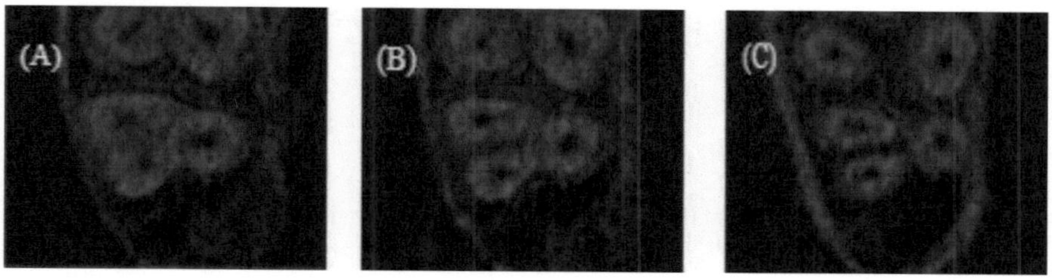

Figure 12.
Maxillary third molar with three roots and four canals (A) coronal third of root canals, (B) middle third of root canal, (C) apical third of root canals.

apical thirds varies per root such as, when the third molar has one root with one canal from the orifice to the apex, the shape of the canal may be oval or long oval in all parts (**Figure 13**). If the one-rooted tooth has two canals, the shape of the canal could be like a ribbon, type I, II, IV, or V by Kim et al. (**Figure 14**). A clinician should pay attention to the root canal shape when preparing and filling the root canal.

4. Root canal morphology of mandibular molars

4.1 Mandibular first molar

This tooth is the most common tooth exposed to caries and frequently requires root canal treatment. It has two roots in the most common form (mesial and distal); occasionally, it has three roots. The mesial root is characterized by a flattened mesiodistal surface and widened buccolingual surface. The distal root is mostly straight. The morphology of mandibular first molar has been investigated in different studies among different populations. The incidence of three-rooted teeth has been reported in some populations: Korea (25.8%) [51], Spain (4.1%) [33], and Turkey (3.6%) [52]; this third root is mostly located distolingually, and it is smaller than the distobuccal root. Root canal system varies from two canals to four canals. The incidence of four canals was reported in some races: in Russia (20.9%) [40], Turkey (15.3%) [52], Spain (52.9%) [33], and Korea (24.3%) (**Figure 15**) [51]. The fourth canal is usually located in the distal root. The mesial root has two separated canals in about 90% of cases (type IV), and in 10 % the two canals are joined into one canal at the apex (type II), while the distal root usually contains one straight oval canal (type I) (**Figure 16**). The incidence of C-shaped root canal is low in this tooth and about 2% [60] (**Table 5** shows the root canal configurations for mandibular first molar in recent studies [30, 33, 51–59]).

4.2 Mandibular second molar

This tooth is similar to the mandibular first molar. Usually, it has two roots (mesial and distal), although it may have one or three roots. The extra root is usually located lingually. The incidence of three-rooted teeth was found in some populations: in Chinese (1.27%) [59], Indian (7.5%) [61], Turkish (0.4%) [52], Spain (6.25%) [33], and Korean (1.1%) [62]. The prevalence of one-rooted mandibular second molar was observed in Russia (0.5%) [40], Spain (16.5%) [33], and Turkey (1.6%) [52]. The most frequent root canal system is three canals (two mesial and one distal) (**Figure 17**). The prevalence of three canals in various populations was in Russia (82.2%) [40], Turkey (86.4%) [52], India (53.5%) [61], and Spain (81.25%) [33]. The mesial root usually has two canals that tend to lie much closer together. The most common root canal configurations in the mesial root are type II

Author(s)	Country (year)	Type of study	Number of teeth	Number of roots				Number of canals					
				1	2	3	4	1	2	3	4	5	6
Sidow et al. [44]	USA (2000)	Clearing	150	15	32	45	7	7.4	3.3	57.3	27.3	2.7	0.7
Ng et al. [48]	Burmese (2001)	Clearing	72	19.4	19.4	55.6	5.6	5.6	25	47.2	22.2	–	–
Alavi et al. [45]	Thai (2002)	Clearing	151	1.3	6.6	88.1	4	9.9	11.3	48.3	29.1	1.3	–
Weng et al. [41]	China (2009)	Clearing	43	–	–	–	–	27.9	11.6	44.2	16.3	–	–
Sert et al. [49]	Turkey (2011)	Clearing	290	35.5	28.6	34.1	1.7	12.4	29.7	46.9	11	–	–
Cosić et al. [47]	Croatia (2013)	Sectioning	56	8.9	5.4	83.9	1.8	7.1	7.1	75	10.8	–	–
Ahmad et al. [46]	Jordan (2016)	Clearing	89	13.5	5.6	74.2	6.7	9	6.7	55.1	27	2.2	–
Zhang et al. [50]	China (2018)	Micro KT	130	51.5	19.2	25.4	3.8	–	–	–	–	–	–
Razumova et al. [40]	Russia (2018)	CBCT	238	47.9	–	52.1	–	13.8	11.8	72.3	2.1	–	–

Table 3.
Number of roots and root canals of maxillary third molars in different populations.

Author(s)	Country (year)	Root	Type (1-1)	Type (2-1)	Type (1-2-1)	Type (2-2)	Type (1-2)	Type (2-1-2)	Type (3-3)	Type (1-2-3)	Type (1-3)	Type (3-2-1)	Type (1-3-2)	Type (3-2)	Type (3-1)
Weng et al. [41]	China (2009) (HAN)	Single	63.2	21	–	–	–	5.3	10.5	–	–	–	–	–	–
		MB	62.5	20.8	4.2	8.3	4.2	–	–	–	–	–	–	–	–
		DB	87.5	–	4.2	–	8.3	–	–	–	–	–	–	–	–
		P	91.6	–	4.2	–	4.2	–	–	–	–	–	–	–	–
Sert et al. [49]	Turkey (2011)	Single	63.1	12.3	7	12.2	3.5	–	–	–	–	–	–	–	1.75
		MB	77.8	13.1	–	5.1	4	–	–	–	–	–	–	–	–
		DB	100	–	–	–	–	–	–	–	–	–	–	–	–
		P	100	–	–	–	–	–	–	–	–	–	–	–	–
Ahmad et al. [46]	Jordan (2016)	Single	66.8	–	8.3	–	8.3	8.3	–	–	8.3	–	–	–	–
		MB	55	5	–	20	15	–	–	5	–	–	–	–	–
		DB	100	–	–	–	–	–	–	–	–	–	–	–	–
		P	100	–	–	–	–	–	–	–	–	–	–	–	–
Zhang et al. [50]	China (2018)	Single	51.4	12.8	5.7	1.4	12.8	–	–	–	1.4	5.7	1.4	1.4	1.4
		MB	72.7	–	–	12.1	12.1	–	3	–	–	–	–	–	–
		DB	100	–	–	–	–	–	–	–	–	–	–	–	–
		P	93.9	–	–	6.1	–	–	–	–	–	–	–	–	–

Table 4.
Root canal configuration of maxillary third molar in different populations.

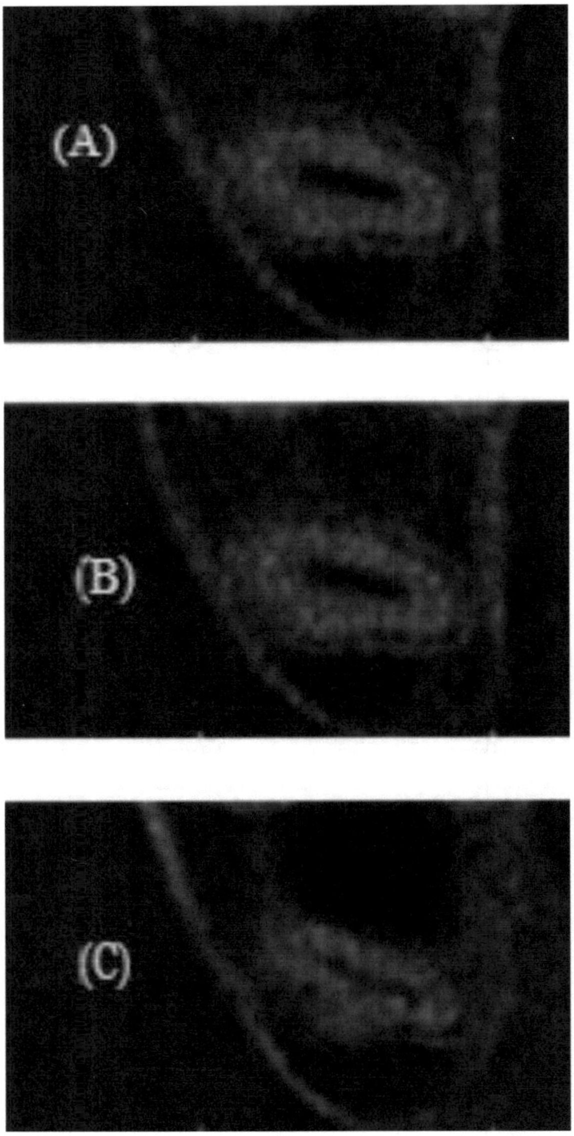

Figure 13.
Maxillary third molar with one root and one long oval canal (A) coronal third of root canals, (B) middle third of root canal, (C) apical third of root canals.

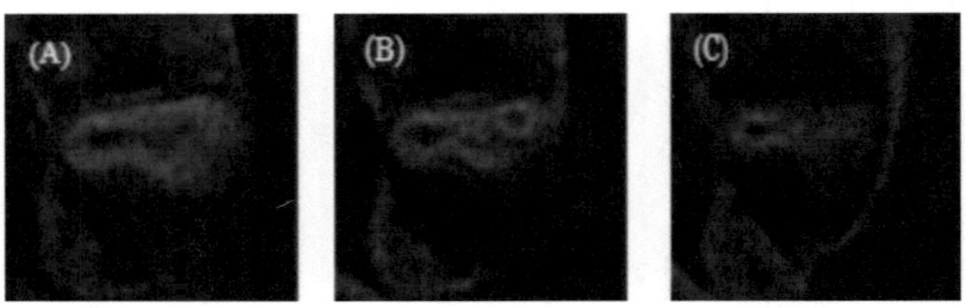

Figure 14.
Maxillary third molar with one root and two canals (A) coronal third of root canals, (B) middle third of root canal, (C) apical third of root canals.

(2-1) and type IV (2-2) (**Table 6**). The distal root has one straight canal with type I (1-1), and the incidence of two canals is less and ranged from 3.5 to 20% [61]. The incidence of C-shaped root canals is higher in this tooth than the other teeth

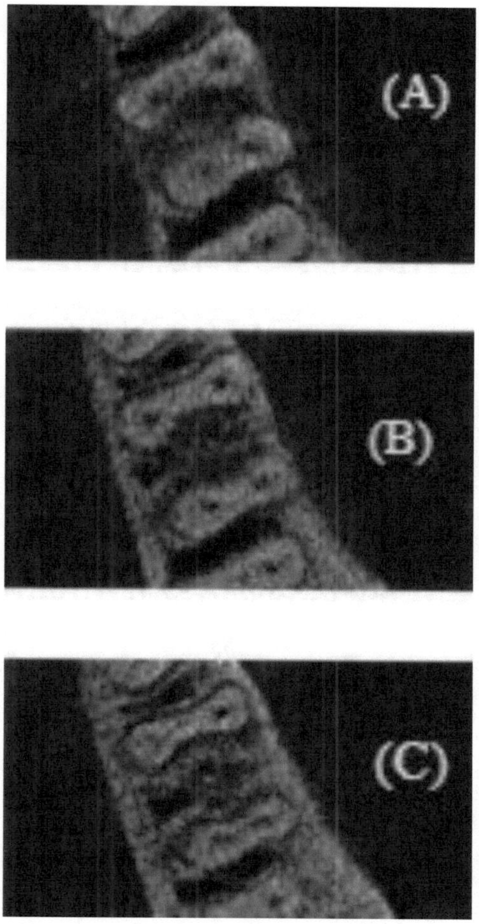

Figure 15.
Mandibular first molar with four canals (two mesial and two distal) (A) coronal third of root canals, (B) middle third of root canal, (C) apical third of root canals.

(**Figure 18**). Several studies have reported the C-shaped canals among various populations: India (13.12%) [61], Korea (40%) [62], Brazil (3.5–15.3%) [63, 64], China (29–39%) [59, 65, 66], Russia (8.5%) [67], Saudi Arabia (9.1%) [60], and Jordan (21.6%) [16]. This variation could be related to ethnic groups. Regarding the root canal shape, mesial roots tend to have ribbon-shape type I or V by Kim et al., and the distal root canal in most cases has an oval shape and round in some cases (**Figure 19**). **Table 6** represents the root canal configurations of two-rooted mandibular second molars.

4.3 Mandibular third molar

This tooth erupts between the ages of 17 and 25 years old. It has morphological radicular variations. Many dental treatment plans work on maintaining this tooth to use it as a strategic abutment when the first and second molars are missed, especially when there is sufficient room in the dental arch. Frequently, it has two roots (mesial and distal). A few studies in various populations found that mandibular third molar could have from one to four roots (**Figures 20** and **21**), which could be related to genetics and race differences; as in Croatia and China, one-rooted third molar was reported in 56% [47] and 48% [50] of cases, respectively (**Figure 22**) (**Table 7**). The root canal system of this tooth is unpredictable;

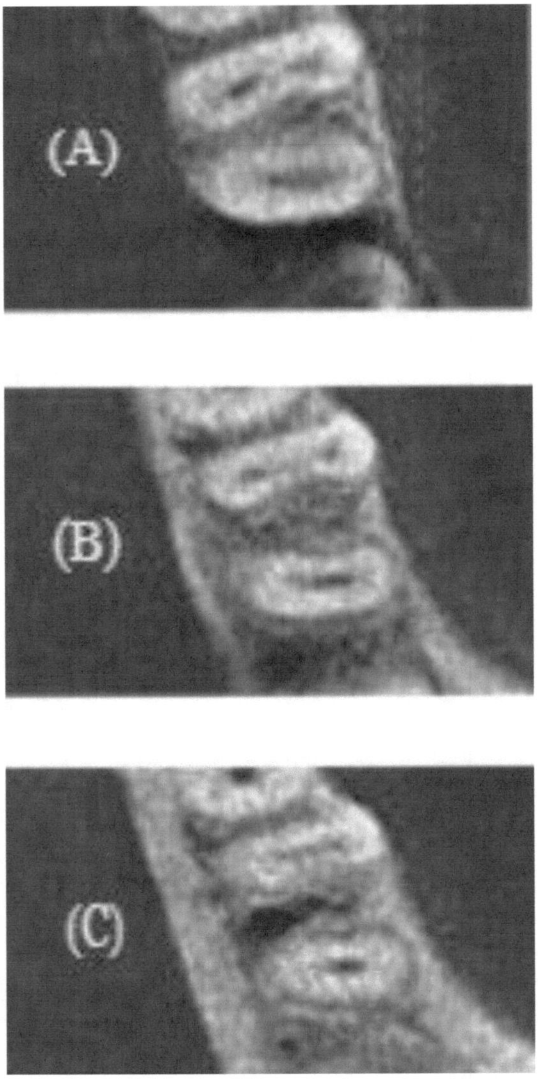

Figure 16.
Mandibular first molar with three canals (two mesial and one distal) the mesial canals shape have the ribbon type I by Kim, while the distal canal shape is long oval (A) coronal third of root canals, (B) middle third of root canal, (C) apical third of root canals.

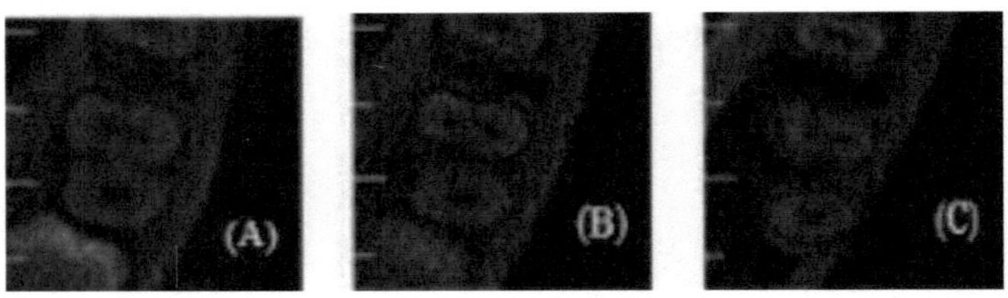

Figure 17.
Mandibular second molar with three canals (two mesial + one distal) (A) coronal third of root canals, (B) middle third of root canal, (C) apical third of root canals.

it could have from one to six canals [44]. The most common form is to have three canals (two mesial canals and one distal canal). **Table 7** presents the root and canal number in different populations. Regarding root canal configurations, type (1-1) prevailed mostly in mesial and distal roots of two-rooted teeth and in

Author(s)	Country (year)	Root	Type (1-1)	Type (2-1)	Type (1-2-1)	Type (2-2)	Type (1-2)	Type (2-1-2)	Type (1-2-1-2)	Type (2-3-1)	Type (2-1-2-1)	Type (3-2)	Type (2-3-2)	Type (3-2-1)	Type (1-2-1-2-1)
Chourasia et al. [52]	India (2012)	M	–	36.6	–	54	0.6	8	0.6	–	–	–	–	–	–
		D	65.3	20.6	1.3	9.3	3.3	–	–	–	–	–	–	–	–
Muriithi et al. [54]	Kenya (2012)	M	3.3	7.9	–	87.3	–	1.1	–	–	–	–	–	–	–
		D	50.3	18.5	1.6	22.2	5.3	–	–	–	–	–	–	–	–
Kim et al. [51]	Korea (2013)	M	1.8	20.2	0.3	76.9	0.5	–	–	–	–	0.1	0.2	–	–
		D	66.6	19	0.3	11.8	2.1	–	–	–	–	–	–	–	–
Zhang et al. [59]	China (2015)	M	0.9	5.6	4.8	87.7	0.9	–	–	–	–	–	–	–	–
		D	65.9	2.4	0.3	9.2	–	–	–	–	–	–	–	–	–
Torres et al. [56]	Chile 2015	M	2.9	19	28.5	21.9	21.9	21.9	3.6	–	–	–	–	–	–
		D	78.8	–	12.4	–	5.8	–	2.9	–	–	–	–	–	–
Torres et al. [56]	Belgium (2015)	M	1.4	5	33.6	16.4	42.9	–	0.7	–	–	–	–	–	–
		D	72.9	–	17.1	–	9.3	–	0.7	–	–	–	–	–	–
Celikten et al. [53]	Turkey (2016)	M	2.4	34.9	–	62.7	–	–	–	–	–	–	–	–	–
		D	84	11.8	0.3	3.4	0.3	0.3	–	–	–	–	–	–	–
Madani et al. [57]	Iran (2017)	M	7.3	31.5	2	57	2	–	–	–	–	–	–	–	–
		D	79.8	10.7	4.6	3.3	1.3	–	–	–	–	–	–	–	–
Martins et al. [30]	Portugal (2017)	M	1.1	46.5	–	41.9	–	4.1	–	–	0.9	2.1	0.2	3.2	–
		D	70.9	12.4	9.6	2.3	3.2	0.9	–	–	0.5	–	–	–	0.2
Pérez-Heredia et al. [33]	Spain (2017)	M	–	51.3	–	37.8	0.8	1.7	–	1.7	–	5.9	–	–	–
		D	72.3	18.5	5.9	2.5	–	–	–	–	–	–	0.8	–	–

Author(s)	Country (year)	Root	Type (1-1)	Type (2-1)	Type (1-2-1)	Type (2-2)	Type (1-2)	Type (2-1-2)	Type (1-2-1-2)	Type (2-3-1)	Type (2-1-2-1)	Type (3-2)	Type (2-3-2)	Type (3-2-1)	Type (1-2-1-2-1)
Gambarini et al. [58]	West Europe (2018)	M		41		59									
		D	100	–	–	–	–	–	–	–	–	–	–	–	–

Table 5.
Root canal configurations of mandibular first molars in different populations.

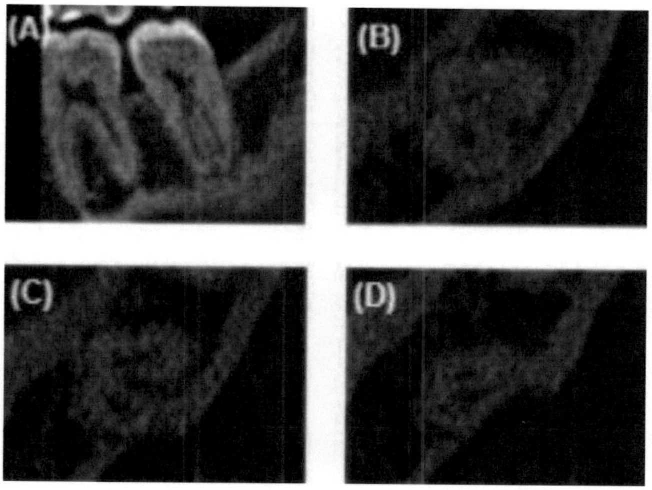

Figure 18.
Mandibular second molar with C-shaped canal (A) Sagittal view of mandibular second molar, (B) coronal third of root canals, (C) middle third of root canal, (D) apical third of root canals.

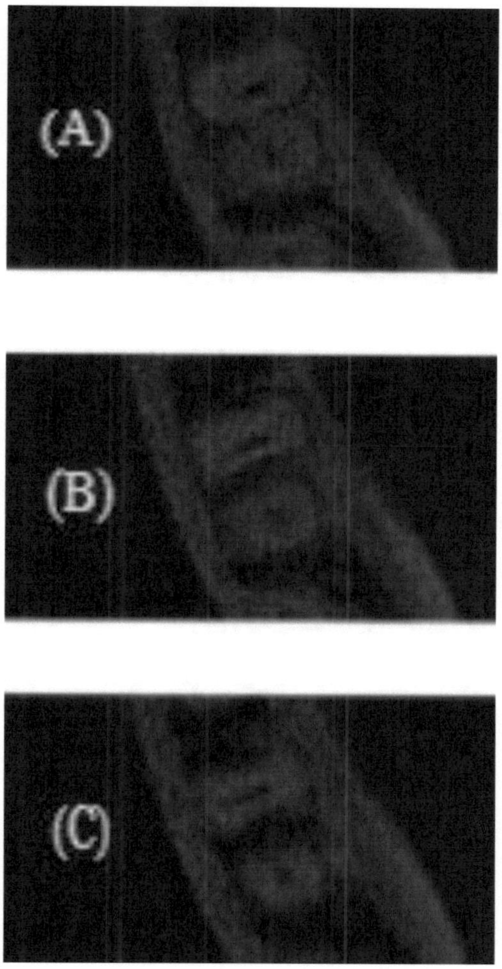

Figure 19.
Mandibular second molar two canals (one oval mesial + one round distal) (A) coronal third of root canals, (B) middle third of root canal, (C) apical third of root canals.

Author(s)	Country (year)	Root	Type (1-1)	Type (2-1)	Type (1-2-1)	Type (2-2)	Type (1-2)	Type (2-1-2)	Type (1-2-1-2)	Type (3-1)	Type (2-1-2-1)	Type (3-2)	Type (2-3-2-1)	Type (3-2-1)	Type (3-2-3-2-1)
Al-Qudah and Awawdeh [16]	Jordan (2009)	M	16.1	32.6	3.5	40.3	3.5	1	0.3	–	–	0.3	–	0.3	–
		D	79	7.7	2.6	4.5	5.5	–	–	–	–	–	–	–	–
Neelakantan et al. [68]	India (2010)	M	8.4	2	1.4	63.1	5.2	–	–	2	–	1.1	–	–	–
		D	64.9	4.6	0.6	11	1.7	–	–	–	–	–	–	–	–
Ceperuelo et al. [69]	Spain (2014)	M	12.5	56.2	18.7	–	6.2	–	–	–	–	–	–	–	–
		D	81.2	6.2	–	6.2	–	–	–	–	–	–	–	–	–
Torres et al. [56]	Chile (2015)	M	17.5	7.2	48.4	4.1	20.6	–	2.1	–	–	–	–	–	–
		D	99	–	–	–	1	–	–	–	–	–	–	–	–
Torres et al. [56]	Belgium (2015)	M	11.7	5.3	37.2	14.9	28.78	–	2.13	–	–	–	–	–	–
		D	98.4	–	–	–	1.06	–	–	–	–	–	–	–	–
Celikten et al. [52]	Turkey (2016)	M	7.1	32.3	0.2	60.3	–	–	–	–	–	–	–	–	–
		D	96.3	2.5	–	1	–	0.2	–	–	–	–	–	–	–
Kim et al. [62]	Korea (2016)	M	13.9	37.7	1.2	44.5	2.6	–	–	–	–	–	–	–	–
		D	96.6	2.1	–	0.9	0.4	–	–	–	–	–	–	–	–
Pérez-Heredia et al. [33]	Spain (2017)	M	3	78.2	–	14.9	1	–	–	1	–	2	–	–	–
		D	92.1	2	3	3	–	–	–	–	–	–	–	–	–
Martins et al. [30]	Portugal (2017)	M	8.1	63.9	5.2	18.1	0.5	1.6	–	–	0.4	0.2	0.4	1.4	0.2
		D	93.5	0.5	4.2	0.4	1.4	–	–	–	–	–	–	–	–
Madani et al. [57]	Iran (2017)	M	18.1	28	5.7	42.9	3.3	0.8	–	–	–	–	–	–	–
		D	91.7	3.3	0.8	1.6	1.6	–	–	–	–	–	–	–	–

Author(s)	Country (year)	Root	Type (1-1)	Type (2-1)	Type (1-2-1)	Type (2-2)	Type (1-2)	Type (2-1-2)	Type (1-2-1-2)	Type (3-1)	Type (2-1-2-1)	Type (3-2)	Type (2-3-2-1)	Type (3-2-1)	Type (3-2-3-2-1)
Pawar et al. [61]	India (2017)	M	7.2	32.5	0.9	45.2	1	–	–	–	–	–	–	–	–
		D	61.1	18.2	–	7.5	–	–	–	–	–	–	–	–	–

Table 6.
Root canal configurations of mandibular second molars in different populations.

Author(s)	Country (year)	Type of study	Number of teeth	Number of roots				Number of canals					
				1	2	3	4	1	2	3	4	5	6
Sidow et al. [44]	USA (2000)	Clearing	150	17	77	5	1	7.3	16.7	55.3	16.7	3.3	0.7
Gulabivala et al. [13]	Burmese (2001)	Clearing	58	–	100	–	–	1.7	51.7	44.8	1.7	–	–
Gulabivala et al. [70]	Thai (2002)	Clearing	173	11.6	86.7	21.2	0.6	6.4	64.1	28.3	5.2	–	–
Sert et al. [49]	Turkey (2011)	Clearing	370	24.9	69.5	5.4	0.3	10.8	52.7	17.3	18.6	0.5	–
Kuzekanani et al. [71]	Iran (2012)	Clearing	150	21.4	72.6	5.3	0.7	10	52	32.7	5.3	–	–
Cosić et al. [47]	Croatia (2013)	Sectioning	50	56	44	–	–	4	6	90	–	–	–
Ahmad et al. [46]	Jordan (2016)	Clearing	70	14.3	74.3	8.6	2.9	7.1	38.6	45.7	8.6	–	–
Zhang et al. [50]	China (2018)	Micro KT	130	47.7	46.1	5.4	0.8	–	–	–	–	–	–
Razumova et al. [40]	Russia (2018)	CBCT	210	20	80	–	–	0.5	40.9	58.6	–	–	–

Table 7.
The number of roots and root canals of mandibular third molars in different populations.

Author(s)	Country (Year)	Root	Type (1-1)	Type (2-1)	Type (1-2-1)	Type (2-2)	Type (1-2)	Type (2-1-2)	Type (3-3)
Sert et al. [49]	Turkey (2011)	Single	65.6	14.7	–	9.8	9.8	–	–
		Mesial	59	24.2	2.7	9.8	3.9	–	–
		Distal	99.2	0.8	–	–	–	–	–
Kuzekanani et al. [71]	Iran (2012)	Single	31.2	21.9	9.4	25	3.1	–	3.1
		Mesial	54.1	17.4	13.8	3.7	7.4	–	–
		Distal	92.7	1.8	2.7	–	–	–	–
Ahmad et al. [46]	Jordan (2016)	Single	55.6	22.2	11.1	–	–	11.1	–
		Mesial	40.6	18.8	3.1	28.1	9.4	–	–
		Distal	93.8	–	–	3.1	3.1	–	–
Zhang et al. [50]	China (2018)	Single	42.7	3.6	–	2.4	2.4	–	–
		Mesial	68.3	5	8.3	3.3	11.7	–	–
		Distal	100	–	–	–	–	–	–

Table 8.
Root canal configuration of maxillary third molar in different populations.

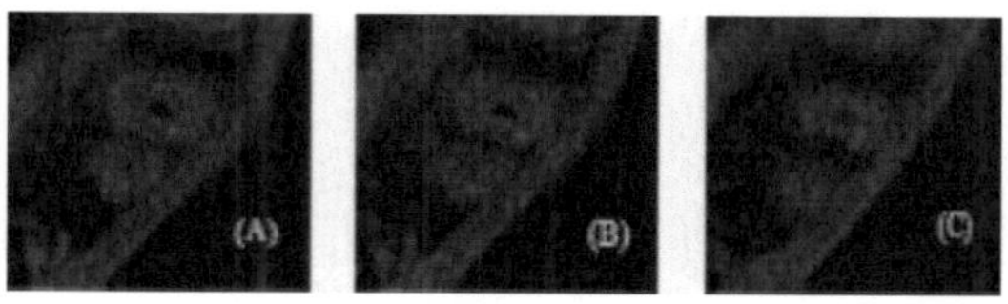

Figure 20.
Mandibular third molar with two roots and two canals(A) coronal third of root canals, (B) middle third of root canal, (C) apical third of root canals.

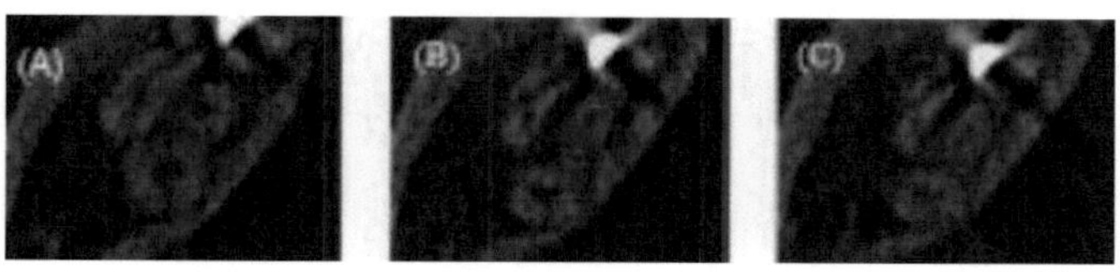

Figure 21.
Mandibular third molar with three roots and three canals(A) coronal third of root canals, (B) middle third of root canal, (C) apical third of root canals.

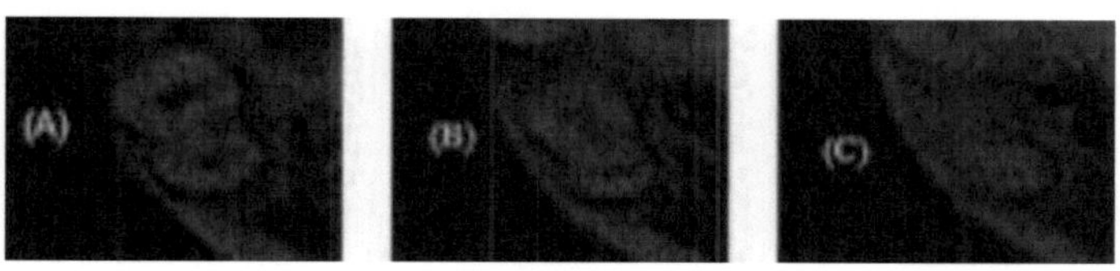

Figure 22.
Mandibular third molar with one root and two canals(A) coronal third of root canals, (B) middle third of root canal, (C) apical third of root canals.

single-rooted third molars (**Table 8**) [46, 49, 50, 71]. The incidence of C-shaped canals was reported in Thailand (11%) [70], Iran (3.3%) [71], and China (3.3%) (**Figure 23**) [50]. Root canal shape of mandibular third molar varies per root.

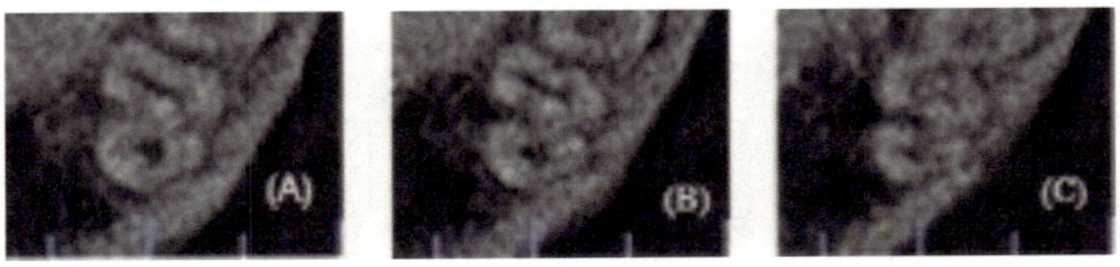

Figure 23.
Mandibular third molar with C-shaped canal(A) coronal third of root canals, (B) middle third of root canal, (C) apical third of root canals.

5. Conclusion

This chapter summarized the root canal system of the maxillary and mandibular molars in different populations. Root canal system of the molar teeth is so complex and unpredictable. It varies among populations and even in individuals in same population. The maxillary first and second molars have in the most common form three roots with four canals. The maxillary third molar may have from one to five roots with different numbers of canals ranging from one to six canals. Mandibular molars in the most common form have two roots with three canals. C-shaped canals are mostly common in mandibular second molars. Clinicians should pay attention to the additional canals and additional configurations when preparing for the root canal treatment, since knowledge of the basic root and root canal morphology as well as possible variation in anatomy of the root canal system is an important factor to achieve successful root canal treatment.

Author details

Svetlana Razumova, Anzhela Brago, Haydar Barakat* and Ammar Howijieh
Department of Propaedeutics of Dental Diseases of Medical Institute,
Peoples' Friendship University of Russia (RUDN University), Moscow, Russia

*Address all correspondence to: dr.haydarbarakat@yahoo.com

References

[1] Rahimi S, Ghasemi N. Maxillary first molar with two root canals. Sultan Qaboos University Medical Journal. 2013;**13**(2):346-349

[2] Blinov VS, Kartashov MV, Zholudev SE, Zornikova OS. Estimation of the cone-beam computed tomography in diagnostics of the molar root system anatomy of the mandible and maxilla. Radiology—Practice. 2016;**59**(5):6-15

[3] Toure B, Faye B, Kane AW, Lo CM, Niang B, Boucher Y. Analysis of reasons for extraction of endodontically treated teeth: A prospective study. Journal of Endodontia. 2011;**37**:1512-1515

[4] Gu Y, Lu Q, Wang H, Ding Y, Wang P, Ni L. Root canal morphology of permanent three rooted mandibular first molars—Part I: Pulp floor and root canal system. Journal of Endodontia. 2010;**36**:1341-1346

[5] Filpo-Perez C, Bramante CM, Villas-Boas MH, Duarte MAH, Versiani MA, Ordinola-Zapata R. Micro-computed tomographic analysis of the root canal morphology of the distal root of mandibular first molars. Journal of Endodontia. 2015;**41**:231-236

[6] Ballullaya SV, Vemuri S, Kumar PR. Variable permanent mandibular first molar: Review of literature. Journal of Conservative Dentistry. 2013;**16**:99-110

[7] Dinakar C, Shetty UA, Salian VV, Shetty P. Root canal morphology of maxillary first premolars using the clearing technique in a south Indian population: An in vitro study. International Journal of Applied & Basic Medical Research. 2018;**8**(3):143-147

[8] Bansal R, Hegde S, Astekar MS. Classification of root canal configurations: A review and a new proposal of nomenclature system for root canal configuration. Journal of Clinical and Diagnostic Research. 2018;**12**(5):ZE01-ZE05

[9] Weine FS, Healey HJ, Gerstein H, Evanson L. Canal configuration in the mesiobuccal root of the maxillary first molar and its endodontic significance. Oral Surgery, Oral Medicine, and Oral Pathology. 1969;**28**:419-425

[10] Vertucci FJ. Root canal anatomy of the human permanent teeth. Oral Surgery, Oral Medicine, and Oral Pathology. 1984;**58**:589-599

[11] Cleghorn BM, Christie WH, Dong CC. The root and root canal morphology of the human mandibular second premolar: A literature review. Journal of Endodontia. 2007;**33**(9):1031-1037

[12] Kartal N, Yanıkoğlu FÇ. Root canal morphology of mandibular incisors. Journal of Endodontia. 1992;**S18**:562-564

[13] Gulabivala K, Aung T, Alavi A, Ng YL. Root and canal morphology of Burmese mandibular molars. International Endodontic Journal. 2001;**34**:359-370

[14] Sert S, Bayirli GS. Evaluation of the root canal configurations of the mandibular and maxillary permanent teeth by gender in the Turkish population. Journal of Endodontia. 2004;**30**:391-398

[15] Peiris H, Pitakotuwage T, Takahashi M, Sasaki K, Kanazawa E. Root canal morphology of mandibular permanent molars at different ages. International Endodontic Journal. 2008;**41**:828-835

[16] Al-Qudah AA, Awawdeh LA. Root and canal morphology of mandibular first and second molar teeth in a Jordanian population. International Endodontic Journal. 2009;**42**:775-784

[17] Kim S, Pecora G, Rubinstein R, Dorscher-Kim J. Color Atlas of Microsurgery in Endodontics. Philadelphia: WB Saunders; 2001

[18] Barbizam JVB, Ribeiro RG. Unusual anatomy of permanent maxillary molars. Journal of Endodontia. 2004;**30**(9):668-671

[19] Alrahabi M, Sohail Zafar M. Evaluation of root canal morphology of maxillary molars using cone beam computed tomography. Pakistan Journal of Medical Sciences. 2015;**31**(2):426-430

[20] Tian XM, Yang XW, Qian L, Wei B, Gong Y. Analysis of the root and canal morphologies in maxillary first and second molars in a Chinese population using cone-beam computed tomography. Journal of Endodontia. 2016;**42**(5):696-701. DOI: 10.1016/j.joen.2016.01.017

[21] Naseri M, Safi Y, Akbarzadeh Baghban A, Khayat A, Eftekhar L. Survey of anatomy and root canal morphology of maxillary first molars regarding age and gender in an Iranian population using cone-beam computed tomography. Iranian Endodontic Journal. 2016;**11**(4):298-303

[22] Zheng QH, Wang Y, Zhou XD, Wang Q, Zheng GN, Huang DM. A cone-beam computed tomography study of maxillary first permanent molar root and canal morphology in a Chinese population. Journal of Endodontia. 2010;**36**(9):1480-1484

[23] Guo J, Vahidnia A, Sedghizadeh P, Enciso R. Evaluation of root and canal morphology of maxillary permanent first molars in a North American population by cone-beam computed tomography. Journal of Endodontia. 2014;**40**(5):635-639

[24] Singh S, Pawar M. Root canal morphology of South Asian Indian maxillary molar teeth. European Journal of Dentistry. 2015;**9**(1):133-144. DOI: 10.4103/1305-7456.149662

[25] Razumova S, Brago A, Khaskhanova L, Barakat H, Howijieh A. Evaluation of anatomy and root canal morphology of the maxillary first molar using the cone-beam computed tomography among residents of the Moscow region. Contemporary Clinical Dentistry. 2018;**9**(Suppl 1):S133-S136

[26] Patil AC, Ramesh HG, Yelamali S. Management of a permanent maxillary first molar with two disto buccal canals with the aid of spiral computed tomography: A case report. Journal of Clinical and Experimental Dentistry. 2010;**2**(3):e153-e156

[27] Cantatore G, Berutti E, Castellucci A. Missed anatomy: Frequency and clinical impact. Endodontic Topics. 2009;**15**:3-31

[28] Olczak K, Pawlicka H. The morphology of maxillary first and second molars analyzed by cone-beam computed tomography in a Polish population. BMC Medical Imaging. 2017;**17**:68

[29] Imura N, Hata GI, Toda T. Two canals in mesiobuccal roots of maxillary molars. International Endodontic Journal. 1998;**3**:410-414

[30] Martins JNR, Marques D, Mata A, Caramês J. Root and root canal morphology of the permanent dentition in a Caucasian population: A cone-beam computed tomography study. International Endodontic Journal. 2017;**50**:1013-1026

[31] Neelakantan P, Subbarao C, Ahuja R, Subbarao CV, Gutmann JL. Cone-beam computed tomography study of root and canal morphology of maxillary first and second molars in an Indian population. Journal of Endodontia. 2010;**36**(10):1622-1627

[32] Ghobashy AM, Nagy MM, Bayoumi AA. Evaluation of root and canal morphology of maxillary permanent molars in an Egyptian population by cone-beam computed tomography. Journal of Endodontia. 2017;**43**(7):1089-1092

[33] Pérez-Heredia M, Ferrer-Luque CM, Bravo M, Castelo-Baz P, Ruíz-Piñón M, Baca P. Cone-beam computed tomographic study of root anatomy and canal configuration of molars in a Spanish population. Journal of Endodontia. 2017;**43**(9):1511-1516. DOI: 10.1016/j.joen.2017.03.026

[34] Ratanajirasut R, Panichuttra A, Panmekiate S. A cone-beam computed tomographic study of root and canal morphology of maxillary first and second permanent molars in a Thai population. Journal of Endodontia. 2018;**44**(1):56-61. DOI: 10.1016/j.joen.2017.08.020

[35] Rezaeian M, Rouhani Tonekaboni M, Iranmanesh F. Evaluating the root canal morphology of permanent maxillary first molars in Iranian population. Iranian Endodontic Journal. 2018;**13**(1):78-82

[36] Zhu Z, Zhao SL. Maxillary second molar with five root canals: A case report. Shanghai Kou Qiang Yi Xue. 2011;**20**:219-221

[37] Kottoor J, Hemamalathi S, Sudha R, et al. Maxillary second molar with 5 roots and 5 canals evaluated using cone beam computerized tomography: A case report. Oral Surgery, Oral Medicine, Oral Pathology, Oral Radiology, and Endodontics. 2010;**109**:e162-e165

[38] Wu D, Zhang G, Liang R, Zhou G, Wu Y, Sun C, et al. Root and canal morphology of maxillary second molars by cone-beam computed tomography in a native Chinese population. The Journal of International Medical Research. 2017;**45**(2):830-842

[39] Ghasemi N, Rahimi S, Shahi S, Samiei M, Frough Reyhani M, Ranjkesh B. A review on root anatomy and canal configuration of the maxillary second molars. Iranian Endodontic Journal. 2017;**12**(1):1-9

[40] Razumova S, Brago A, Khaskhanova L, Howijieh A, Barakat H, Manvelyan A. A cone-beam computed tomography scanning of the root canal system of permanent teeth among the Moscow population. International Journal of Dentistry. 2018;**2018**:2615746

[41] Weng XL, Yu SB, Zhao SL, Wang HG, Mu T, Tang RY, et al. Root canal morphology of permanent maxillary teeth in the Han nationality in Chinese Guanzhong area: A new modified root canal staining technique. Journal of Endodontia. 2009;**35**(5):651-656

[42] Kalender A, Celikten B, Tufenkci P, Aksoy U, Basmacı F, Kelahmet U, et al. Cone beam computed tomography evaluation of maxillary molar root canal morphology in a Turkish Cypriot population. Biotechnology & Biotechnological Equipment. 2016;**30**(1):145-150

[43] Naseri M, Ali Mozayeni M, Safi Y, Heidarnia M, Akbarzadeh Baghban A, Norouzi N. Root canal morphology of maxillary second molars according to age and gender in a selected Iranian population: A cone-beam computed tomography evaluation. Iranian Endodontic Journal. 2018;**13**(3):373-380

[44] Sidow SJ, West LA, Liewehr FR, Loushine RJ. Root canal morphology of human maxillary and mandibular third molars. Journal of Endodontia. 2000;**26**(11):675-678

[45] Alavi AM, Opasanon A, Ng YL, Gulabivala K. Root and canal morphology of Thai maxillary molars. International Endodontic Journal. 2002;**35**:478-485

[46] Ahmad IA, Azzeh MM, Zwiri AM, Abu Haija MS, Diab MM. Root and root canal morphology of third molars in a Jordanian subpopulation. Saudi Endodontic Journal. 2016;**6**:113-121

[47] Cosić J, Galić N, Vodanović M, Njemirovskij V, Segović S, Pavelić B, et al. An in vitro morphological investigation of the endodontic spaces of third molars. Collegium Antropologicum. 2013;**37**(2):437-442

[48] Ng YL, Aung TH, Alavi A, Gulabivala K. Root and canal morphology of Burmese maxillary molars. International Endodontic Journal. 2001;**34**:620-630

[49] Sert S, Sahinkesen G, Topçu FT, Eroglu SE, Oktay EA. Root canal configurations of third molar teeth. A comparison with first and second molars in the Turkish population. Australian Endodontic Journal. 2011;**37**:109-117

[50] Zhang W, Tang Y, Liu C, Shen Y, Feng X, Gu Y. Root and root canal variations of the human maxillary and mandibular third molars in a Chinese population: A micro-computed tomographic study. Archives of Oral Biology. 2018;**95**:134-140. DOI: 10.1016

[51] Kim SY, Kim BS, Woo J, Kim Y. Morphology of mandibular first molars analyzed by cone-beam computed tomography in a Korean population: Variations in the number of roots and canal. Journal of Endodontia. 2013;**39**(12):1516-1521

[52] Celikten B, Tufenkci P, Aksoy U, Kalender A, Kermeoglu F, Dabaj P, et al. Cone beam CT evaluation of mandibular molar root canal morphology in a Turkish Cypriot population. Clinical Oral Investigations. 2016;**20**(8):2221-2226

[53] Chourasia HR, Meshram GK, Warhadpande M, Dakshindas D. Root canal morphology of mandibular first permanent molars in an Indian population. International Journal of Dentistry. 2012;**2012**:745152

[54] Muriithi NJ, Maina SW, Okoth J, Gathece LW. Internal root morphology in mandibular first permanent molars in a Kenyan population. East African Medical Journal. 2012;**89**(5):166-171

[55] Zhang X, Xiong S, Ma Y, et al. A cone-beam computed tomographic study on mandibular first molars in a Chinese subpopulation. PLoS One. 2015;**10**(8):e0134919. DOI: 10.1371/journal.pone.0134919

[56] Torres A, Jacobs R, Lembrechts P, Brizuela C, Cabrera C, Concha G, et al. Characterization of mandibular molar root and canal morphology using cone beam computed tomography and its variability in Belgian and Chilean population samples. Imaging Science in Dentistry. 2015;**45**:95-101

[57] Madani ZS, Mehraban N, Moudi E, Bijani A. Root and canal morphology of mandibular molars in a selected Iranian population using cone-beam computed tomography. Iranian Endodontic Journal. 2017;**12**(2):143-148

[58] Gambarini G, Piasecki L, Ropini P, Miccoli G, Di Nardo D, Testarelli L. Cone-beam computed tomographic analysis on root and canal morphology of mandibular first permanent molar among multiracial population in Western European population. European Journal of Dentistry. 2018;**12**(3):434-438

[59] Zhang R, Wang H, Tian YY, Yu X, Hu T, Dummer PM. Use of cone-beam computed tomography to evaluate root and canal morphology of mandibular molars in Chinese individuals. International Endodontic

Journal. 2011;**44**(11):990-999. DOI: 10.1111/j.1365-2591.2011.01904.x

[60] Alfawaz H, Alqedairi A, Alkhayyal AK, Almobarak AA, Alhusain MF, Martins JNR. Prevalence of C-shaped canal system in mandibular first and second molars in a Saudi population assessed via cone beam computed tomography: A retrospective study. Clinical Oral Investigations. Jan 2019;**23**(1):107-112

[61] Pawar AM, Pawar M, Kfir A, Singh S, Salve P, Thakur B, et al. Root canal morphology and variations in mandibular second molar teeth of an Indian population: An in vivo cone-beam computed tomography analysis. Clinical Oral Investigations. 2017;**21**(9):2801-2809

[62] Kim SY, Kim BS, Kim Y. Mandibular second molar root canal morphology and variants in a Korean subpopulation. International Endodontic Journal. 2016;**49**(2):136-144

[63] Silva EJ, Nejaim Y, Silva AV, Haiter-Neto F, Cohenca N. Evaluation of root canal configuration of mandibular molars in a Brazilian population by using cone-beam computed tomography: An in vivo study. Journal of Endodontia. 2013;**39**:849-852

[64] Ladeira DB, Cruz AD, Freitas DQ, Almeida SM. Prevalence of C-shaped root canal in a Brazilian subpopulation: A cone-beam computed tomography analysis. Brazilian Oral Research. 2014;**28**:39-45

[65] Scarfe WC, Levin MD, Gane D, Farman AG. Use of cone beam computed tomography in endodontics. International Journal of Dentistry. 2010;**2009**:634567

[66] Kim Y, Perinpanayagam H, Lee JK, et al. Comparison of mandibular first molar mesial root canal morphology using microcomputed tomography and clearing technique. Acta Odontologica Scandinavica. 2015;**73**:427-432

[67] Rogazkyn D, Metzger Z, Solomonov M. The prevalence and asymmetry of C-shaped root canals in second mandibular molars in a European-Russian population: A cone-beam computed tomography study in vivo. International Journal of Endodontic Rehabilitation. 2016;**2**:12-16

[68] Neelakantan P, Subbarao C, Subbarao CV, Ravindranath M. Root and canal morphology of mandibular second molars in an Indian population. Journal of Endodontia. 2010;**36**(8):1319-1322. DOI: 10.1016/j.joen.2010.04.001

[69] Ceperuelo D, Lozano M, Duran-Sindreu F, Mercade M. Root canal morphology of chalcolithic and early bronze age human populations of el mirador cave (sierra de atapuerca, Spain). The Anatomical Record. 2014;**297**:2342-2348

[70] Gulabivala K, Opasanon A, Ng YL, Alavi A. Root and canal morphology of Thai mandibular molars. International Endodontic Journal. 2002;**35**:56-62

[71] Kuzekanani M, Haghani J, Nosrati H. Root and canal morphology of mandibular third molars in an Iranian population. Journal of Dental Research, Dental Clinics, Dental Prospects. 2012;**6**:85-88

Chapter 9

Root Canal Morphology and Anatomy

Esra Pamukcu Guven

Abstract

Success in root canal treatment depends on the proper application of all procedures of root canal treatment. This wholistic approach includes leakproof crown restoration, following ideal instrumentation, irrigation and hermetic obturation. Therefore, the first step of root canal treatment begins with understanding the tooth morphology in detail. The teeth vary according to their localization at the jaws and the gender and race of people. Detection of the extra canals, canal curvatures, isthmuses and lateral and accessory canals plays an important role in the success of root canal treatment. With all this, the academic knowledge and proficiency of the dentist and/or endodontist enable tooth morphology to be more clearly understandable.

Keywords: tooth morphology, root canal morphology, dental anatomy, technologic devices, illumination and magnification systems

1. Introduction

Understanding the anatomy of the root canal system is essential for a successful root canal treatment. Complexity of root canals depends on reasons such as ethnicity, gender, age, the existence of lateral/accessory canals, isthmuses, the location of the teeth at the jaws and anomalies of the teeth (dens invaginatus, dens evaginatus, fusion, gemination, dens in dente). Besides all of these, some physiological alterations occur in enamel and dentin with age. Mineralization of dentin results in calcification of dentinal tubules; thus, dentin becomes sclerotic. Several difficulties occur during root canal treatment in such cases. The utilization of novel technologic equipments for magnification and lightning of the root canal system like dental microscope, loupe, radiographic visualization systems and cone beam computed tomography (CBCT) in dentistry enlightens endodontic treatment [1].

2. Maxillary incisor teeth

Maxillary central teeth have one root and one main canal [2]. Rarely, at 6% rate one canal of maxillary central teeth is divided into two parts at the apical foramina which can be classified as Vertucci type V (**Figure 1**). Apical root canal anatomy should be regarded because of its main effect on the success of root canal treatment (**Figure 2**). In the study of Adorno et al. [3], accessory canals in the apical 3 mm at Japanese population were found in 46% of the specimens.

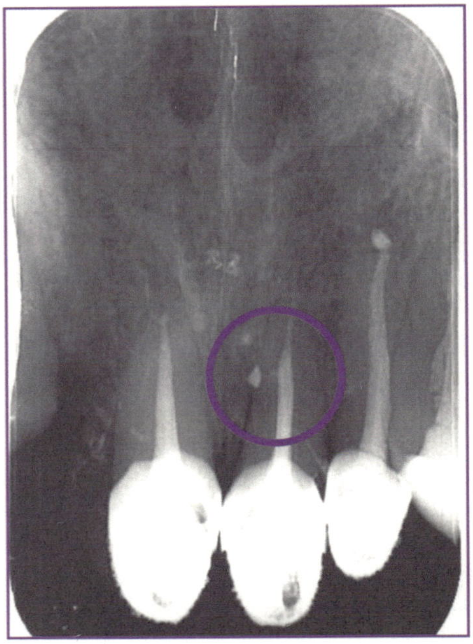

Figure 1.
Endodontic treatment of a maxillary left first incisor tooth with lateral canal.

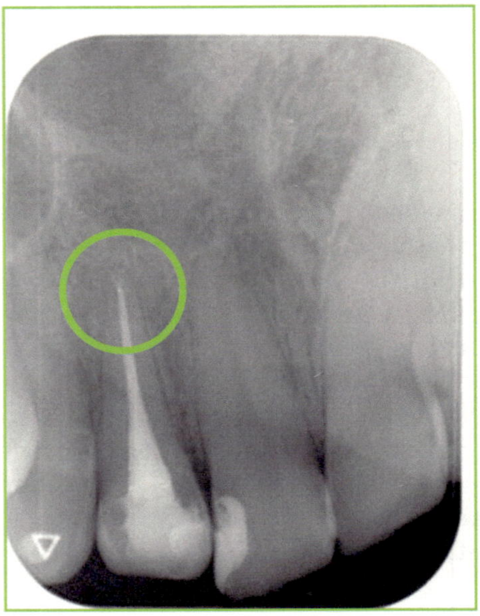

Figure 2.
Accessory canals in the apical 3 mm of the root.

According to Vertucci's classification, maxillary lateral incisor teeth have one main canal (100%) [2]. Generally, maxillary lateral incisor teeth are single-rooted with a single canal [4]. The apex of the maxillary lateral teeth is positioned at the palatal side. In the study of Adorno et al. [3], among Japanese population, accessory canals in the apical 3 mm were found in 29% of the specimens.

3. Maxillary canine teeth

According to Vertucci's classification, maxillary canine teeth have one main canal (100%) [2]. In the study of Adorno et al. [3], among Japanese population, accessory canals in the apical 3 mm related with the maxillary canine teeth were found in 38% of the specimens. The endodontic cavity should be prepared at the palatal side of the tooth in oval shape in these teeth.

4. Maxillary premolar teeth

In the study of Tian et al. [5], it was found that in Chinese population, 66% of the premolar teeth had one root, 33% had two roots and 1% had three roots. According to Vertucci's classification, root canal morphology is classified into eight types:

Type I: One canal extending to the apex.

Type II: One canal beginning from the pulp chamber, dividing into two parts at the 1/3 middle of the root and then ending in one part at the apex.

Type III: One canal leaving the pulp chamber, dividing into two and ending as one canal by merging.

Type IV: Two canals leaving the pulp chamber and ending as two separate canals.

Type V: One canal leaving the pulp chamber and dividing into two distinct canals with separate apical foramina.

Type VI: Two separate canals leaving the pulp chamber, merging in the 1/3 of the root canal and then separating to exist as two distinct canals.

Type VII: One canal leaving the pulp chamber, merging in the 1/3 of the root canal and then separating to exist as two distinct canals.

Type VIII: Three separate, distinct canals extend from the pulp chamber to the apex.

According to Weine (1976), the classifications are divided into four groups as:

Type I: One canal extending as one canal to the apex.

Type II: Two separate canals leaving from the pulp chamber and merging at the 1/3 of the apex.

Type III: Two canals leaving the pulp chamber and extending as two canals to the foramen.

Type IV: One canal leaving from the pulp chamber, dividing into two parts at the 1/3 middle of the root and extending as two canals to the apex.

In the study of Pan et al. [6], the prevalence of maxillary first premolar teeth with one main root canal was 67.8%, with two roots was 31.9% and with two canals was 88.2%. In Malaysian population, according to Vertucci's classification, second premolars were detected to be single-rooted with type I in the 58.2% incidence [2]. Based on the detection of premolars in molar shape, the endodontic cavity of the maxillary premolar teeth should begin to be prepared as "T-shaped" on the occlusal surface instead of oval shape. In these teeth, two root canal orifices are at the buccal side, and one is at the palatal side [7].

5. Maxillary molar teeth

The upper first molar teeth have three roots and three or four canals (palatal, mesiobuccal 1 (MB1), mesiobuccal 2 (MB2) and disto-buccal (DB)). In the study of Kumar et al. [8], the upper molar teeth were shown to have seven canals. At Burmese population, the prevalence of two canals in mesiobuccal roots of the upper first molar teeth decreases towards the upper third molar teeth. Around 85.2% of

270 roots of the upper molar teeth have one canal in one root at the apex, 14% have two canals at the apex and 0.8% have three canals at the apex [9]. According to Pan et al. [6], a second palatal canal was detected in 0.9% in the maxillary first molar teeth in Malaysian population. Ninety-one percent of mesiobuccal roots of maxillary first molars was detected to have accessory canals [10, 11]. Accessory canals with 85% of incidence were found to be located in the apical third of the roots [10]. According to micro-computed tomography analysis of the mesiobuccal root canal anatomy referring to second mesiobuccal canals of maxillary first molar tooth, the results were in 60% in accordance with Weine et al.'s (1969) classification and in 70% with Vertucci's (1984) classification [10].

Mikrogeorgis et al. [12] determined two root canals in conjunction with the apexIn addition, as the morphological differences determined related with the mesiobuccal root of upper molar teeth, distal root has also been detected to have two seperate canals; distobuccal 1(DB1) & distobuccal 2 (DB2) as shown in **Figure 3**.

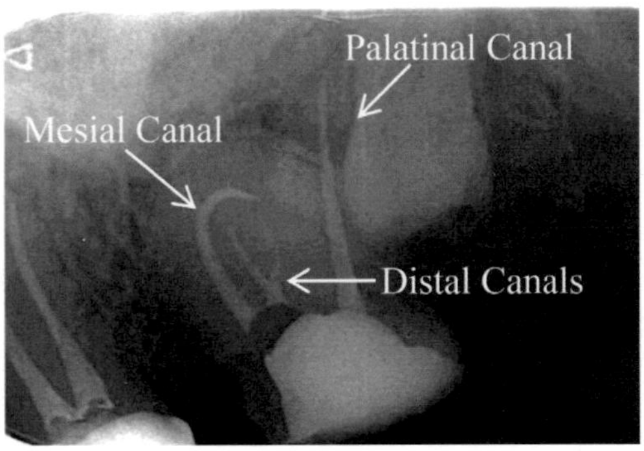

Figure 3.
The radiograph of a maxillary second molar tooth with two distal canals.

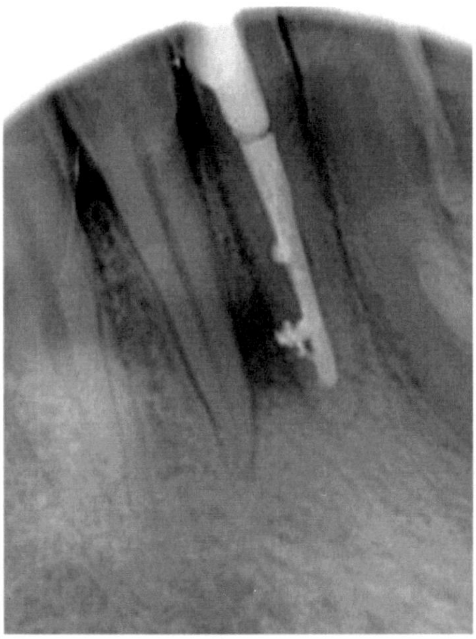

Figure 4.
Endodontic treatment of a mandibular right first incisor tooth with a lateral canal.

6. Mandibular incisors

In the study of Sert et al. [17], in Turkish population, it was pointed out that 68% of mandibular central incisors have two canals and 6.5% have lateral canals. In addition, in the same study, it was pointed out that 63% of mandibular lateral incisors had two canals and the prevalence of lateral canals was 13% in Turkish population. Mandibular first incisor tooth with a lateral canal is seen in **Figure 4**.

7. Mandibular canine teeth

According to a morphological study of Soleymani et al. [18], in the Iranian population, 89.7% of the mandibular canine teeth were found to have type I, 5.7% had type III, 3.7% had type II and 1% had type V morphology.

8. Mandibular premolar teeth

The endodontic cavity has to be prepared in oval shape on the occlusal surface of the premolar teeth regarding the localization of root canal orifices. In Turkish population, 62% of the mandibular premolar teeth have one main root canal [17]. Vertucci found out a second canal in 26% of the mandibular first premolars and 3% at the second premolars [2]. In Turkish population, 71% of the mandibular second premolars have one main root canal [17].

9. Mandibular Molar teeth

According to Vertucci's classification, 44% of the mesial roots of the mandibular first molar teeth were found to be type I, whilst 54% were type II. Al-Qudah et al. [16] reported that in Jordanian population, the mandibular first molar teeth had three canals (48%) and four canals (46%). The frequency of the mesial root canals' combination in the first (56, 34%) and second (67, 41%) mandibular molars is more common in three-rooted teeth than four-rooted teeth [19]. Huang et al. [20] pointed out that the incidence of mandibular first molars with two, three and four roots was 55.5, 26.5 and 18.0%, respectively. They also added that double-rooted distal root was associated with two mesial canals. In a CBCT assessment study of mandibular molars, the distance from the apex to the canal orifice is found to be 13.15 mm [21]. The existence of isthmus is a type of morphological difference seen in mandibular molar teeth. Endodontic treatment of a mandibular right first molar tooth with an isthmus located between the mesiobuccal and the mesiolingual canals is seen in **Figure 5**.

The results of a study evaluating the root canals of the mandibular second molar teeth showed that 76% of the two-rooted mandibular second molars had a single distal canal and 87.5% had two mesial canals that combined apically with the prevalence of 53% [17]. In South Asian Pakistani population, the mesial roots of the mandibular molar teeth were found to have two canals (97%), whereas the distal roots had single canals (50%) [22]. In the study of Al-Qudah et al. [16], the incidence of three canals in Jordanian mandibular second molars was reported as 58%, two canals as 19% and four canals as 17%. Gulabivala et al. [23] reported that 68% of Thai mandibular molars had two distinct roots and 20% had fused roots.

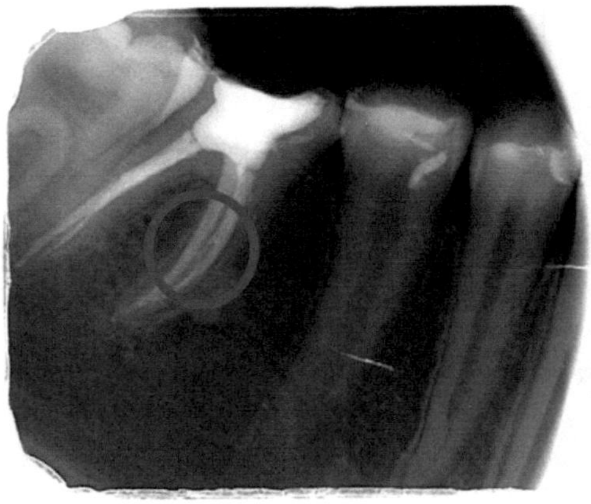

Figure 5.
Endodontic treatment of a mandibular right first molar tooth with an isthmus located between the mesiobuccal and the mesiolingual canals.

10. C-shaped root Canals

C-shaped root canals' anatomy is defined as the connection of two distal roots internally and C-shaped appearance panoramically. C-shaped root canals can be observed in the upper and lower first and second molar teeth. They are seen at high rates in the mandibular second molar teeth in Asian population. The treatment of C-shaped root canals needs more care because of their wide, oval and complex anatomy and the bleeding potential of wide pulpal tissue. In the study of Kim et al. [13], the problems with the treatment of C-shaped root canals were found as unsuccessful sealing ability of the canal (45.2%), overlooked canal (9.5%), overfilling (7.1%) and iatrogenic problems (7.1%).

Irrigation protocols have significant importance for removing pulpal remnants and hard tissue debris, especially for the unreachable points in the root canals [4]. The morphology of C-shaped root canals may result in elbows during root canal shaping in curved canals. The percentages of elbow formation were reported as 42.1% in C form canals, 40.0% in J form canals and 19.3% in straight form canals. Zip formation was observed in 83.5% of C form canals [14]. Eighty percent of C-shaped root canals were found to have 1–3 apical foramina [15]. In Malaysian population, the C-shaped root canals were found to have 48.7% of incidence [6]. In Jordanian population the mandibular second molar teeth had C-shaped roots in 10% of incidence [16].

11. Dental anomalies

Dental morphological anomalies accompany some growth and developmental abnormalities. Dens invaginatus, dens evaginatus, dens in dente, fusion and gemination are among the often seen dental anomalies. Dental anomalies could also be associated with syndromes, such as Down syndrome.

Dens invaginatus is determined as an infolding of dentin and enamel extending into the pulp chamber. In a case report of Kottoor et al. [24], a maxillary lateral incisor was found to have four main canals called distal, labial, mesial and lingual in a dens invaginatus case. Dens invaginatus is more often characterized with an immature tooth with a periapical lesion. The decision on treatment type depends on the tooth's morphological situation. This pathology is treated by regenerative procedures in which root dentin thickness and newly developed apical foramina are expected.

In a morphology study conducted among individuals with Down syndrome, it was reported that all teeth, except mandibular first premolars, showed significantly shorter crown and root lengths [25]. This information is valuable during making a decision of the crown restoration type regarding the crown-root proportions.

12. Conclusion

Focusing on the tooth morphology considering root canal complexity allows dentists to perform successful root canal treatment. Besides the dentists' knowledge and interest in root canal morphology and anatomy, proficiency on root canal treatment and the tendency to use novel technological devices enable prosperous endodontic treatment. The novel tooth morphology classification presented by Ahmed and Dummer, based on the simplicity and clarity respecting tooth number, number of roots and root canal configuration types, is the prominent leading literature for dentistry [26].

Author details

Esra Pamukcu Guven
Faculty of Dentistry, Department of Endodontics, Istanbul Okan University, Istanbul, Turkey

*Address all correspondence to: esra.pamukcu@okan.edu.tr

References

[1] Peters OA, Laib A, Göhring TN, Barbakow F. Changes in root canal geometry after preparation assessed by high resolution computed tomography. Journal of Endodontia. 2001;**27**:1-6

[2] Vertucci FJ. Root canal anatomy of the human permanent teeth. Oral Surgery, Oral Medicine, and Oral Pathology. 1984;**58**:589-599

[3] Adorno CG, Yoshioka T, Suda H. Incidence of accessory canals in Japanese anterior maxillary teeth following root canal filling *ex vivo*. International Endodontic Journal. 2010;**43**:370-376

[4] Konstantinidi E, Psimma Z, Chavez de Paz LE, Boutsioukis C. Apical negative pressure irrigation versus syringe irrigation: A systematic review of cleaning and disinfection of the root canal system. International Endodontic Journal. 2017;**50**:1034-1054

[5] Tian Y-Y, Guo B, Zhang R, Yu X, Wang H, Hu T, et al. Root and canal morphology of maxillary first premolars in a Chinese subpopulation evaluated using cone-beam computed tomography. International Endodontic Journal. 2012;**45**:996-1003

[6] Pan JYY, Parolia A, Chuah SR, Bhatia S, Mutalik S, Pau A. Root canal morphology of permanent teeth in a Malaysian subpopulation using cone beam computed tomography. BMC Oral Health. 2019;**14**:1-15

[7] Sieraski SM, Taylor GT, Kohn RA. Identification and endodontic management of three-canalled maxillary premolars. Journal of Endodontia. 1989;**15**:29-32

[8] Kumar R. Report of a rare case: A maxillary first molar with seven canals confirmed with cone-beam computed tomography. Iranian Endodontic Journal. 2014;**9**(2):153-157

[9] Ng Y-L, Aung TH, Alavi A, Gulabivala K. Root and canal morphology of Burmese maxillary molars. International Endodontic Journal. 2001;**34**:620-630

[10] Verma P, Love RM. A micro CT study of the mesiobuccal root canal morphology of the maxillary first molar tooth. International Endodontic Journal. 2011;**44**:210-217

[11] Gu Y, Lee JK, Spangberg LS, Lee Y, Park CM, Seo DG, et al. Minimum-intensity projection for in depth morphology study of mesiobuccal root. Oral Surgery, Oral Medicine, Oral Pathology, Oral Radiology, and Endodontics. 2011;**112**:671-677

[12] Mikrogeorgis G, Lyroudia KL, Nikopoulos N, Pitas I, Molyvdas I, Lambrianidis TH. 3D computer-aided reconstruction of six teeth with morphological abnormalities. International Endodontic Journal. 1999;**32**:88-93

[13] Kim Y, Lee D, Kim DV, Kim SY. Analysis of cause of endodontic failure of C-shaped root canals. Scanning. 2018:1-7. DOI: 10.1155/2018/2516832

[14] Nagy CD, Bartha K, Berna M, Verdes E, Szabo J. The effect of root canal morphology on canal shape following instrumentation using different techniques. International Endodontic Journal. 1997;**30**:133-140

[15] Cheung GSP, Yang J, Fan B. Morphometric study of the apical anatomy of C-shaped root canal systems in mandibular second molars. International Endodontic Journal. 2007;**40**:239-246

[16] Al-Qudah AA, Awawdeh LA. Root and canal morphology of mandibular first and second molar teeth in a Jordanian population. International Endodontic Journal. 2009;**42**:775-784

[17] Sert S, Aslanalp V, Tanalp J. Investigation of the root canal configurations of mandibular permanent teeth in the Turkish population. International Endodontic Journal. 2004;**37**:494-499

[18] Soleymani A, Namaryan N, Moudi E, Gholinia A. Root canal morphology of mandibular canine in an Iranian population: A CBCT assessment. Iranian Endodontic Journal. 2017;**12**(1):78-82

[19] Furri M. Differences in the confluence of mesial canals in mandibular molar teeth with three or four root canals. International Endodontic Journal. 2008;**41**:777-780

[20] Huang R-Y, Cheng W-C, Chen C-J, Lin C-D, Lai T-M, Shen E-C, et al. Three-dimensional analysis of the root morphology of mandibular first molars with Disto-lingual roots. International Endodontic Journal. 2010;**43**:478-484

[21] Gambarini G, Ropini P, Piasecki L, Costantini R, Carneiro E, Testarelli L, et al. A preliminary assessment of a new dedicated endodontic software for use with CBCT images to evaluate the canal complexity of mandibular molars. International Endodontic Journal. 2018;**51**:259-268

[22] Wasti F, Shearer AC, Wilson NHF. Root canal systems of the mandibular and maxillary first permanent molar teeth of south Asian Pakistanis. International Endodontic Journal. 2001;**34**:263-266

[23] Gulabivala K, Opasanon A, Ng Y-L, Alavi A. Root and canal morphology of Thai mandibular molars. International Endodontic Journal. 2002;**35**:56-62

[24] Kottoor J, Murugesan R, Albuquerque DV. A maxillary lateral incisor with four root canals. International Endodontic Journal. 2012;**45**:393-397

[25] Kelsen AE, Love RM, Kieser JA, Herbison P. Root canal anatomy of anterior and premolar teeth in Down's syndrome. International Endodontic Journal. 1999;**32**:211-216

[26] Ahmed HMA, Dummer PMH. A new system for classifying tooth, root and canal anomalies. International Endodontic Journal. 2018;**51**:389-404

Chapter 10

The C-Shaped Root Canal

Jesús Alejandro Quiñones Pedraza

Abstract

A thorough understanding of root canal anatomy is of paramount importance in the field of dentistry. The C-shaped root canal is an anatomical variation occurring mostly in mandibular second molars. In a transverse section, the shape of this canal is observed as the letter C. The presence of a fin or web connecting the individual root canals is another anatomic feature. Due to its complex anatomy, different classifications have been proposed through the years for a better comprehension. In endodontic literature, the C-shaped root canal has been of high interest and its prevalence is reported in different regions of the world. Additionally, its endodontic management has been widely described and analyzed.

Keywords: C-shaped root canal, anatomy, anatomical variation, canal configuration, human teeth

1. Introduction

The C-shaped root canal is considered an anatomical variation in human teeth [1] and was firstly documented in endodontic literature by Cooke and Cox in 1979 [2]. This anatomical variation has been widely studied. Additionally, several case reports have described its endodontic management [3–5].

The main cause of a C-shaped root is due to the failure of the Hertwig's epithelial root seath to fuse on the lingual or buccal root surface [1]. The roots of human molars with C-shaped canals may be conical and fused. For these characteristics, studies suggested that C-shaped root canals could be identified based on preoperative radiographs [6, 7]. However, not all conical roots have a C-shaped canal and various reports stated that a C-shaped root canal is not easily seen using only radiographs [6]. On the other hand, additional reports have demonstrated that a

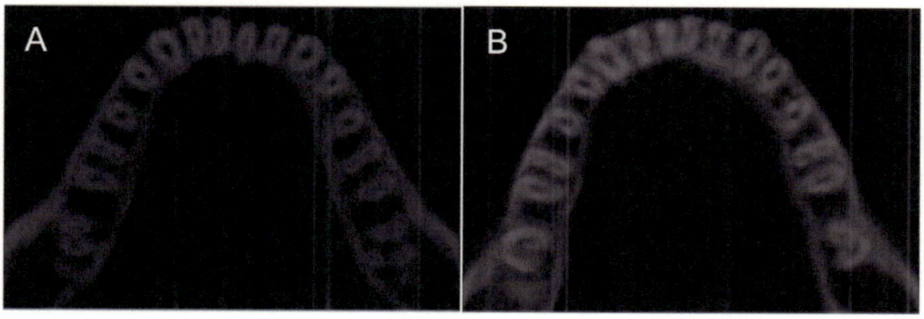

Figure 1.
(A) Unilateral C-shaped root canal in mandibular second molar; (B) bilateral C-shaped root canal in mandibular second molar.

C-shaped canal may be bilateral [8] (i.e., when it is present on one side, it can also be present in the contralateral tooth) (**Figure 1**).

The C-shaped root canal has been found in mandibular and maxillary molars [9, 10], mandibular premolars [11], and even in some incisors [12]. However, it is most commonly present in mandibular second molars [3]. As other anatomical variations, its prevalence has been associated with ethnicity. Interestingly, the prevalence of this canal in Asian populations has been higher than other populations [13].

2. Classification

Different techniques have been used to analyze the morphology of C-shaped root canals [14, 15]. In a transverse section of a tooth with this morphology, the shape of the canal is observed as the letter C (**Figure 2**) and different patterns may be present along the canal. The presence of fins connecting the individual root canals is other anatomical feature [1]. Likewise, the shape of the letter C may be interrupted and observed as separate canals [16]; for this reason, different anatomical classifications have been proposed through the years for a better understanding [17, 18].

Although there are different classifications, the following [18] has been commonly cited and well accepted by clinicians (**Figure 3**):

- Category I (C1): the shape was an uninterrupted “C” with no separation or division.

- Category II (C2): the canal shape resembled a semicolumn resulting from a discontinuation of the “C” outline, but either angle alpha or beta was no less than 60°.

- Category III (C3): two or three separated canals and both angles, alpha and beta, were less than 60°.

- Category IV (C4): only one round or oval canal in that cross-section.

- Category V (C5): no canal lumen could be observed (which was usually seen near the apex only).

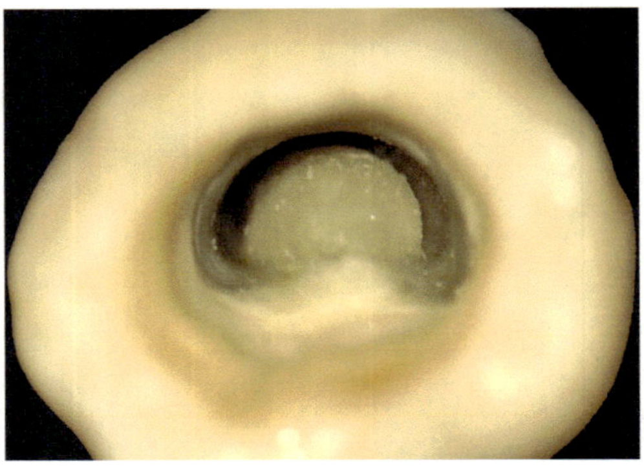

Figure 2.
C-shaped root canal, the shape of the canal is observed as the letter “C.”

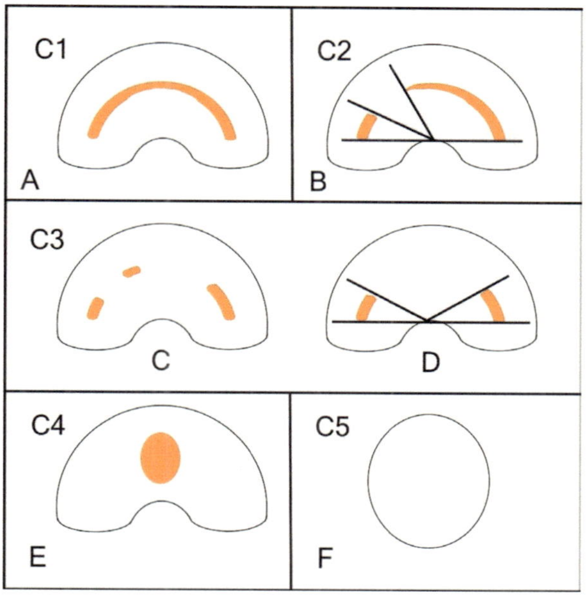

Figure 3.
This representative illustration explains the classification of C-shaped root canal. (A) Category I; (B) category II; (C) and (D) category III; (E) category IV and (F) category V.

3. Endodontic management

In the field of dentistry, the C-shaped root canal has been of high interest, especially in endodontics. Lack of knowledge regarding root canal anatomy may lead to deficient endodontic treatments [19]. Irregular areas in a C-shaped canal can keep remnants of soft tissue, debris, and infected tissue or may be a source of bleeding during a root canal treatment [20, 21]. Therefore, root canal treatments in these cases may require specific skills.

In 1979, the first case reports of C-shaped root canals were documented [2]. Clinical images were presented where the C shape was evident in mandibular and maxillary molars. Since then, numerous case reports have described their clinical management [22].

The chemomechanical preparation and obturation of C-shaped canals have been challenging in some cases [23]. Sodium hypochlorite has been the most used endodontic irrigant because of its antimicrobial properties and tissue-dissolving capabilities [24]. Obturation techniques with warm condensation have been indicated in some cases of C-shaped root canals [25]. Likewise, the use of manual, rotary, and reciprocating files has resulted effective in mechanical preparation of teeth with aberrant anatomies [26].

The disinfection process is affected for isthmuses and other irregularities. Careful exploration with a small, precurved file may be helpful to locate additional canals. Although it is not possible to carry out an appropriate negotiation in all the canals, the penetration of sodium hypochlorite with ultrasonics may allow an effective disinfection process [27].

4. Conclusions

A thorough understanding of root canal anatomy is of paramount importance in the field of dentistry. Variations in the number of roots and root canal system anatomy are not uncommon in human teeth. The C-shaped root canal represents an important and challenging anatomical variation. Likewise, knowledge of the different morphologies of C-shaped root canals can help avoid complications during endodontic treatments.

Acknowledgements

The author denies any conflict of interest related to this study.

Author details

Jesús Alejandro Quiñones Pedraza
Department of Endodontics, Intracanal, Monterrey, Nuevo León, México

*Address all correspondence to: aqp.endo@gmail.com

References

[1] Jafarzadeh H, Wu YN. The C-shaped root canal configuration: A review. Journal of Endodontics. 2007;**33**:517-523

[2] Cooke HG 3rd, Cox FL. C-shaped canal configurations in mandibular molars. Journal of the American Dental Association. 1979;**99**:836-839

[3] Kato A, Ziegler A, Higuchi K, Nakamura H, Ohno N. Aetiology, incidence and morphology of the C-shaped root canal system and its impact on clinical endodontics. International Endodontic Journal. 2014;**47**:1012-1033

[4] Martins JN, Quaresma S, Quaresma MC, Frisbie Teel J. C-shaped maxillary permanent first molar: A case report and literature review. Journal of Endodontics. 2013;**39**:1649-1653

[5] Zheng Q, Zhang L, Zhou X, Wang Q, Wang Y, Tang L, et al. C-shaped root canal system in mandibular second molars in a chinese population evaluated by cone-beam computed tomography. International Endodontic Journal. 2011;**44**:857-862

[6] Sinanoglu A, Helvacioglu-Yigit D. Analysis of C-shaped canals by panoramic radiography and cone-beam computed tomography: Root type specificity by longitudinal distribution. Journal of Endodontics. 2014;**40**:917-921

[7] Fan B, Cheung GS, Fan M, Gutman JL, Fan W. C-shaped canal system in mandibular second molars: Part II-radiographic features. Journal of Endodontics. 2004;**30**:904-908

[8] Dankner E, Friedman S, Stabholz A. Bilateral C shape configuration in maxillary first molars. Journal of Endodontics. 1990;**16**:601-603

[9] Martins JN, Mata A, Marques D, Anderson C, Caramês J. Prevalence and characteristics of the maxillary C-shaped molar. Journal of Endodontics. 2016;**42**:383-389

[10] Weine FS. The C-shaped mandibular second molar: Incidence and other considerations. Journal of Endodontics. 1998;**24**:372-375

[11] Martins JNR, Francisco H, Ordinola-Zapata R. Prevalence of C-shaped configurations in the mandibular first and second premolars: A cone-beam computed tomographic in vivo study. Journal of Endodontics. 2017;**43**:890-895

[12] Boveda C, Fajardo M, Millan B. Root canal treatment of an invaginated maxillary lateral incisor with a C-shaped canal. Quintessence International. 1999;**30**:707-711

[13] von Zuben M, Martins JNR, Berti L, Cassim I, Flynn D, Gonzalez JA, et al. Worldwide prevalence of mandibular second molar C-shaped morphologies evaluated by cone-beam computed tomography. Journal of Endodontics. 2017;**43**:1442-1447

[14] Helvacioglu-Yigit D, Sinanoglu A. Use of cone-beam computed tomography to evaluate C-shaped root canal systems in mandibular second molars in a Turkish subpopulation: A retrospective study. International Endodontic Journal. 2013;**46**:1032-1038

[15] Seo MS, Park DS. C-shaped root canals of mandibular second molars in Korean population: Clinical observation and in vitro analysis. International Endodontic Journal. 2004;**37**:139-144

[16] Amoroso-Silva PA, Ordinola-Zapata R, Duarte MA, Gutman JL, del Carpio-Perochena A, Bramante CM, et al. Micro-computed tomographic analysis of mandibular second molars with C-shaped root canals. Journal of Endodontics. 2015;**41**:890-895

[17] Melton DC, Krell KV, Fuller MW. Anatomical and histological features of C-shaped canals in mandibular second molars. Journal of Endodontics. 1991;**17**:384-388

[18] Fan B, Cheung GS, Fan M, Gutmann JL, Bian Z. C-shaped canal system in mandibular second molars: Part I-anatomical features. Journal of Endodontics. 2004;**30**:899-903

[19] Nair PN. On the causes of persistent apical periodontitis: A review. International Endodontic Journal. 2006;**39**:249-281

[20] Ordinola-Zapata R, Bramante CM, de Moraes IG. Analysis of the gutta-percha filled area in C-shaped mandibular molars obturated with modified mocroseal technique. International Endodontic Journal. 2009;**42**:186-197

[21] Gok T, Capar ID, Akcay I, Keles A. Evaluation of different techniques for filling simulated C-shaped canals of 3-dimensional printed resin teeth. Journal of Endodontics. 2017;**43**:1559-1564

[22] Ring J, Ring KC. Rare root canal configuration of mandibular second premolar using cone-beam computed tomographic scanning. Journal of Endodontics. 2017;**43**:1897-1900

[23] Walid N. The use of two pluggers for the obturation of an uncommon C-shaped canal. Journal of Endodontics. 2000;**26**:422-424

[24] Zhender M. Root canal irrigants. Journal of Endodontics. 2006;**32**:389-398

[25] Liewehr FR, Kulild JC, Primack PD. Obturation of a C-shaped canal using an improved method of a warm lateral condensation. Journal of Endodontics. 1993;**19**:474-477

[26] Solomonov M, Paqué F, Fan B, Eliat Y, Berman LH. The challenge of C-shaped canal systems: A comparative study of the self-adjusting file and protaper. Journal of Endodontics. 2012;**38**:209-214

[27] Fan B, Min Y, Lu G, Yang J, Cheung GSP, Gutman JL. Negotiation of C-shaped canal systems in mandibular second molars. Journal of Endodontics. 2009;**35**:1003-1008

Section 3

Pathology and Clinical Considerations

Chapter 11

Pathology and Abnormality of the First Permanent Molar among Children

Mouna Hamza, Amal Chlyah, Bouchra Bousfiha, Bouchra Badre, Maria Mtalsi, Hasna Saih and Samira El Arabi

Abstract

The first permanent molar (FPM) plays an essential role in the masticatory function by contributing to the implementation and the maintenance of the occlusion. However, it is considered as the most frequently affected and the earliest affected tooth by caries; 27.4% of the 6–8 years old children have developed at least one cavity on one of the four first permanent molars, according to a study conducted among 3276 school children in Casablanca .Therefore, the FPM should benefit from special vigilance on the part of the practitioner to ensure that any early carious lesion is intercepted. In addition, the FPM, due to its period of mineralization coinciding with early childhood diseases, can erupt with a structural abnormality. Molar incisor hypomineralization (MIH) is considered to be the most common defects observed on first permanent molars among children. A study conducted among 1077 children aged 7–10 years enrolled in schools in Casablanca showed that 7.9% of children were affected with MIH. About 84.7% of the children had the four molars affected. Children with HIM had a significantly higher prevalence of caries: 78.8 versus 33.5%.These structural abnormalities of the enamel must be carried out earlier to ensure that the coronary anatomy is the least compromised.

Keywords: molar, dental caries, risk factors, therapeutic, prevention measures, molar incisor hypomineralization, tooth abnormalities, dental care for children, Morocco

1. Introduction

The first permanent molar (FPM) is considered as the most important tooth for the dentition and dental development with a key role in occlusion. It participates in the maxillary growth and physiology of the mandibular system.

However, it is considered to be the most and earliest affected tooth by cavities. Indeed, the early time of its eruption when hygiene is difficult and poorly controlled makes it particularly vulnerable to carious disease.

In addition, FPM, due to its period of mineralization coinciding with early childhood diseases, can erupt with a structural abnormality. Molar incisor hypomineralization is considered to be the most common defect observed on FPM in children.

Other uncommon abnormalities can affect the FPM such as shape, size, or eruption abnormalities. The early diagnosis of lesions on this tooth allows in a large number of cases to avoid complications and the systematic use of endodontic and prosthetic treatments and sometimes even tooth extraction.

The purpose of this chapter is to review the main pathologies and abnormalities of the first permanent molar. Epidemiological data, risk factors, clinical aspects, therapeutic, and preventive approach are described and illustrated by clinical cases treated at the Casablanca Pedodontics Department.

2. Carious pathology of the first permanent molar

2.1 Epidemiology and risk factors

The importance of the carious pathology of the first permanent molar has been known clinically for a long time. Epidemiological surveys carried out in several countries have shown the extent of this problem [1–5]. In France, in 2007, a survey on the oral health of 12–15 years old children attending school in the southern province revealed that 52.4% of children had already carious disease and 11.9% have four FPM affected teeth [1]. In 2015, Xue et al. reported, in Tangshan (China), a prevalence of caries of 47.49% on the FPM. Another study conducted among Sudanese children showed a prevalence of 6-year-old tooth disease of 61% [2, 3].

In Morocco, epidemiological surveys were carried out to determine the state of the FPM among schoolchildren and consultants in the Pedodontic Department in the Universities of Hassan II of Casablanca and Souissi of Rabat. They all showed a high rate of decay in the FPM [6, 7].

Indeed, a descriptive cross-sectional study of 3276 children aged 6–8 years enrolled in school in Casablanca revealed that 27.4% had at least one cavity in one of the four FPMs [6].

A survey of 216 children aged 6–13 years old who were consultants in the Pedodontics Department in the University of Hassan II of Casablanca showed that 73.14% of subjects had at least one FPM affected by cavities and 12.65% of subjects had all four teeth affected [8]. As in the Pedodontics Department of the University of Suissy of Rabat, 65% of children aged 6–15 years had at least one carious FPM [7]. The prevalence of caries increases with age, and this is in accordance with studies carried out by Al-Samadani and Ahmad [2] and Aldossary et al. [9] in Saudi Arabia. Most of these studies showed that the first mandibular molars were statistically more affected than their maxillary counterparts ($p < 0.01$) [8, 9].

In the permanent dentition, first permanent molar was observed to be highly susceptible to carious lesions in its occlusal aspect due to the early time of its eruption, to its morphological characteristics and to its positioning in the oral cavity [10–12].

First permanent molar is the first permanent tooth appearing in the child's mouth; most parents are unaware that these teeth are the first permanent teeth and often neglect its importance considering it a primary insignificant tooth [13]. Sometimes, parents think that the first permanent molar is a deciduous tooth, and instead of restoring it, they extract the tooth and deprive the child of the right to permanent teeth in the future [14].

Regarding parents of children consulting in the Pedodontic Department in the University of Hassan II of Casablanca, only 19% of them know that this tooth is permanent. The others do not know when it erupted and confuse it with a temporary molar [8]. According to the study by Heydari et al., most parents are unaware of the presence of FPMs in their children's oral cavity [14].

The first permanent molar has a longer eruption time. Carvalho and Abernathy found that the first permanent molars were more susceptible to caries during the first 1–3 years after the eruption and the occlusal aspects of the first permanent molars were particularly vulnerable to the caries development at the age of 6 [15].

The complicated pits and fissures and the operculum covering the distal half of the first permanent molars allow for the accumulation and retention of bacterial plaque [16–18]. Favorable conditions for biofilm accumulation during tooth eruption are likely to explain, at least in part, the present findings. First, the amount of biofilm accumulated on the occlusal aspects has been shown to be higher in partially erupted molars than in fully erupted molars. In addition, Brailsford et al. showed the qualitative differences in the biofilm composition, with partially erupted teeth having higher counts of non-mutans streptococci and Actinomyces israelii than fully erupted teeth [19].

Besides, first permanent molar exhibits an increased susceptibility to caries due to its positioning in the oral cavity in the posterior region of the child's mouth which makes it further difficult for the child to properly clean this area [19, 20].

The first permanent molars are at greater risk of damage and loss, because of their special morphology. Pits and fissures on occlusal aspects of permanent teeth are particularly susceptible to the development of tooth decay. This susceptibility to tooth decay is related with the individual morphology of the tooth's pits and fissures, which can be prosperous shelters for microorganisms and make the oral hygiene procedures of these areas more difficult, allowing greater plaque accumulation [21].

Many surveys have reported a preferred site of mainly occlusal caries: 90% of caries occurs at this level in children and adolescents [22]. The same results were found at the Pedodontics Department in the University of Hassan II of Casablanca, where 87.7% of the FPM caries were found in the occlusal grooves [8].

The occlusal fissured surface of the first permanent molars and their lower buccal and upper lingual pits are among the most susceptible sites for caries.

Waterman and Knutson believed that first permanent molars especially lower molars among the other teeth are most susceptible to caries [13].

In the survey of Alwayli et al., the caries prevalence in the mandibular FPMs was significantly higher than the caries prevalence in the maxillary FPMs. This finding is in agreement with other studies [23, 25]. The reason expected behind this finding is the difference in the morphology and the earlier eruption time of mandibular compared with maxillary FPMs.

On the other hand, caries in primary molars is an important indicator for the development of cavities in the permanent dentition, particularly in the first molar teeth [24, 25]. The severity of the caries of primary molars may also increase the risk of caries in the early erupting stage of the first permanent molars [26]. According to Gray et al., the presence of three or more deciduous molars with caries at the age of 5 years was the best predictor of caries experience in the first permanent molars at the age of 7 years [27].

The increase in the prevalence of dental caries is a result of dietary changes, including frequent consumption of high-energy, low-cost foods that are poor in nutrients and rich in sugar and fat and unbalanced consumption of sugar content. The consumption rate of sweet foods for children aged 6–11 years increased from 23.1% in 2002 to 43.9% in 2012 [28, 29].

2.2 Clinical forms and complications

The caries of FPM in children is characterized by its precocity and speed of evolution, due to the immaturity of the tissues that compose it. The carious lesions, often active in children, will evolve insidiously towards the chronic inflammation of the pulp and eventually towards the pulp necrosis, which can compromise the root edification. As a result, early diagnosis is essential [30].

The clinical examination includes both a visual examination under good lighting and a tactile examination. Visual examination can detect advanced lesions, initial lesions usually go unnoticed. Tactile examination allows sounding, useful for the detection of dentinal hardness of cavitary lesions, but is found to be iatrogenic in the detection of initial lesions [31].

In 2005, a consensus conference proposed to rationalize the visual signs of detection of carious lesions in the form of a codified system, the ICDAS (International Caries Detection and Assessment System), which gives an idea of the demineralized tissues and which, therefore, allows a therapeutic adapted to the tissue damage [32]. This system contains seven codes from 0 (healthy tooth) to 6 (extended dentin caries) [33] (http://www.icdas.org) (**Table 1**).

The ICDAS classification allows a visual diagnosis. However, it should not be limited to this criterion alone; an assessment of lesion activity is required. It is based mainly on two clinical indicators; the presence of plaque related to the localization of the lesion and the tactile sensation to the sounding [33–36].

FPM caries are mainly located on the occlusal aspects of the tooth. There are, in particular, two clinical forms of predominant carious lesions: cavities in grooves, pits, and fissures, and hidden or surprise carie. At the proximal level, more rarely, another form of caries called stopped is observed [37, 38].

The decay of grooves, pits, and cracks begins at the bottom of the crevice. The complex anatomy of pits and fissures and the presence of discoloration can complicate both clinical examination and diagnosis. Indeed, early lesions may not be clinically and radiographically visible, and their early diagnosis will require new diagnostic techniques based on fluorescence [34–37].

Hidden carie is the characteristic of immature FPM. It is located on the occlusal aspect of the tooth and develops in the pulpal direction by extending in width under the surface of the enamel, which appears intact. This evolution is very often done without painful clinical signs. Detection, often very late, is done during a routine clinical examination, when a small pertuis attaches to the probe. The radiograph reveals, in a surprising way, the extent of the dentinal damage compared with the usual clinical aspect of the caries [38, 39] (**Figure 1**).

Mesial caries is often related to the progressive caries of the distal surface of the second temporary molar. The fall or loss of this molar will allow a better hygiene of the region and the initial carious lesion by remineralizing it which can be transformed into an arrested lesion [39, 40] (**Figure 2**).

In the absence of treatment of the active carious lesions, the inflammation insidiously gains the young pulp and evolves rapidly towards the necrosis. This necrotic state compromises the continuation of root edification. Infectious problems can settle and spread to the cellulo-adipous tissues. The evolution of cellulitis can be acute or chronic.

Serious cellulitis is the initial essentially inflammatory stage. It is characterized by an important swelling, a feeling of impasto and diffuse heat, a spontaneous pain, a trismus, a very painful percussion, and a positive buccal palpation.

Suppurative acute cellulitis is the progressive form of serious cellulitis in the absence of treatment. It is characterized by the abcedation with appearance of general signs: trismus, insomnia, difficult feeding, asthenia, sometimes aches, paleness, fever, throbbing pain accompanied by headache, and feeling of beatings at the swelling. The collection can be fistulized to the oral mucosa or to the skin. It can also spread to nearby anatomical compartments and become a diffuse cellulitis that is life-threatening [41, 42].

	ICDAS classification	Histological involvement	
0		No demineralization	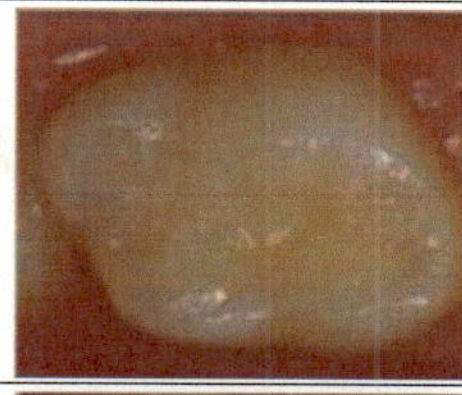
1	Visible change after drying	Demineralization limited to the external half of the enamel	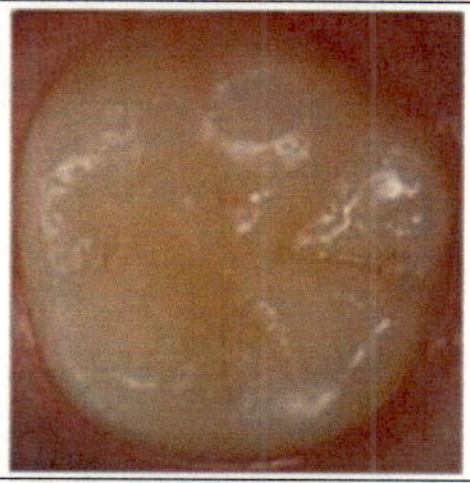
2	Visible change without drying	Demineralization limited to the internal half of the enamel	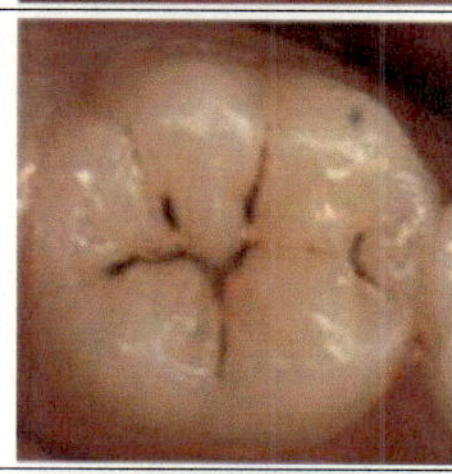
3	Localized rupture of the enamel without demineralization of the underlying visible dentin	Damage of the dentino enamel junction. Start of external demineralization of dentin	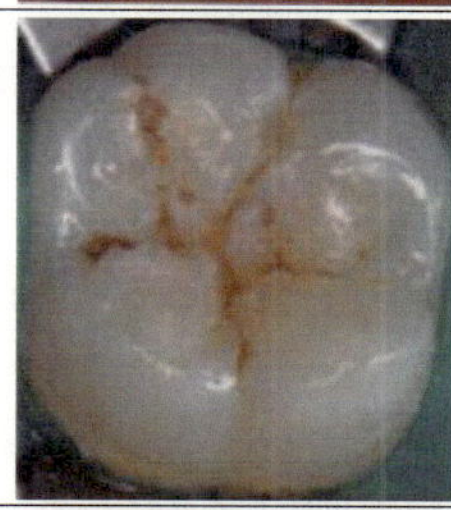
4	Carious dentin visible by transparency with or without localized rupture of the enamel	external demineralization of dentin	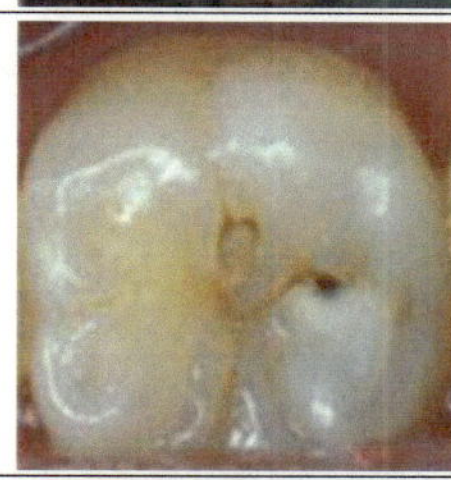
5	Visible micro-cavity with visible dentin	demineralization of the middle third of dentin	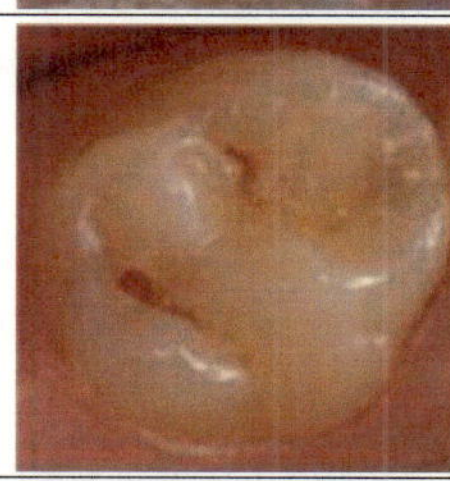
6	Extended dentin caries	Demineralization of the deep third of dentin	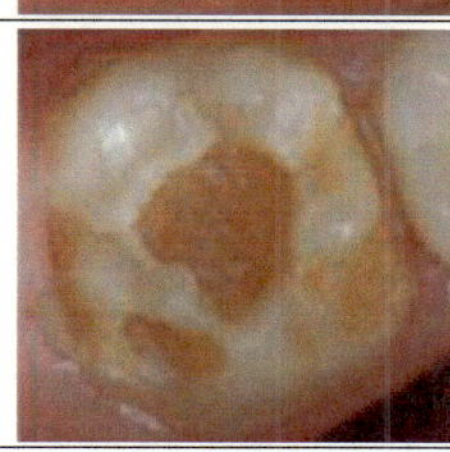

Table 1.
ICDAS classification.

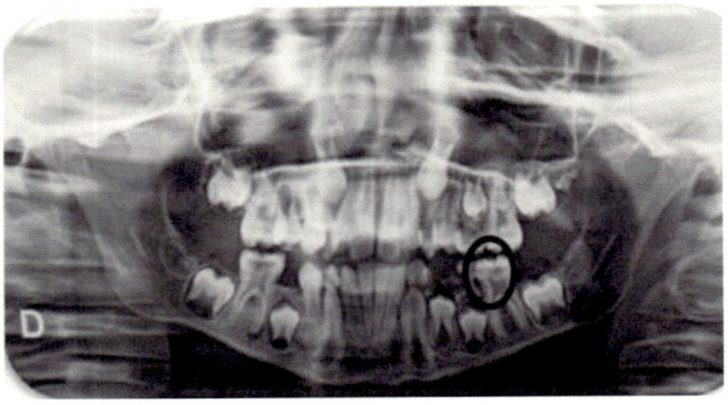

Figure 1.
Hidden carie on the tooth 36, with preservation of an enamel veil.

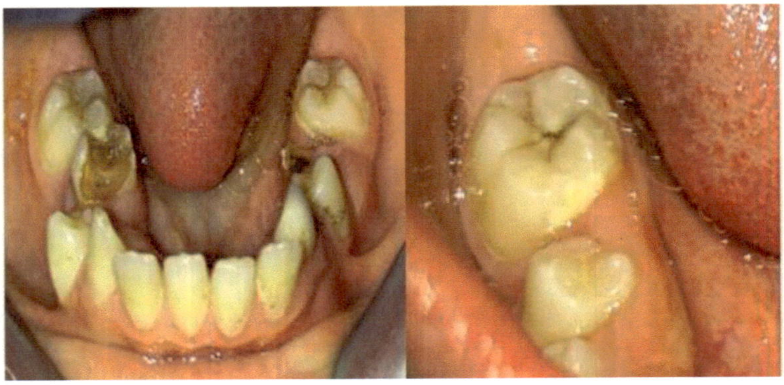

Figure 2.
Stoped caries: initial caries in mesial of the 46, likely to remineralize after the fall of the 85.

The evolution towards chronicity can be following a badly treated bad cellulitis. It is characterized by a painless swelling on palpation, adhering to the skin with the presence of an indurated cord. Chronic cellulitis evolves irreversibly, with no general or functional signs [42] (**Figure 3**).

2.3 Therapeutic approach

The therapeutic management of caries of FPM should be done according to the principle of tissue economy to respect the healthy hard tissue and to preserve pulp vitality in case of deep carious lesions.

Nowadays, the evolution of dental restoration techniques and materials provides us different therapeutic possibilities to deal with the carious lesions. The International Caries Detection and Assessment System (ICDAS) allows a treatment adapted to tissue involvement according to the dental demineralization degree [43].

- Remineralization techniques will be performed on ICDAS 1 and 2 by topical application of fluoride on smooth surfaces and furrow sealing in grooves [44].

- For cavitary lesions (ICDAS 3 and 4), the treatment will involve minimally invasive dentistry by using microdrills, aeroabrasion for occlusal cavities, and sonoabrasion for inter-proximal cavities. The filling materials used are fluwable composite resins (small cavities) or micro-hybrids (wider cavities).

- For ICDAS 5 and 6, the symptomatology must be taken into consideration for the therapeutic management of these lesions.

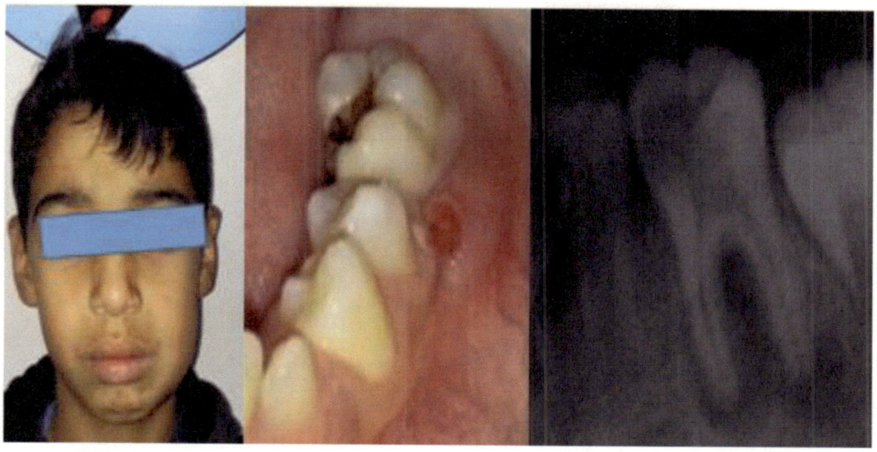

Figure 3.
Chronic cellulitis related to necrotic 36 in a 9-year-old child.

In case of deep decay that does not reach the pulp with the absence of clinical signs, the treatment of choice is indirect pulp capping which can be done in one step by removing the external area of the infected dentin, leaving a layer of firm internal affected dentin in order to avoid pulp exposure during caries removal. A calcium hydroxide is used as a base followed by a final coronal restoration [45].

Another approach can also be proposed, the "stepwise excavation" technique. It consists in cleaning the cavity in two steps with 3–6 months interval [45]. The tooth decay is incompletely removed at the bottom of the cavity, a calcium hydroxide is placed then a temporary, and hermetic sealing is performed by permitting the remineralization and the development of tertiary dentin [46]. A few months later, in a second step, the intervention will remove the remaining carious tissue and leaving the place for a harder dentin with the characteristics of an inactive lesion [45–47]. Stepwise excavation decreases the risk of pulp exposure compared with direct complete excavation.

In a randomized clinical trial Bjorndal et al. (2010), it showed a survival rate of 74% after 1 year of SW compared with 62.4% after selective removal to firm dentin [48].

If a pulp exposure occurs following dental excavation, a direct pulp capping will be indicated in case of a spontaneous bleeding stop [46] (**Figures 4** and **5**). Calcium hydroxide was widely used, but currently, the mineral trioxide aggregate and Biodentine are recommended with excellent clinical and radiographic results up to 6 months, 1 year, and even 2–3 years for some studies [49–51].

If the FPM is symptomatic, pulp vitality is compromised and a pulp treatment should be interesting either part or all of the cameral pulp. These pulp treatments are universally accepted on young permanent teeth [46, 52].

The pulpotomy procedure involves removing pulp tissue that has inflammatory, leaving intact the remaining vital non-inflammed tissue, which is covered with a pulp capping agent to promote healing at the amputation site. Usually, pulpotomy consists in removing the entire coronal pulp up to the cervical area. Today, the depth of tissue removal is based on a clinical view, only tissue with profuse bleeding judged to be inflamed or infected should be removed, and the capping material should be placed on healthy tissue. MTA and biodentine seem to be the treatment of choice to stimulate dentin bridge formation in young permanent teeth with exposed pulps [51–53].

There is a controversy as to the indications for performing root canal treatment after root maturation. Prophylactic endodontic treatment is not recommended because of the low percentage of pulp necrosis [54]. It is important to perform a permanent restoration to prevent bacterial leakage and ensure the success of the treatment.

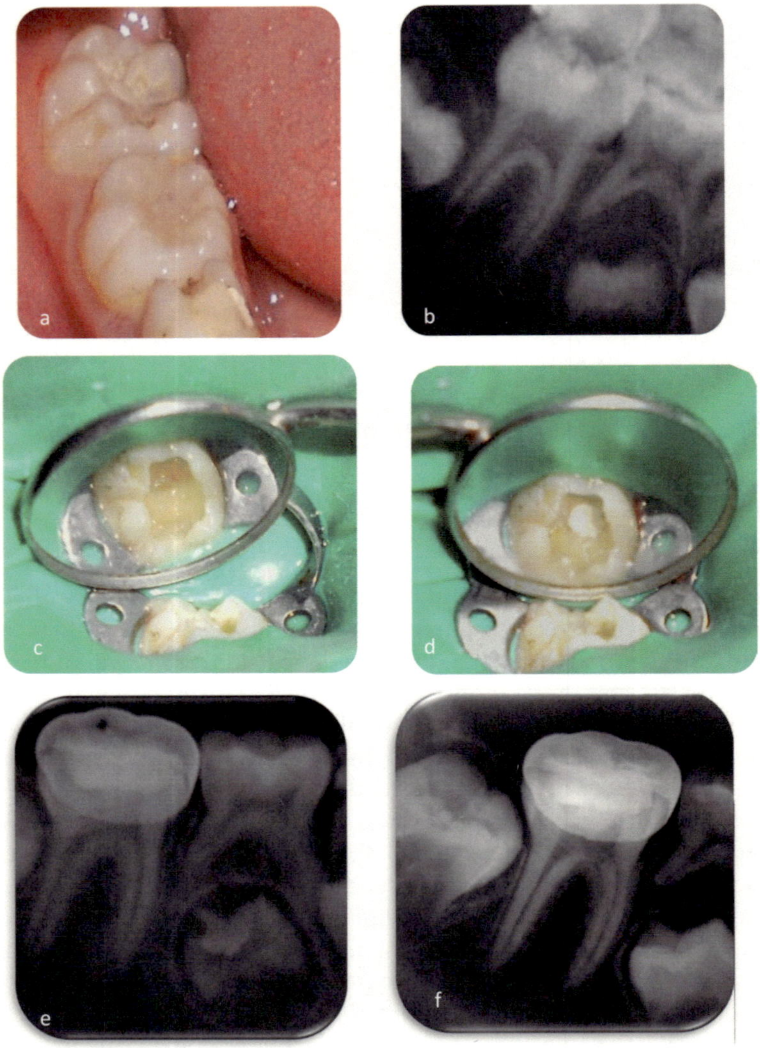

Figure 4.
Direct pulp capping on the right first permanent immature molar. (a, b) Deep caries close to the pulp. (c, d) Direct pulp capping with calcium hydroxide after pulp exposure. (e, f) Radiographs after 6 and 18 months of treatment showing good evolution and apexogenesis.

There should be no adverse clinical signs or symptoms such as sensitivity, pain, or swelling. There should be no radiographic sign of internal or external resorption, abnormal canal calcification, or periapical radiolucency post-operatively. Teeth having immature roots should continue normal root development and apexogenesis.

For the first immature permanent molars whose pulp is no longer vital or necrotic, apexification treatment is undertaken to induce development and apical closure. It can be achieved in two manners, either as a long-term procedure using calcium hydroxide dressing to allow the formation of a hard tissue barrier (**Figure 6**), or as a short-term procedure creating an apical plug of MTA [52]. Although calcium hydroxide has properties including bactericidal action on aerobic and anaerobic germs to heal periapical lesions [55, 56] (**Figure 7**), it has some inconveniences relied to a long-term treatment and a high-risk of root fracture of permanent immature teeth.

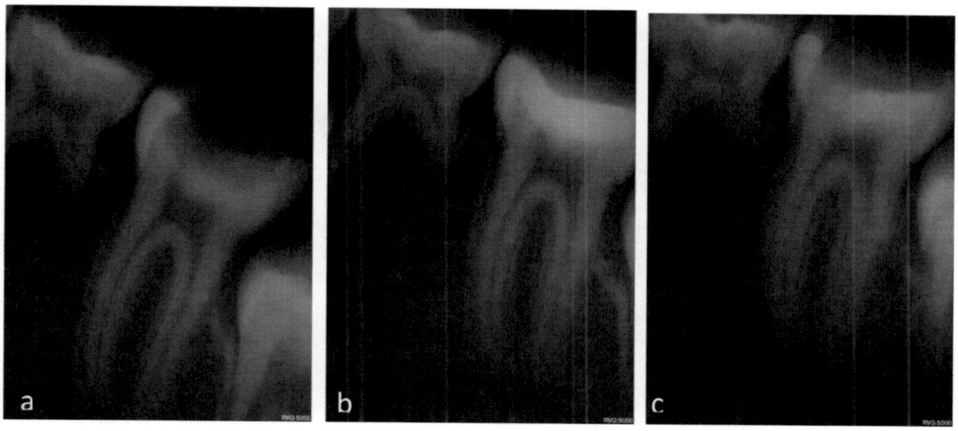

Figure 5.
Direct pulp capping on the left first permanent molar. (a) Deep caries with pulpal involvement on the 36 asymptomatic. (b) Direct pulp capping with biodentine. (c) Radiograph after 6 months of treatment showing favorable evolution.

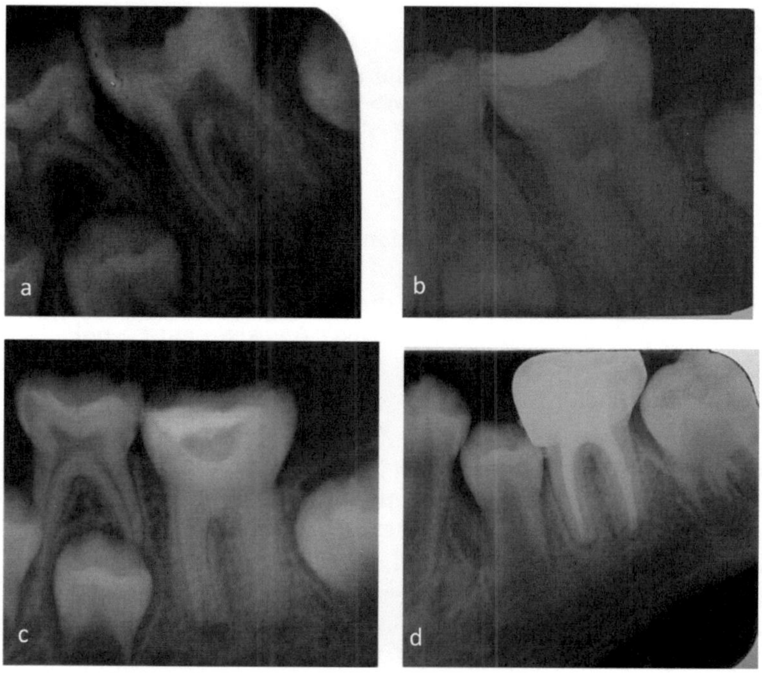

Figure 6.
Apexification of the 36. (a) Deep caries reaching the pulp with peripical apical lesions on the immature tooth. (b) Endodontic treatment and root canal filling with calcium hydroxide. (c) Radiograph after 6 months of treatment showing the favorable evolution and regression of periapical lesions. (d) Final root canal treatment with gutta-percha after apical closure achieved after 2 years.

Despite the success of apexification, the canal walls remain short and thin increasing the fracture risk of the tooth.

Recently, revascularization has been proposed as an alternative procedure to treat the necrotic immature permanent teeth with open apex regardless the periapical pathology. It is based on the elimination and the replacement of infected necrotic pulp by a neoformed tissue. Indeed, the use of the capacity of stem cell

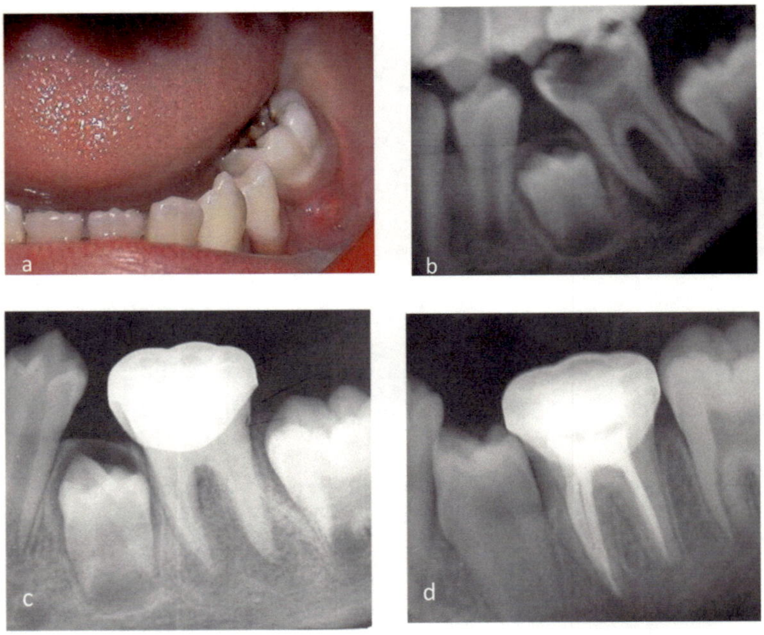

Figure 7.
Treatment of peripical lesions of the left first permanent molar. (a) Deep occlusal caries on 36 with abscess facing the tooth. (b) Retro alveolar showing pulpal involvement by decay and significant periapical lesions on the mature tooth. (c) At 3 weeks of root canal treatment with calcium hydroxide, regression of periapical lesions. (d) Final root canal treatment.

differentiation could allow a reconstruction of dental structures, root development, and apical closure [57–59] (**Figure 8**).

Early diagnosis of carious lesions and the application of appropriate preventive measures will avoid the use of heavy and often expensive dentine-pulpal treatments.

2.4 Preventive approach

The time between the eruption of the first permanent molars and the establishment of functional occlusion is a critical period to protect the permanent teeth from caries. Prevention should begin as soon as the first permanent molar erupts rather than wait until the eruption is completed.

These facts dictate the need for caries-prevention technology, targeted at the most susceptible tooth surfaces in the most susceptible members of the population. First permanent molars need special attention; thus, careful preventive strategies include fissure sealant, topical fluoride applications, and meticulous home care [60, 61].

Fissure sealants used on occlusal tooth surfaces were introduced in 1960s for protecting pits and fissures from dental caries. Such sealants prevent the growth of bacteria that promote decay in pits and fissures in teeth (**Figures 9** and **10**).

The application of fissure sealants should be complemented with oral health education for children, adolescents, and their families to assimilate adequate oral hygiene habits and understand the need of regular dental appointments for primary prevention and early diagnosis of oral diseases [21].

There is an agreement that in high-risk populations, all children should receive sealants [62, 63].

Several sealant materials are available. Currently, the two pre-dominant types of dental sealant nowadays are resin-based and glass ionomer cement (GIC) sealants.

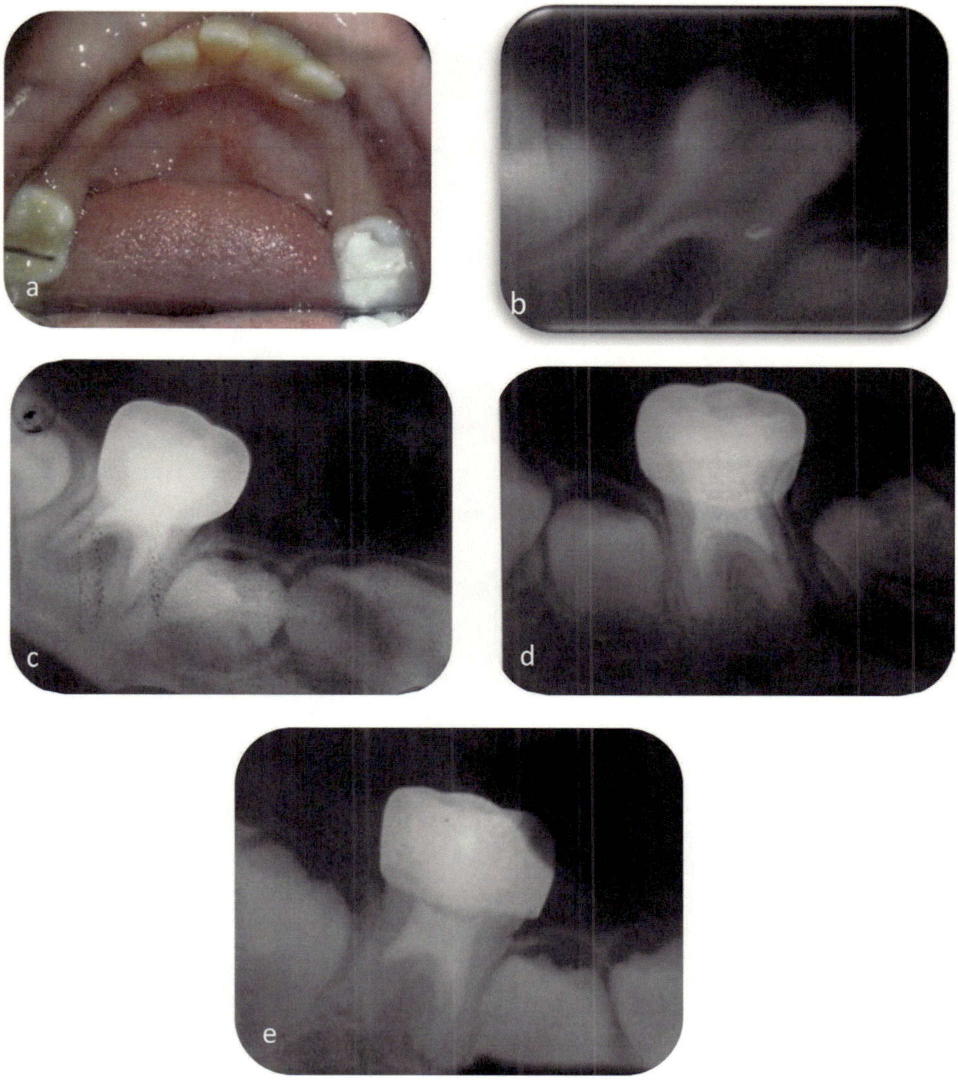

Figure 8.
Revascularization treatment on the left first permanent molar [58]. (a) Clinical status of the 36 with temporary coronal obturation. (b) Peroperative radiography: short immature roots with periapical radiolucency. (c) 3 weeks after canal disinfection and blood clot, MTA was applied and stainless steel crown was placed. (d) 10 months follow-up, periodontal healing, with the disappearance of radiolucency from the mesial root canal. (e) 14 months follow-up: thickening of the root and beginning of canal obliteration.

For high-quality resin sealant placement, electrically powered dental equipment and good clinical conditions are required. However, this may be difficult to achieve in regions, where access to modern dental clinics is limited. This problem may be overcome by using GIC sealants because they can be placed without the use of electrically powered dental equipment [64].

When considering fissure sealants, the earlier the application is performed, the more effective they are. Therefore, in children, fissure sealants are recommended to be applied soon after tooth eruption, mainly at the level of the first permanent molars. Studies have shown that fissure sealants applied both in clinics and schools are highly effective in preventing dental caries, reducing caries in pits and fissures up to 60% for 2–5 years after its implementation [65].

Numerous studies have investigated the clinical effectiveness of fissure sealants, and this has been the subject of a Cochrane review. A meta-analysis of seven studies

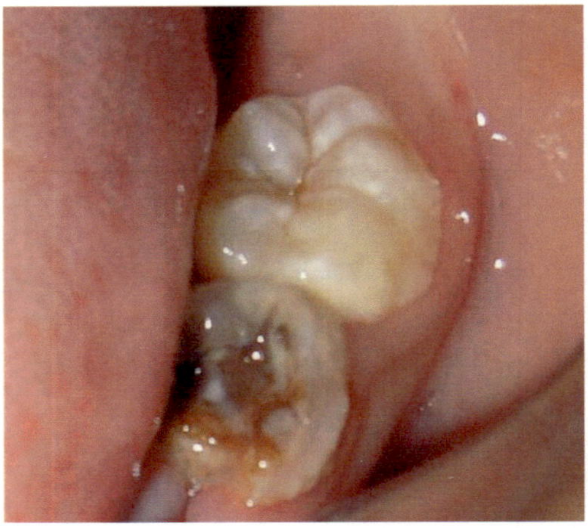

Figure 9.
First permanent molar with deep pits and fissures and important accumulation of plaque.

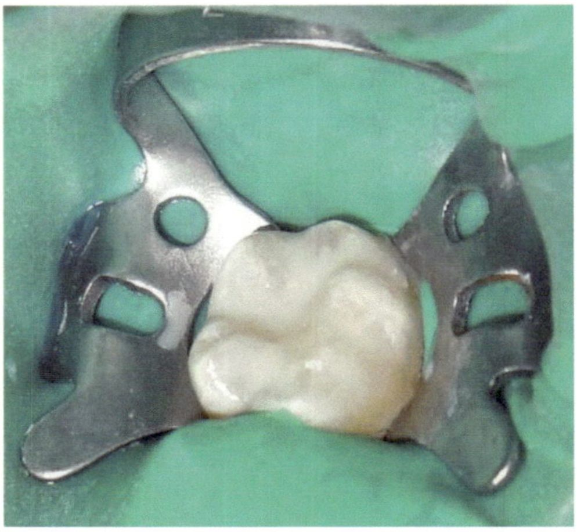

Figure 10.
After sealant application.

comparing sealed teeth to untreated controls demonstrated caries reductions ranging from 87% at 12 months to 60% at 48–54 months [66].

Several studies have demonstrated that the effectiveness of fissure sealants depends on the longevity of sealant coverage, that is, clinical retention [20].

In terms of retention and the need to reassess sealants within a year after placement, it is very important to adequately isolate the teeth. Salivary contamination is the major cause of sealants loss in the first year [67, 68].

The retention of resin sealants was good on average in all studies at each follow-up. After 12 months of follow-up, resin sealants were retained completely in 79–92% of cases. The corresponding retention after 24 and 36 months of follow-ups for resin sealants was 71–85 and 61–80%. There is an evidence in the literature regarding fissure sealants' effectiveness in caries prevention and control, for both individual and community-based interventions for children and adolescents [20, 69–71].

In field conditions where isolation control is difficult, using a material less affected by humidity, it gives significant advantage [72]. In fact, fissure restorers with glass-ionomer-based chemical hardening feature applied in recent years in field conditions displayed a better cavity prevention performance compared with antiresins [73].

Fluoride varnishes have also been marketed since 1960s and comprise a topical medication, which is painted onto the tooth surface. They contain a high concentration of fluoride (22,600 ppm) and are licensed for application by dental professionals. The varnish forms a quick-setting base which subsequently releases fluoride.

The aim of topical fluoride varnish application is to treat hard tooth surfaces in such a way that caries is arrested or reversed. Fluoride acts to prevent caries in three ways: by inhibiting the demineralization and promoting the remineralization of dental enamel, and by inhibiting acid formation by bacterial plaque especially before the complete eruption of the teeth.

Sometimes, topical fluoride has been combined with sealant application to strengthen overall effectiveness in the prevention of dental caries [74].

At the end of 4 year period, Songpaisan et al. based on a study conducted in Thailand found that pit and fissure restorers provided a much more superior protection than fluoride protocols applied individually. It was also seen that glass ionomer fissure restorers provided a better protection than the fluoride gel [75].

Data from three randomized controlled trials suggest that in children and adolescents with sound occlusal surfaces, the use of pit and fissure sealants compared with fluoride varnishes may reduce the incidence of occlusal carious lesions in permanent molars by 73% after 2–3 years of follow-up (OR, 0.27; 95% CI, 0.11–0.69) [76].

3. First permanent molar abnormalities

Several factors can disrupt the development of PMP. Depending on when these disturbances occur, anomalies in number, shape, size, or structure may be observed.

Among these, MIH remains the most commonly encountered and described anomaly today.

3.1 Molar-incisor hypomineralization

3.1.1 Epidemiology

Molar incisor hypomineralization, conventionally known by the acronym MIH, corresponds to the qualitative defects of the enamel, of systemic origin, affecting one or more first permanent molars, often associated with defects on one or more incisors [77].

The involvement of the second temporary molars and cuspidian tip of the permanent canines has also been described [78].

The prevalence of MIH varies considerably according to studies ranging from 2.4% in Germany [79] to 2.5% in China [80] and to 40% in the United Kingdom [81]. In Africa, studies in Libya, Morocco, Kenya, and Nigeria reported the prevalences of 2.9, 7.9, 13.7, and 17.7%, respectively [82–85]. According to a recent meta-analysis published in 2018 [86], the global average prevalence is 13.1% with 17.5 million new cases estimated in 2016, of which 4.8 million require management.

While the prevalence of MIH is comparable between the two sexes [82, 87], the location of defects by arch and by sector remains variable. It seems that the risk of incisor damage increases with the number of molars affected. Cho et al. reported, in 2008 [80], an incisor participation of 62.5% for cases with the four affected molars versus 36% for children with single molar involvement. In a study conducted in Casablanca [82], the high number of children with the first four permanent molars affected (84.7%) may explain the high incisor participation found (92.94%).

3.1.2 Risk factors

The precise etiology of MIH stills unknown. The probable systemic origin is probably multifactorial and with a possible genetic component. The pre-natal factors involved are urinary tract infections, vitamin D deficiency, and the use of antiepileptic medications during pregnancy. In the perinatal period, we could note cesarean delivery, delayed delivery, and prematurity. Post-natal causes are related not only to early childhood diseases such as repeated fevers, ear infections, pneumonia, asthma, and gastrointestinal disorders, but also the exposure to bisphenol A or dioxin and frequent use of antibiotics [88–90].

3.1.3 Diagnosis

The clinical aspect of the lesions is characteristic. These lesions are white, yellow, or brown opacities, well-defined with a clear demarcation between the affected enamel and the healthy one. They are located in the occlusal and/or incisal third, which may extend over a more or less important area of the coronary surface. These lesions are asymmetrical and the severity of the lesions is very variable. In severe cases, the affected molars suffer from masticatory forces, a post-eruptive fracture of the fragile enamel resulting in substance loss, hypersensitivity, and the development of carious lesions. Affected incisors, often unsightly, have fewer complications [77, 78, 91] (**Figure 11**).

In order to standardize and facilitate the diagnosis of MIH, the European Association of Pediatric Dentistry (EAPD) has been adopted, since 2003, five criteria that are the presence of delimited opacities, post-eruptive enamel loss, atypical restorations, extraction of first molars associated with incisor damage in a patient at low risk of caries, and the absence or delay of eruption of first molars or permanent incisors [92].

Since 2016, an international working group, the Wurzburg MIH work group, has been introduced the MIH treatment need index (MIH TNI) to assess the severity of MIH with a score based on the presence or absence of sensitivity and the extent of clinical destruction with the ultimate objective of proposing a therapeutic approach based on this index [93].

The MIH should not be confused with other structural abnormalities of the enamel, whether of hereditary or acquired origin, namely imperfect amelogenesis, fluorosis, and especially enamel hypoplasia, for which the limits of substance loss are rounded and bordered by a well-mineralized enamel, unlike the MIH where the edges of substance loss are sharp and bordered by a hyperomineralized enamel [94].

3.1.4 Treatment

The management of MIH is a real challenge for the practitioner for several reasons. The affected teeth are difficult to anesthetize because the pulp has histological

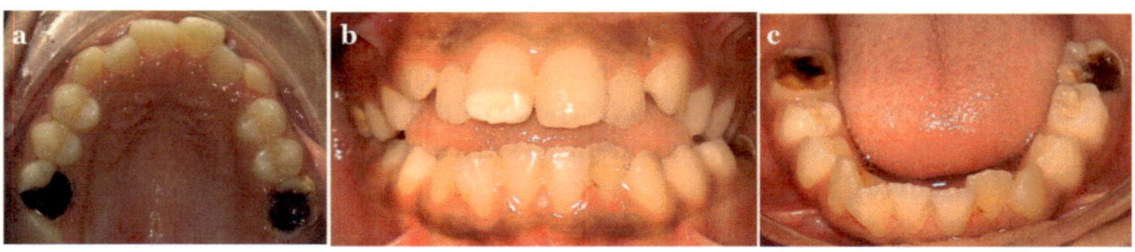

Figure 11.
(a, c) MIH involving the four FPM with post-eruptive fracture and carious complication in an 11-year-old patient suffering from a digestive disease. (b) Asymmetrical lesion of tooth 11 with white opacities, well-defined and located in the incisal third of coronary surface.

features responsible for chronic inflammation, most often requiring the use of truncular, intra-ligamentary, or transcortical anesthesia. The limits of the preparation during caries excavation are difficult to determine since the practitioner remains divided between the desire not to be too invasive and the need to remove all the hypomineralized enamel to ensure the durability of the restorations. The anxiety of patients suffering, on the one hand from hypersensitivity to hot, cold, and tooth brushing and on the other hand from repeated care due to the more delicate adherence to the enamel structure, remains difficult to manage and often involves the use of conscious inhalation sedation [78, 95].

Several therapeutic options are possible depending on the patient's age and cooperation, the severity of the disease, pulp involvement, orthodontic diagnosis, long-term prognosis, and the cost of treatment [96].

For mild abnormalities with a smooth enamel surface, the application of fluoride varnish and sealing of the grooves is recommended (**Figure 12**). When abnormalities are moderate with one or both affected surfaces without affecting the cusps, the teeth are restored with the composite by direct method [97].

In the case of severe MIH, direct restoration has certain mechanical limitations and perfect restoration of the tooth anatomy is difficult to achieve. Preformed pedodontic copings (PPC) and bonded indirect partial restorations (BIPR) in the form of onlays, overlays, or inlays are then indicated (**Figure 13**). PPCs remain simpler to implement, less expensive with a high success rate. However, they must be replaced by a peripheral crown in adulthood. For BIPRs, they are made using composite or ceramic materials in two stages or even in a single session if computer-aided design and manufacturing (CAD/CAM) is used. In young patients, composite BIPRs are preferred because it allow repairs by direct composite addition, allow thinner restorations, present less risk of fracture, and their esthetic appearance remains satisfactory [96].

For very severe abnormalities, it is sometimes more appropriate to extract the tooth. Nevertheless, it will be necessary to choose the ideal moment to allow the second permanent molar to make a spontaneous mesial eruption instead of the first extracted molar. This moment corresponds to the period of formation of the furcation zone of the second permanent molar visible on a panoramic radiograph. However, orthodontic consultation is recommended [98, 99].

The MIH remains a frequent, progressive abnormality that can lead, in the absence of treatment, to the total destruction of the tooth. Thus, only early diagnosis, adequate care, and regular follow-up can keep the 6-year-old tooth on the arch and allow it to play its full role in children.

3.2 Other abnormalities of the first permanent molar

The FPM may be affected by other rare abnormalities: anatomical, eruptive, or agenesis.

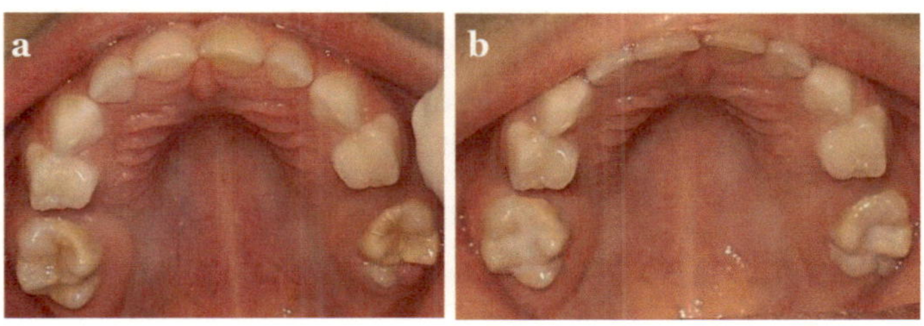

Figure 12.
(a) MIH involving the upper FPM in a 6-year-old patient with HIV infection. (b) Sealing of the grooves and application of fluoride varnish.

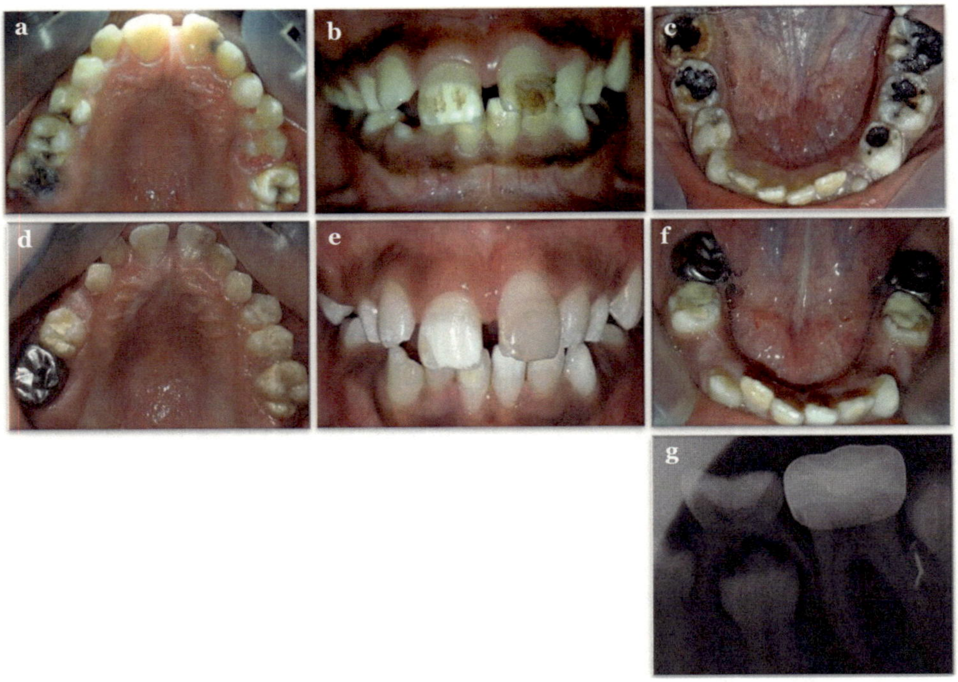

Figure 13.
(a–c) Severe MIH with incisive involvement in an adolescent with mental retardation. The four FPM are affected with post-eruptive fracture on 16, 36, 46, and carious complication. (d–f) Reconstruction under conscious sedation of teeth 16, 36, and 46 using preformed pedodontics caps after the preservation of pulpal vitality by indirect capping. Restoration of teeth 21 and 26 with the composite by direct method. (g) Radiographic control of lower left sector.

3.2.1 Anatomical abnormalities

The first upper molar has a very stable anatomy with strongly expressed anatomical characteristics. However, some variations have been described for the Carabelli's tubercle; mesio-distal accessory cuspidian tubercle can have a high variability in shape and volume [100].

The Bölk tubercle, which is sometimes present on the buccal aspect of the tooth or at the mesio-buccal angle of the second upper molar, can exceptionally be observed on the upper FPM (**Figure 14**). The presence of an accessory root can be associated with a large Bölk tubercle (**Figure 14b**).

As for the lower FPM, it may have anatomical variabilities that mainly concern the number of cusps, which can vary from four to seven cusps instead of the usual five cusps [100] (**Figure 15**).

These morphological abnormalities can interfere with good oral hygiene and are a factor in susceptibility to carious disease. Early diagnosis allows the implementation of preventive measures based on sealant.

Root abnormalities are quite numerous, either in direction and number or in shape and size. Taurodontism is also a particular variety of root-shaped abnormalities (**Figure 16**).

3.2.2 Eruption abnormalities

Ectopic eruption of the FPM is a phenomenon that affects 3–4% of the population and is mainly observed in the upper FPMs [101].

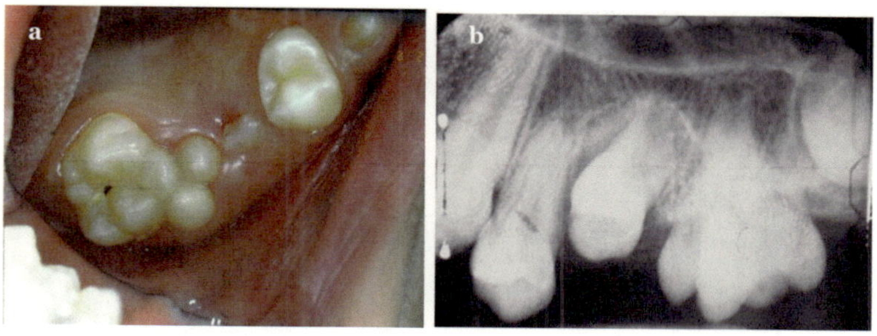

Figure 14.
(a) Very developed Bôlk tubercle on the mesio-buccal angle of the upper FPM in an 11-year-old girl. (b) Accessory root associated with this wide tubercle.

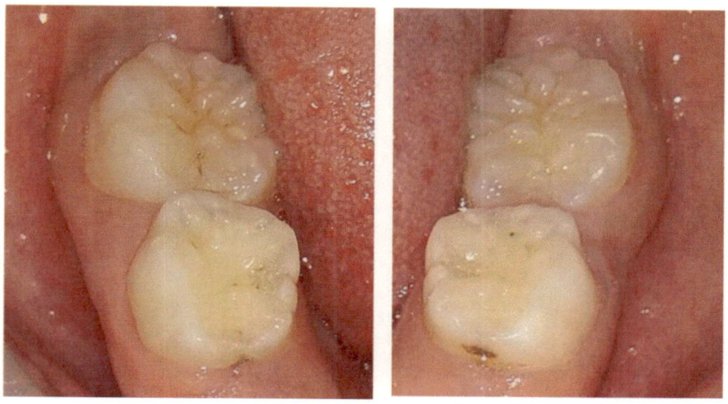

Figure 15.
Lower FPM with an unusual number of cusps and grooves.

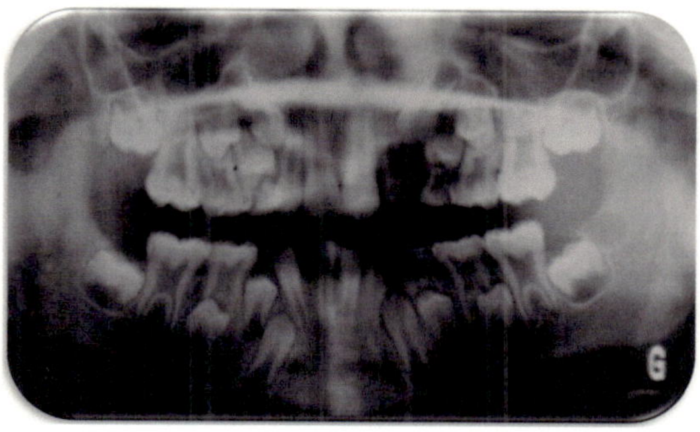

Figure 16.
The four FPMs and the second temporary molars have taurodontism.

It corresponds to an evolution according to an abnormal mesial trajectory, thus causing the pathological resorption of the disto-buccal root of the adjacent second temporary molar.

Interception of the ectopic eruption of the FPMs is essential to avoid permanent tooth blockage and the loss of space prejudicial to the eruption of adjacent premolars causing malocclusions [102].

Inclusion is the most common eruption abnormalities encountered. Its incidence varies from 5.6 to 18.8%. The upper canines, FPMs, and lower lateral incisors are the most prone to inclusion [103]. The inclusion of FPMs can be isolated or associated with complex syndromes (**Figure 17**).

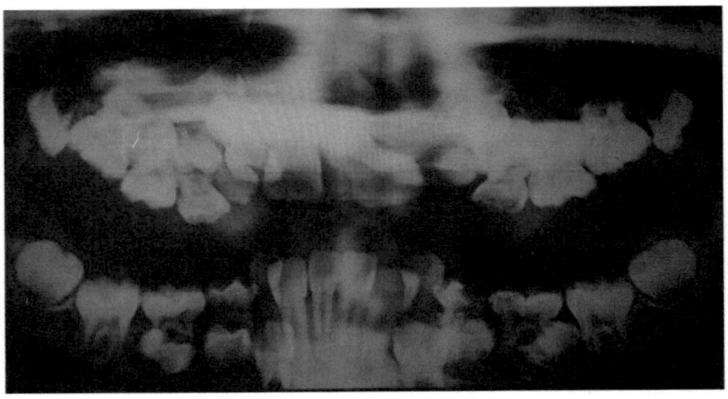

Figure 17.
Retention of FPMs in an 8-year-old girl with an unlabeled syndrome.

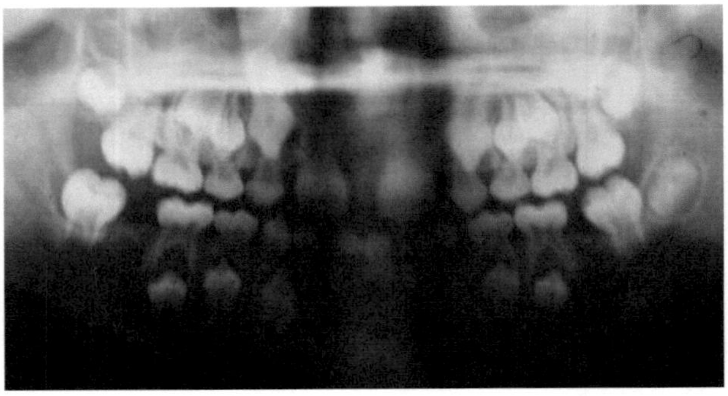

Figure 18.
12-year-old patient with agenesis of lower FPM, lower incisors, and upper lateral incisors.

3.2.3 Agenesis

Agenesis consists in the absence of the development of a dental germ. The prevalence of dental agenesis varies from 3.4 to 10.1% depending on the country. It mainly affects the permanent teeth. The most frequently affected teeth are the lower second premolars, upper lateral incisors, and upper second premolars.

The agenesis of superior FPMs is rare with a prevalence of 0.01–0.04% [104]. It can be observed in the context of oligodontics associated with rare diseases (**Figure 18**).

4. Conclusion

The vulnerability of the first permanent molar exposes it very early to carious disease and its complications.

Therefore, in children, this tooth must be given special attention by the practitioner in order to assess the carious risk, detect and intercept any early lesion, provide appropriate treatment, and ensure regular follow-up.

Collective prevention measures in schools are also needed to reduce the prevalence of carious disease.

Conflict of interest

There is no conflict of interest.

Author details

Mouna Hamza*, Amal Chlyah, Bouchra Bousfiha, Bouchra Badre, Maria Mtalsi, Hasna Saih and Samira El Arabi
Faculty of dentistry of Casablanca, University Hassan II, Morocco

*Address all correspondence to: mounahamza22@gmail.com

References

[1] Cerba O, Gillet P. Survey on the EBD of 12- and 15-year-old children attending school in the province of South France in 2007. Available from: https://www.ass.nc/publication/doc_download/106

[2] Al-Samadani KH, Ahmad MS. Prevalence of first permanent molar caries in and its relationship to the dental knowledge of 9-12-year olds from Jeddah, Kingdom of Saudi Arabia. ISRN Dentistry. 2012. 6 p. ID: 391068. DOI: 10.5402/2012/391068

[3] Sadeghi M. Prevalence and bilateral occurrence of first permanent molar caries in 12-year-old students. Journal of Dental Research, Dental Clinics, Dental Prospects. 2007;**1**(2):86-92. DOI: 10.5681/joddd.2007.015

[4] Xue Y, Lin W, Jie L, Qing D. Caries status of the first permanent molar among 7- to 9-year-old children in Tangshan city and their correlation. Hua Xi Kou Qiang Yi Xue Za Zhi. 2015;**33**(1):54-57

[5] Abuaffan AH, Hayder S, Hussen AA. Prevalence of dental caries of the first permanent molars among 6-14 years old Sudanese children. Indian Journal of Dental Education. 2018;**11**(1):13-16

[6] Ziani H. Prevalence of tooth decay in 6-year-old teeth in the Greater Casablanca region (doctoral thesis in dental medicine). 2016

[7] Zouaidi K, Chala S, Ameziane R, Chhoul H. First permanent molar caries: A case study of Moroccan children between 6 and 15 year-old. Odonto-stomatologie Tropicale. 2012;**35**(140):5-10

[8] Kadim FZ, Hajjou S. Pathology of the six-year-old tooth: Survey in the pedodontics and emergency department at the Casablanca dental consultation and treatment centre [doctoral thesis in dental medicine]. 2015

[9] Aldossary MS, Alamri AA, Alshiha SA, Hattan MA, Alfraih YK, Alwayli HM. Prevalence of dental caries and fissure sealants in the first permanent molars among male children in Riyadh, Kingdom of Saudi Arabia. International Journal of Clinical Pediatric Dentistry. 2018;**11**(5):365-370. DOI: 10.5005/jp-journals-10005-1541

[10] Alwayli HM, Alshiha SA, Alfraih YK, Hattan MA, Alamri AA, Aldossary MS. A survey of fissure sealants and dental caries prevalence in the first permanent molars among primary school girls in Riyadh, Saudi Arabia. European Journal of Dentistry. 2017;**11**(4):455-460. DOI: 10.4103/ejd.ejd_189_17

[11] Batchelor PA, Sheiham A. Grouping of tooth surfaces by susceptibility to caries: A study in 516 year old children. BMC Oral Health. 2004;**4**(1):2. DOI: 10.1186/1472-6831-4-2

[12] Beauchamp J, Caufield PW, Crall JJ, Donly K, Feigal R, Gooch B, et al. American dental association council on scientific affairs. Evidence based clinical recommendations for the use of pit and fissure sealants: A report of the American dental association council on scientific affairs. The Journal of the American Dental Association. 2008;**139**(3):257-268. DOI: 10.14219/ jada.archive.2008.0155

[13] Bassir L, Khanehmasjedi M. Survey on the condition of first permanent molars in 15-year-old students in Ahwaz, Iran in 2005. Journal of Dental Research, Dental Clinics, Dental Prospect. 2008;**2**(2):58-62. DOI: 10.5681/joddd.2008.012

[14] Heydari A, Shahrabi M, Sha zadeh M, Anaraki EA, Aref M. Parental knowledge and awareness of the

first permanent molar. International Journal of Clinical Pediatric Dentistry. 2018;**11**(5):382-385. DOI: 10.5005/jp-journals-10005-1544

[15] Carvalho JC, Ekstrand KR, Thylstrup A. Dental plaque and caries on occlusal surfaces of first permanent molars in relation to stage of eruption. The Journal of Dental Research. 1989;**68**(5):773-779. DOI: 10.1177/00220345890680050401

[16] Wang Z, Rong W, Zhang Y, Zeng X, Li Z, Liu Z. Prevalence and contributing factors of dental caries of 6-year-old children in four regions of China. Peer Journal. 2019;7:e6997. DOI: 10.7717/peerj.6997

[17] Ekstrand KR, Christiansen J, Christiansen ME. Time and duration of eruption of first and second permanent molars: A longitudinal investigation. Community Dentistry and Oral Epidemiology. 2003;**31**(5):344-350

[18] Quaglio JM, Sousa MB, Ardenghi TM, Mendes FM, Imparato JCP, Pinheiro SL. Association between clinical parameters and the presence of active caries lesions in first permanent molars. Brazilian Oral Research. 2006;**20**(4):358-363

[19] Alves LS, Zenkner JE, Wagner MB, Damé-Teixeira N, Susin C, Maltz M. Eruption stage of permanent molars and occlusal caries activity/arrest. The Journal of Dental Research. 2014;**93**(7 Suppl):114S-119S. DOI: 10.1177/0022034514537646

[20] Ahovuo-Saloranta A, Forss H, Walsh T, Hiiri A, Nordblad A, Mäkelä M, et al. Sealants for preventing dental decay in the permanent teeth. Cochrane Database of Systematic Reviews. 2013;**28**(3):CD001830. DOI: 10.1002/14651858.CD001830.pub4

[21] Veiga NJ, Pereira CM, Ferreira PC, Correia IJ. Prevalence of dental caries and fissure sealants in a Portuguese sample of adolescents. PLoS One. 2015;**10**(3):e0121299. DOI: 10.1371/journal.pone.0121299

[22] Ebrahimi M, Ajami BA, Sarraf Shirazi AR, Afzal Aghaee M, Rashidi S. Dental treatment needs of permanent first molars in Mashhad schoolchildren. Journal of Dental Research, Dental Clinics, Dental Prospects. 2010;**4**(2):52-55. DOI: 10.5681/joddd.2010.014

[23] Togoo RA, Yaseen SM, Zakirulla M, Al Garni F, Khoraj A, Meer A. Prevalence of first permanent molar caries among 7-10 years old school going boys in Abha city, Saudi Arabia. Journal of International Oral Health. 2011;**3**(5):29-34

[24] Srinivasan D, Louis CJ. Evaluation of caries in deciduous second molar and adjacent permanent molar in mixed dentition. Journal of Pharmacy and Bioallied Sciences. 2015;7(Suppl 2):S572-S575. DOI: 10.4103/0975-7406.163544

[25] Leroy R, Bogaerts K, Lesaffre E, Declerck D. Effect of caries experience in primary molars on cavity formation in the adjacent permanent first molar. Caries Research. 2005;**39**(5):342-349. DOI: 10.1159/000086839

[26] Skeie MS, Raadal M, Strand GV, Espelid I. The relationship between caries in the primary dentition at 5 years of age and permanent dentition at 10 years of age—A longitudinal study. The International Journal of Paediatric Dentistry. 2006;**16**(3):152-160. DOI: 10.1111/j.1365-263X.2006.00720.x

[27] Baginska J, Rodakowska E, Milewski R, Kierklo A. Dental caries in primary and permanent molars in 7-8-year-old schoolchildren evaluated with caries assessment Spectrum and treatment (CAST) index. BMC Oral Health. 2014;**14**:74. DOI: 10.1186/1472-6831-14-74

[28] Dhamo B, Elezi B, Kragt L, Wolvius EB, Ongkosuwito EM. Does dental caries affect dental development in children and adolescents? Bosnian Journal of Basic Medical Sciences. 2018;**18**(2):198-205. DOI: 10.17305/bjbms.2018.2841

[29] Mobley C, Marshall TA, Milgrom P, Coldwell SE. The contribution of dietary factors to dental caries and disparities in caries. Academic Pediatrics. 2009;**9**(6):410-414. DOI: 10.1016/j.acap.2009.09.008

[30] Lussi A, Hotz P, Stich H. Les caries de sillons. Rev Mens Suisse Odontostomal. 1999;**9**:105-107

[31] Blique M. La prophylaxie dentaire individualisée. Réal Clin. 1999;**10**:541-556

[32] Vital S. Formation and physiology of the immature permanent tooth: Clinical implications. Réalités Cliniques. 2012;**23**(4):253-259

[33] Braga M, Mendes F, Ekstrand K. Detection activity assessment and diagnosis of dental caries lesions. Dental Clinics of North America. 2010;**54**:479-493. DOI: 10.1016/j.cden.2010.03.006

[34] Tassery H, Levallois B, Terrer E. Use of new minimum intervention dentistry technologies in caries management. Australian Dental Journal. 2013;**58** (1 Suppl):40-59. DOI: 10.1111/adj.12049

[35] Gomez J. Detection and diagnosis of the early caries lesion. BMC Oral Health. 2015;**15**(Suppl 1):1-7

[36] Abogazalah N, Ando M. Alternative methods to visual and radiographic examinations for approximal caries detection. Journal of Oral Science. 2017;**59**(3):315-322. DOI: 10.2334/josnusd.16-0595

[37] Duruturk L, ÇiftÇi A, Baharoglu S. Clinical evaluation of diagnodent in detection of occlusal caries in newly erupted noncavitated first permanent molars in caries-active children. Operative Dentistry. 2011;**36**(4):348-355. DOI: 10.2341/10-309-C

[38] Kudiyirickal M, Ivančaková R. Early enamel lesion part I classification and detection. ActaMedica (Hradec Králové). 2008;**51**(3):145-149. DOI: 10.14712/18059694.2017.16

[39] Roopa KS, Pathak S, Poornima P, Neena IE. White spot lesions: A literature review. Journal of Pediatric Dentistry. 2015;**3**:1-7

[40] Satish V, Prabhadevi CM, Hegde KV. Occult caries: The hidden truth. International Journal of Clinical Pediatric Dentistry. 2010;**3**(3):225-229. DOI: 10.5005/jp-journals-10005-1083i

[41] Lakouichmi M, Tourabi K, Abir BE. Les cellulites cervico-faciales graves, facteurs et critères de gravité. Pan African Medical Journal. 2014;**18**:57. DOI: 10.11604/pamj.2014.18.57.3702

[42] Gaetti-Jardim E Jr, Landucci LF, de Oliveira KL, Costa I, Ranieri RV, Okamoto AC, et al. Microbiota associated with infections of the jaws. International Journal of Dentistry. 2012;**2012**:369751. DOI: 10.1155/2012/369751

[43] International Caries Detection and Assessment System. 2018. Available from: http://www.icdas.org

[44] Hackmyer SP, Orpheus L. Conservative caries treatment. Decisions in Dentistry. 2017;**3**(6):22-27

[45] Ricketts DNJ, Innes NPT. In: Splieth CH, editor. Revolutions in Pediatric Dentistry. London: Quintessence Publishing; 2011. pp. 120-133

[46] American Academy of Pediatric Dentistry: Pulp Therapy for Primary

and Immature Permanent Teeth. Recommendations Best Practices. 2014. Available from: https://www.aapd.org/globalassets/guidelines/bp_pulptherapy.pdf

[47] Carvalho JC, Dige I, Machiulskiene V, Qvist V, Bakhshandeh A, Fatturi-Parolo C, et al. Occlusal caries diagnosis and management. Caries Research. 2016;**50**:527-542. DOI: 10.1159/000448662

[48] Bjørndal L, Reit C, Bruun G, Markvart M, Kjaeldgaard M, Näsman P, et al. Treatment of deep caries lesions in adults: Randomized clinical trials comparing stepwise vs. direct complete excavation, and direct pulp capping vs. partial pulpotomy. European Journal of Oral Sciences. 2010;**118**(3):290-297. DOI: 10.1111/j.1600-0722.2010.00731

[49] Katge FA, Patil DP. Comparative analysis of 2 calcium silicate-based cements (biodentine and mineral trioxide aggregate) as direct pulp-capping agent in young permanent molars: A split mouth study. Journal of Endodontia. 2017;**43**(4):507-513. DOI: 10.1016/j.joen.2016.11.026

[50] Brizuela C, Ormeño A, Cabrera C, Cabezas R, Silva CI, Ramírez V, et al. Direct pulp capping with calcium hydroxide, mineral trioxide aggregate, and biodentine in permanent young teeth with caries: A randomized clinical trial. Journal of Endodontia. 2017;**43**(11):1776-1780. DOI: 10.1016/j.joen.2017.06.031

[51] Awawdeh L, Al-Qudah A, Hamouri H, Chakra RJ. Outcomes of vital pulp therapy using mineral trioxide aggregate or biodentine: A prospective randomized clinical trial. Journal of Endodontia. 2018;**44**(11):1603-1609. DOI: 10.1016/j.joen.2018.08.004

[52] Fuks A, Kupietzki A, Guelmann M. Pulp therapy for the young permanent dentition. In: Casamassimo PS, Fields HW, Mc- Tigue DJ, Nowak A, editors. Pediatric Dentistry: Infancy through Adolescence. 5th ed. St. Louis, Mo: Elsevier/Saunders; 2013. pp. 490-502

[53] Taha NA, Abdulkhader SZ. Full pulpotomy with biodentine in symptomatic young permanent teeth with carious exposure. Journal of Endodontics. 2018;**44**(6):932-937. DOI: 10.1016/j.joen.2018.03.003

[54] Oginnini AO, Adekoya-Sofowora CA, Kolawole KA. Evaluation of radiographs, clinical signs and symptoms associated with pulp canal obliteration: An aid to treatment decision. Dental Traumatology. 2009;**25**:620-625. DOI: 10.1111/j.1600-9657.2009.00819.x

[55] Cwikla SJ, Bélanger M, Ciguère S. Dentinal tubule disinfection using three calcium hydroxide formulations. Journal of Endodontics. 2005;**31**(1):50-52

[56] Gimbel M, Correa A, Lin LM. Calcium hydroxide as a temporary filling of post space in root-filled teeth. Oral Surgery, Oral Medicine, Oral Pathology, and Oral Radiology. 2002;**94**:98-102

[57] Chen YP, Jovani-Sancho Mdel M, Sheth CC. Is revascularisation of immature permanent teeth an effective and reproducible technique? Dental Traumatology. 2015;**31**:429-436. DOI: 10.1111/edt.12214

[58] Wigler R, Kaufman AY, Lin S, Steinbock N, Hazan-Molina H, Torneck CD. Revascularisation: A treatment for permanent teeth with necrotic pulp and incomplete root development. Journal of Endodontics. 2013;**39**(3):319-326. DOI: 10.1016/j.joen.2012.11.014

[59] Mtalsi M, Rahmaoui M, Benkirane L, Elarabi S. Pulp revascularization of the first necrotic immature molar: Clinical

case report and development. Revue francophone d'odontologie pédiatrique. 2017;**12**(4):166-167

[60] Al-Samadani KH, Ahmad MS. Prevalence of first permanent molar caries in and its relationship to the dental knowledge of 9-12-year olds from Jeddah, Kingdom of Saudi Arabia. ISRN Dentistry. 2012;**2012**:391068. DOI: 10.5402/2012/391068

[61] Chestnutt IG, Chadwick BL, Hutchings S, Playle R, Pickles T, Lisles C, et al. Protocol for "seal or varnish?" (SoV) trial: A randomised controlled trial to measure the relative cost and effectiveness of pit and fissure sealants and fluoride varnish in preventing dental decay. BMC Oral Health. 2012;**12**:51. DOI: 10.1186/1472-6831-12-51

[62] Azarpazhooh A, Main PA. Pit and fissure sealants in the prevention of dental caries in children and adolescents: A systematic review. Journal of the Canadian Dental Association. 2008;**74**(2):171-177

[63] Flório FM, Pereira AC, Meneghim Mde C, Ramacciato JC. Evaluation of non-invasive treatment applied to occlusal surfaces. ASDC Journal of Dentistry for Children. 2001;**68** (5-6):326-331, 301

[64] Liu BY, Xiao Y, Chu CH, Lo EC. Glass ionomer ART sealant and fluoride-releasing resin sealant in fissure caries prevention—Results from a randomized clinical trial. BMC Oral Health. 2014;**14**:54. DOI: 10.1186/1472-6831-14-54

[65] Michalaki M, Sifakaki M, Oulis CJ, Lygidakis NA. Attitudes, knowledge and utilization of ssure sealants among Greek dentists: A national survey. European Archives of Paediatric Dentistry. 2010;**11**(6):287-293

[66] Ahovuo-Saloranta A, Hiiri A, Nordblad A, Worthington HV, Mäkelä M. Pit and fissure sealants for preventing dental decay in the permanent teeth of children and adolescents. Cochrane Database of Systematic Reviews. 2004;**3**:CD001830

[67] Jokovic A, Locker D. Evidence-based recommendations for the use of pit and fissure sealants in Ontario's Public Dental Health Programs. In: Locker D, editor. Quality Assurance Report #21: Community Dental Health Services Research Unit (CDHSRU). University of Toronto; 2001. Available: www.caphd-acsdp.org/PDF/ebd-seal.pdf

[68] Feigal RJ, Musherure P, Gillespie B, Levy-Polack M, Quelhas I, Hebling J. Improved sealant retention with bonding agents: A clinical study of two bottle and single-bottle systems. The Journal of Dental Research. 2000;**79**(11):1850-1856

[69] Wendt LK, Koch G, Birkhed D. Long-term evaluation of a fissure sealing programme in public dental service clinics in Sweden. Swedish Dental Journal. 2001;**25**(2):61-65

[70] Wright JT, Tampi MP, Graham L, Estrich C, Crall JJ, Fontana M, et al. Sealants for preventing and arresting pit-and- ssure occlusal caries in primary and permanent molars. Pediatric Dentistry. 2016;**38**(4):282-308

[71] Baldini V, Tagliaferro EP, Ambrosano GM, Meneghim Mde C, Pereira AC. Use of occlusal sealant in a community program and caries incidence in high- and low-risk children. Journal of Applied Oral Science. 2011;**19**(4):396-402

[72] Dulgergil CT, Ercan E, Colak H. Evaluation of school-based prevention program in Turkey: Results of a 24-month study. European Journal of Dentistry. 2016;**10**(2):245-249. DOI: 10.4103/1305-7456.178312

[73] Beiruti N, Frencken JE, van't Hof MA, Taifour D, van Palenstein Helderman WH. Caries-preventive effect of a one-time application of composite resin and glass ionomer sealants after 5 years. Caries Research. 2006;**40**(1):52-59

[74] Ahovuo-Saloranta A, Forss H, Hiiri A, Nordblad A, Mäkelä M. Pit and fissure sealants versus fluoride varnishes for preventing dental decay in the permanent teeth of children and adolescents. Cochrane Database of Systematic Reviews. 2016;**1**:CD003067. DOI: 10.1002/14651858.CD003067.pub4

[75] Songpaisan Y, Bratthall D, Phantumvanit P, Somridhivej Y. Effects of glass ionomer cement, resin based pit and fissure sealant and HF applications on occlusal caries in a developing country field trial. Community Dentistry and Oral Epidemiology. 1995;**23**(1):25-29

[76] Wright JT, Crall JJ, Fontana M, Gillette EJ, Nov BB, Dhar V, et al. Evidence-based clinical practice guideline for the use of pit-and-fissure sealants: A report of the American Dental Association and the American Academy of Pediatric Dentistry. The Journal of the American Dental Association. 2016;**147**(8):672-682.e12. DOI: 10.1016/j.adaj.2016.06.001

[77] Weerheijm KL, Jalevik B, Alaluusua S. Molar-incisor hypomineralisation. Caries Research. 2001;**35**(5):390-391. DOI: 10.1159/000047479

[78] Jedeon K, Maupile S, Babajko S. Les hypominéralisations molaires–incisives (MIH): prévalence, étiologie et pratique médicale. Revue d'Odonto-Stomatologie. 2016;**45**:234-250

[79] Dietrich G, Sperling S, Hetzer G. Molar incisor hypomineralization in a group of children and adolescents living in Dresden (Germany). European Journal of Paediatric Dentistry. 2003;**4**(3):133-137

[80] Cho SY, Ki Y, Chu V. Molar incisor hypomineralization in Hong Kong Chinese children. The International Journal of Paediatric Dentistry. 2008;**18**:348-352. DOI: 10.1111/j.1365263 X.2008.00927.x

[81] Jalevik B. Prevalence and diagnosis of molar-incisor-hypomineralisation (MIH): A systematic review. European Archives of Paediatric Dentistry. 2010;**11**(2):59-64. DOI: 10.1007/ BF03262714

[82] Benkirane L, Boukhari S, Gridech FZ. Prévalence de l'hypominéralisation incisive et molaire chez les enfants scolarisés de Casablanca. Odontostomatologie tropicale. 2017;**40**(159):46-52

[83] Fteita D, Ali A, Alaluusua S. Molar incisor hypomineralization in a group of school aged children in Benghazi, Libya. European Archives of Paediatric Dentistry. 2006;**7**(2):92-95

[84] Kemoli A. Prevalence of molar-incisor hypomineralization in six to eightyear old in two rural divisions in Kenya. East African Medical Journal. 2008;**85**:514-519

[85] Oyedele TA, Folayan MO, Adekoya-Sofowora CA. Prevalence, pattern and severity of MIH in 8- to 10- year- old school children in Ile-Ife, NIgeria. European Archives of Paediatric Dentistry. 2015;**16**(3):277-282. DOI: 10.1007/ s40368-015-0175-y

[86] Schwendicke F, Elhennawy K, Reda S. Global burden of molar incisor hypomineralization. Journal of Dentistry. 2018;**68**:10-18

[87] Kevrekidou A, Kosma I, Arapostathis K. Molar incisor hypomineralization of eight- and 14-year-old children: Prevalence,

severity, and defect characteristics. Pediatric Dentistry. 2015;**37**(5):455-461

[88] Alaluussua S. Aetioloy of molar-incisor hypomineralization: A systematic review. European Archives of Paediatric Dentistry. 2010;**11**(2):53-58

[89] Jacobsen PE, Henriksen TB, Haubek D. Developmental enamel defects in children prenatally exposed to anti-epileptic drugs. PLoS One. 2013;**8**(3):e58213. DOI: 10.1371/journal.pone.0058213

[90] Lygidakis NA, Dimou G, Griseniou E. Molar incisor hypomineralization, aretrospective clinical study in greek children II. Possible medical aetiological factors. European Archives of Paediatric Dentistry. 2009;**9**(4):207-217. DOI: 10.1007/BF03262637

[91] Americano GC, Jacobsen PE, Soviero VM. A systematic review on the association between molar incisor hypomineralization and dental caries. The International Journal of Paediatric Dentistry. 2017;**27**(1):11-21

[92] Weerheijm KL, Duggal M, Mejàre I. Judgement criteria for molar-incisor hypomineralization (MIH) in epidemiologic studies: A summary of the European meeting on MIH held in Athens 2003. European Journal of Paediatric Dentistry. 2003;**4**:110-113

[93] Steffen R, Kramer N, Bekes K. The Wurzburg MIH concept: The MIH treatment need index (MIH TNI): A new index to assess and plan treatment in patients with molar incisor hypomineralisation (MIH). European Archives of Paediatric Dentistry. 2017;**18**:355-361. DOI: 10.1007/s40368-017-0301-0

[94] Garot E, Veschambre CC, Manton DJ. Differential diagnoses of enamel hypomineralisation in an archaeological context: A post-medieval skeletal collection reassessment. International Journal of Osteoarchaeology. 2019. DOI: 10.1002/oa.2785 (Version of Record online:28 June 2019)

[95] Jalevic B, Klingberg GA. Dental treatment, dental fear and behavior management problems in children with severe enamel hypomieralization of their permanent first molars. The International Journal of Paediatric Dentistry. 2002;**12**(1):24-32. DOI: 10.1046/j.0960-7439.2001.00318.x

[96] Lagarde M, Pujade C, Wulfman C. Les hypominéralisations molaires-incisives (MIH): quelle restauration pour les PMP en cas d'atteinte sévère? RFOP. 2019;**14**(1):9-17

[97] Almuallem Z, Busuttil NA. Molar incisor hypomineralization (MIH)—An overview. The British Dental Journal. 2018;**225**:601-609

[98] Lygidakis NA, Wong F, Jalevick B. Best clinical practice guidance for clinicians dealing with children presenting with MIH: An EAPD policy document. European Archives of Paediatric Dentistry. 2010;**11**(2):75-81. DOI: 10.1007/BF03262716

[99] Elhennawy K, Schwendicke F. Managing molar-incisor hypo-mineralization: A systematic review. Journal of Dentistry. 2016;**55**:16-24. DOI: 10.1016/j.jdent.2016.09.012

[100] Tilotta F, Lautrou A, Lévy G. Anatomie dentaire. Elsevier Masson; 2018

[101] Kennedy DB. Management of an ectopically erupting permanent mandibular molar: A case report. Pediatric Dentistry. 2008;**30**(1):63-65

[102] Yaseen SM, Naik S, Uloopi KS. Ectopic eruption—A review and case report. Contemporary Clinical

Dentistry. 2011;**2**(1):3-7. DOI: 10.4103/0976-237X.79289

[103] Frank CA. Treatment options for impacted teeth. The Journal of the American Dental Association. 2000;**131**(5):623-632

[104] Polder BJ, Van't Hof MA, Van der Linden FP, Kuijpers-Jagtman AM. A meta-analysis of the prevalence of dental agenesis of permanent teeth. Community Dentistry and Oral Epidemiology. 2004;**32**(3):217-226

Chapter 12

Orthodontic Management of Residual Spaces of Missing Molars: Decision Factors

Hakima Aghoutan, Sanaa Alami, Amal El Aouame and Farid El Quars

Abstract

In the daily practice, the orthodontist may be confronted with particular clinical situations with one or more missing teeth. This can complicate the therapeutic plan and influence the choice of possible extractions imposed by treatment requirements. In case of permanent molar absence, making decision becomes even more delicate. The practitioner must use his/her critical sense and clinical common sense to make the right choice between closing and redeveloping the residual spaces. Its choice must meet the patient's expectations and correct the clinical problem without risking overtreatment, or extending duration care. Several factors guide the therapeutic decision, ranging from the patient's age to economic factors, not to mention the technical complexity, therapeutic predictability, and patient comfort, which determine proper compliance and therefore success. In this chapter, we will focus on these decision-making factors by determining the scientific evidence level in terms of success, survival, and patient-centered outcomes (quality of life and functional efficiency).

Keywords: missing permanent molars, first permanent molar, second permanent molar, orthodontic management, decision factors, adult, children, space closure, space reopening, multidisciplinary treatment

1. Introduction

Orthodontic treatment aims globally to improve dentofacial esthetic and stomatognathic system functions in harmony with the patient's wishes. To achieve these objectives, inter- and intra-arch occlusion is the guiding field of action. Therefore, any orthodontic movement must be carefully considered including in the molar area. Indeed, permanent molars are considered as significant determinants for normal tooth development and facial growth [1, 2]. They play a central role in the mastication of food, in supporting the vertical dimension of the face, and as anchorage teeth against orthodontic forces [3]. Moreover, posterior dental contacts are important to adapt and coordinate growth between the mandible and maxilla and a lack of chewing function in children will disrupt their maxillofacial growth [1, 4]. Hence, every orthodontist must ensure a well-thought-out management of missing molar spaces mostly in children.

IntechOpen

The molar missing may be primary, due to the agenesis phenomenon, or secondary to extraction not compensated by prosthetic rehabilitation. It complicates decision-making process, since the orthodontist's first vocation is to balance dentofacial pattern with a better cost-benefit ratio, especially in young patients. What is more, molar absence is generally accompanied with other complicated dental and skeletal problems, which affect treatment planning and outcomes.

Molar agenesis may be an isolated anomaly or associated with particular syndromes. It is an uncommon clinical condition not well documented in the literature. Moreover, it has also been reported that anterior agenesis may depend more on genes while posterior missing might be sporadic [5]. Its prevalence rate has been reported to fluctuate between 0 and 0.05% in the general population for the first permanent molar (FPM) [1] and to revolve around 0.8% for the second permanent molar (SPM) [4]. This phenomenon was reported to be associated with a higher prevalence of other permanent tooth agenesis and advanced tooth agenesis [3]. Consequently, when treating patients with molar agenesis, the orthodontist should consider that observed alterations of craniofacial dimensions might occur beyond the variations associated with age and gender [6].

On the other hand, in case of acquired lack of molars, many factors can be incriminated. Carious lesions, dental hypoplasia including molar-incisor hypomineralization (MIH), and periodontal disease are the major concerns [7, 8]. Several authors have dealt with the best time to extract first permanent molar when this is unavoidable in the young patient. There is only little scientific evidence about the extraction timing in order to minimize unwanted negative effects. In a recent meta-analysis [6], authors suggested that it is when the second permanent molar is at Demirjian stage E. Otherwise, several consequences can occur and if orthodontic need arises, the treatment plan can be complicated or modified to adapt to these modifications, especially in adults.

In this section, we will address the main etiologies and dentoskeletal consequences of molar missing and focus on decision-making factors related to orthodontic management of residual space of one or several missing molars. We will discuss some clinical situations to illustrate this topic.

2. Problem statement

The consequences of permanent molar extraction and all consequences and treatment considerations have been largely discussed in the literature for the first molar. Second molar is less commonly addressed. Currently, the majority of first permanent molars are extracted because of dental caries [9]. The eruption of the first permanent molar occurs, as its name suggests, around the age of 6 years. Its early eruption, as well as the immaturity of its histological components and its occlusal anatomy (grooves, pits, and fissures), makes it vulnerable to various microbial, periodontal, or structural pathologies, and more prone to possible premature extraction before 15 years [6, 10]. The period between the eruption of the tooth and the definitive maturation of its histological components, especially that of the enamel, is considered to be cario-susceptible.

As said above, permanent molars act as a guide for the permanent teeth since they control the establishment of dental occlusion and participate in the maxillary growth and physiology of the mandibular apparatus. Therefore, loss of permanent molars without any remedy could disturb the developing dentition, generate numerous malocclusions, and affect dental health [6]. It typically leads to occlusal disturbances by pathological migration of neighboring teeth and periodontal lesions as alveolar melting or false periodontal pocket adjacent to the tipped teeth which is induced by bone contour remodeling following the cementoenamel junction [11] (**Figures 1–3**).

These complications are all the more serious, as the period of molar absence on the arch is extended; hence, the importance of the multidisciplinary approach with a large communication between the pediatric dentist and the orthodontist in order to establish the best care and to plan potential extraction, which is useful to correct discrepancies and prevent the development of malocclusions [10].

For managing this space problem, the orthodontist can adopt two therapeutic strategies including space reopening or space closing. The orthodontist ought to use his/her critical sense and clinical common sense to make the right choice, which must not only take into consideration dental arch length and occlusion [12] but also all the technical and biological specificities of treated case. Space can be reopened for implant insertion, autotransplantation, and prosthetic restoration; while space closing can be undertaken to correct the other associate malocclusions. Either way, his/her choice must meet the patient's expectations and correct the clinical problem

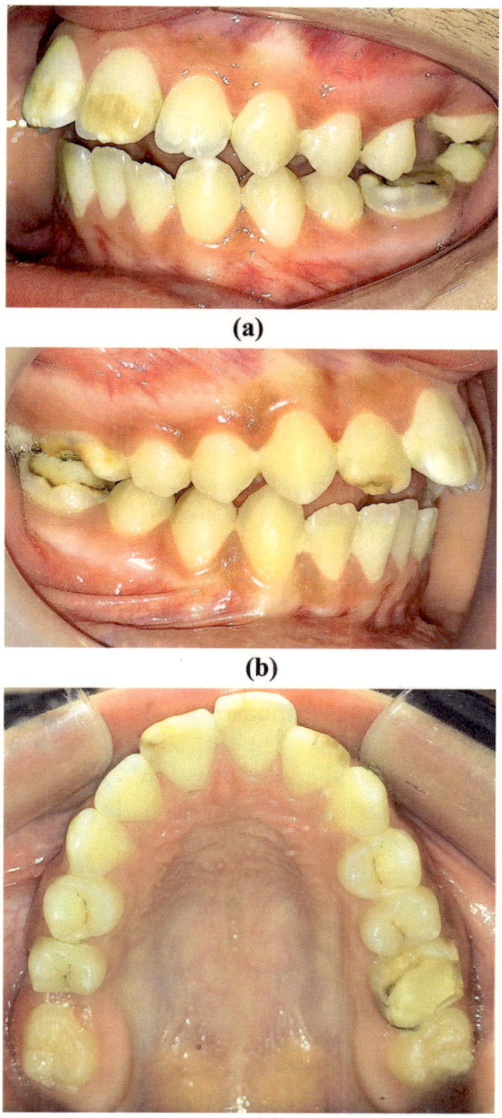

(a)

(b)

(c)

Figure 1.
Case of MIH in a 11-year-old boy, with severe molar damage and loss of 26. We can observe displacement of second left upper molar: (a and b) lateral occlusion views; (c) occlusal view of maxillary arch.

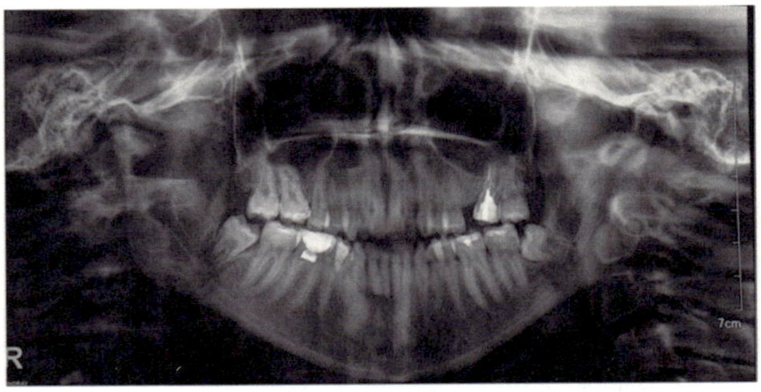

Figure 2.
Orthopantomogram (OPG) of an adult showing the absence of 16 and 26 with version and false periodontal pocket in the mesial side of 17 and 27. We can note the low floor level of the right maxillary sinus, which may complicate orthodontic mesial movement of posterior teeth.

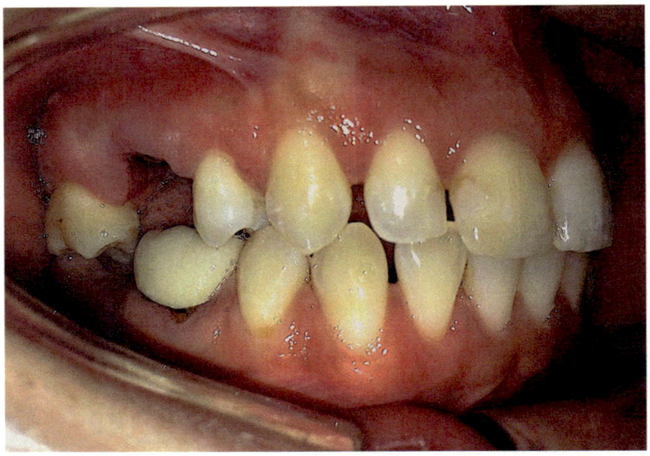

Figure 3.
Case of an adult with multiple molars missing. The over eruption of 17 is due to no-compensated extraction of 47.

without risking overtreatment, or extending duration care, especially since patients with missing molars often need a compensatory treatment in the opposite arch.

Besides, some authors [11, 13, 14] claim that space closure by molar orthodontic movement is time-consuming and more problematic mainly in the mandibular arch and in atrophic extraction sites exhibiting a reduction in vertical height and a decrease in width of the residual ridge. The orthodontist must avoid teeth tipping, damage of the gingiva and marginal bone. Hence, this decision requires confrontation with the alternative prosthetic treatment especially in old adults who usually show less bone apposition around moved molars into the narrowed space, and poor stability of the closed space, leading in some, if not several, cases to an orthodontic compromise. Nevertheless, fixed appliances can achieve excellent outcomes at different ages following permanent molars' loss particularly with the advent of temporary anchorage devices. Studies have reported that posterior spaces have been closed by protracting posterior teeth, which prevent detrimental effects without reopening of the edentulous spaces or increased pocket depth in the follow-up period [15]. In case of related orthodontic abnormalities, it is necessary to use all or part of the space given by molar extraction to correct the dysmorphy. A golden rule is to determine the anchorage value and location as well as any associated auxiliary devices.

On the other hand, before any prosthetic rehabilitation succeeding space redevelopment, the practitioner has to upright and to parallelize the adjacent teeth in order to gain sufficient space, even apically at the root level [14]. Moreover, in these cases, wisdom teeth are often removed [16]. Consequently, the orthodontist has always to wonder which of the two options is better: (a) close residual molar space to control the wisdom tooth positioning or (b) remove the third molar and place a prosthesis on the missing molar, which is more expensive. Obviously other biomechanical considerations must be taken into account, to be explained later.

On another note, over the years of craniofacial growth, teeth and their supporting tissues are able to adapt to functional demands. Thus, continuous changes are observed after tooth missing, and the orthodontist has to choose optimal treatment for his/her patient taking into account several decision factors. In his literature review [14], Thilander has shown that both closure and space opening alternatives have their advantages as well as disadvantages, but the evidence base is weak, with currently no randomized trials reporting on the outcome of different interventions [9]. More research is needed with relevant clinical follow-up, varying craniofacial morphology, different ages, and large sample. This will be of great value for comprehension of tissue reaction to orthodontic space management and continuous changes of the dentition and its supporting tissues. From then on, treatment choice can be standardized.

3. Clinical features

The direct consequence of molar extraction is the creation of a 10- to 12-mm diastema. The movements of the neighboring and antagonistic teeth will cause occlusal and periodontal imbalance. It was reported that post-extraction migration occurred in the following ways: over eruption of opposing teeth, horizontal migration of neighboring teeth, space reduced by tipping, dual drift (horizontal and vertical), or complete space closure [6]. In addition to this, authors investigated contour changes of the alveolar processes of posterior extraction sites and demonstrated a reduction in width of the residual alveolar ridge of up to 50% during a 12-month healing period, of which two-thirds of the reduction occurred within the first 3 months of healing in [17]. In case of an extraction on one arch, the opposing tooth can significantly over erupt (**Figures 4** and **5**). In general terms, malocclusions are complicated by the early loss of a first permanent molar without treatment [10].

Moreover, sinus pneumatization was identified after extraction of maxillary posterior teeth. This phenomenon occurs within 4–6 months of healing duration, and is caused by atrophy associated with the replacement of dental socket by non-functional bone [18, 19]. The expansion of the sinus was larger following extraction of teeth enveloped by a superiorly curving sinus floor, extraction of several adjacent posterior teeth, and extraction of second molars in comparison with first molars [19].

A systematic review reported that the post-extraction space of first permanent molar was closed mostly by the SPM rather than by the second premolar [6]. For certain authors [20, 21], no significant relation was found between patient Angle's Classification or the timing of FPM extraction based upon SPM development stage and complete spontaneous space closure in both arches, contrary to the usual recommendations indicating that the ideal time for FPM extraction, with fewer undesirable consequences, is when the SPM is at Demirjian stage E (early bifurcation) [6, 9]. For these authors, apart from extraction timing of the FPM, the presence of the third permanent molar, mesioangulation of the SPM in relation to the FPM, and the engagement of second premolar in the bifurcation of the second primary molar are better predictors of spontaneous space closure of the FPM mainly in mandibular arch where closure space is more problematical and leads frequently to mesial tipping and distobuccal rotation of the SPM or angulation and distal movement of the second premolar. This might be due to the differences in the eruption paths of SPM in the mandible and maxilla [10].

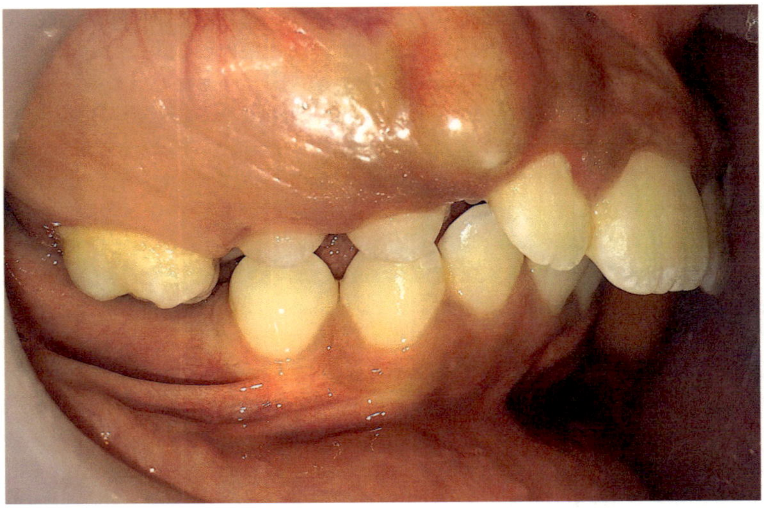

Figure 4.
Over eruption of tooth 16 after extraction of tooth 46.

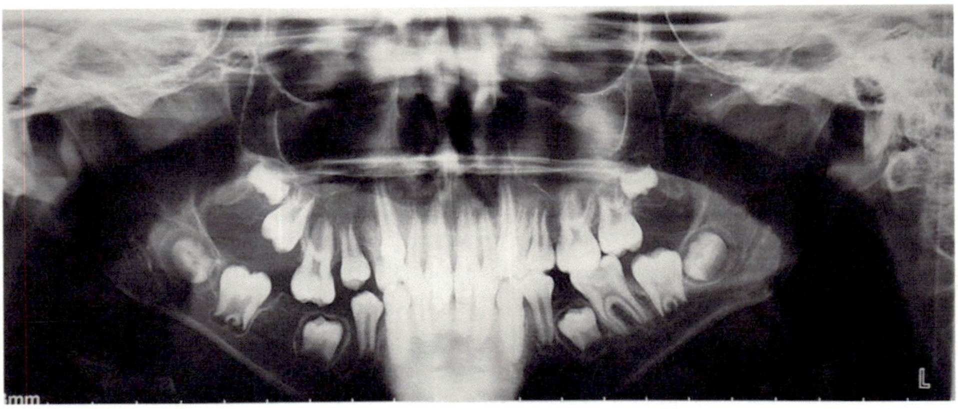

Figure 5.
OPG of the same patient showing the consequences of extraction of tooth 46: over eruption of 16, distal displacement of 45 germ and slight mesial displacement of 47.

The occlusal and skeletal consequences in the vertical direction after extraction of FPM were much discussed. Some authors noted counterclockwise rotation of the occlusal plane and an improvement in infraclusion [6, 13] but most studies did not notice a significant influence on the vertical dimension [6]. Also, there was no significant effect described on the maxillomandibular relationship in the anteroposterior direction.

Furthermore, it was stated that the FPM and SPM extraction accelerated significantly the development and eruption of the third molars when a posterior space is created [13, 22–24] and led to lingual tipping and retrusion of incisors mostly in lower arch [6]. However, some authors have discussed the effect of various extraction patterns on provision of space both anteriorly and posteriorly within the arch and they highlighted the fact that FPM extraction seems to have less effect on the profile than premolar extraction [13].

Finally, in the aforementioned systematic review, the authors concluded that the published studies have too many weaknesses to draw sufficient evidence. Therefore, further prospective studies are needed to investigate the consequences of FPM extraction and to confirm the ideal time of this extraction.

4. Treatment choices

In patients with missing molar, a standard treatment plan does not exist. There are essentially two orthodontic treatment approaches to manage this problem, which are space closure or reopening for prosthetic replacements, and implant or autotransplantation. Several elements guide the therapeutic decision, ranging from the patient's age to economic possibilities, not to mention the technical complexity, therapeutic predictability, and patient comfort, which determine proper compliance and therefore success.

Patients with missing molars often manifest with many underlying skeletal and dental problems and a multidisciplinary approach is recommended and depends on several factors. The amount of crowding, type of malocclusion, facial profile, age of the patient, periodontal conditions, bone volume in alveolar process, vertical or horizontal growth pattern, the number of missing teeth, and the available space should be considered in treatment plan [5]. Moreover, all the consequences that occurred after an old extraction must also be taken into account since they determine the choice of the biomechanical system.

The main advantage of the space closure resides in the fact that the whole treatment can be finished immediately after completion of orthodontics. When possible, it must be systematically preferred because better longer term outcomes can be achieved without growth-related infraocclusion, blue coloring of the gingiva, or periodontal problems as the tooth has displaced along with its supporting tissues [5]. Additionally, orthodontic space closure will reduce the financial expenses for the patient along with resolving arch crowding or anteroposterior malocclusion. Nevertheless, space closure is one of the most challenging approaches to molar extraction cases [13]. Like any treatment, this procedure presents indications and contraindications that have to be rigorously considered. For example, in hypodivergent patients, the closure of the space cannot be indicated due to the muscular and cortical anchoring, making it difficult or impossible to move the molars horizontally and to reduce the overbite [25]. Likewise, the practice of compensating and balancing the extraction of lost permanent molars along with space closing should be discussed. It aims to preserve occlusal relationships and arch symmetry within the whole dentition. A compensating extraction is the removal of a permanent molar from the opposing quadrant, while a balancing extraction signifies the extraction of a permanent molar from the opposite side of the same dental arch [9]. The long-term prognosis of the remaining permanent molars, the developmental status of the dentition including third molars as well as the underlying malocclusion were the main decision factors for or against balancing and compensating treatment [9, 13].

As regards patient age, this result is of great interest for a young adult or an adolescent by guiding the erupting teeth into a stable occlusion and can be considered a cost-effective alternative to complex restorations that require replacement over the life span [20]. Indeed, despite cessation of statural growth, vertical growth of the face permits continued teeth eruption past puberty and could adversely affect the alignment of teeth after orthodontic therapy. Facial growth in the horizontal plane is ended significantly sooner than growth in the vertical plane predominantly in patients with vertical growth patterns [26]. Accordingly, if an implant is placed before growth and eruption completion, it will become in infraocclusion, as it behaves like ankylosed teeth while the adjacent teeth continue to erupt. The magnitude of the vertical changes after age 20 seems to have little clinical importance [26].

In other words, in case of residual molar space in children, it is largely indicated to choose closure option in order to avoid all restrictions related to the periodontal immaturity. In other cases where the extraction space is preserved in growing children, autotransplantation of the tooth is preferable to the implant option [25]. However, other parameters must be studied before deciding treatment plan.

On the other hand, in adults undergoing comprehensive orthodontic therapy, coexisting dental and periodontal problems require multidisciplinary treatment approaches to manage malocclusions often complicated by the migration of adjacent teeth into the extraction sites. Periodontal defects, multiple missing teeth, and atrophic extraction sites make it difficult to close all the extraction spaces, which require remodeling of cortical bone [11]. Also, adults show less bone apposition when moving molars into the narrowed space, poor maintenance of the closed space, and, in some cases, resorption of the second molar roots when moved in place of first molar [11]. Duration of treatment has to be considered and adapted to patient needs. For these reasons, the placement of an implant may be the treatment of choice for adults with missing molars. Be that as it may, this proposition may be in some instances valid for an adult patient whose biological and biomechanical therapeutic specificities must be kept in mind. Precise 3-D control of tooth movement during closure of extraction spaces is very important in meeting treatment goals. Second molar protraction is time-consuming and relatively difficult. Therefore, this treatment option may be justified only when the periodontal health of the protracted second molar is not compromised [24]. Protracting the molars may be advantageous for the patient by increasing alveolar ridge width that had previously been lost in the edentulous space. It should ideally be done before significant vertical bone resorption occurs [27]. In respect of orthodontic force system, bodily movement of molars can be obtained by using temporary skeletal anchorage devices and rational biomechanics [24]. Several authors have reported some useful clinical tips and tricks that surround providing this therapy [11, 13, 15, 27]: a long buccal hook, an uprighting spring, a toe-in bend in the posterior portion of the archwire with constriction, or a balancing lingual force can be used to prevent side effects such as posterior tooth tipping, mesial rotation, and buccal sweep.

Regardless of the chosen option, the fate of wisdom teeth must be assessed. The final success of the treatment depends on its satisfactory positioning [16]. So, it is important to evaluate angulation, eruption space, root developmental stage, and periodontal status of this tooth before deciding to close molar space [27]. Actually, space reopening is indicated when the wisdom tooth is absent.

Furthermore, closure can be difficult, in the maxillary posterior area with sinus proximity, because tooth movement through the maxillary sinus is limited. The increased difficulty of moving teeth in the maxillary sinus is similar to moving a tooth in the atrophic posterior mandibular ridge. In severe cases, the pneumatization can extend completely to the alveolar bone adjacent to the gap. This not only makes it difficult to move teeth through the sinus but also to place an implant without sinus wall lifting surgery [18, 19]. Closing the space should not be chosen as the usual treatment method, as it extends the duration of the treatment without predictable results.

5. Clinical cases

In this section, we will review some clinical cases with one or more missing molars and will justify our therapeutic choices for each situation.

5.1 Case presentation

Case no. 1 (**Figures 6–9**).

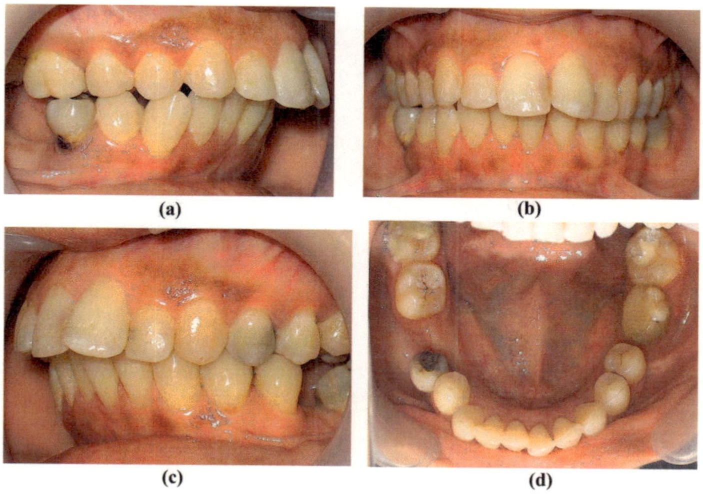

Figure 6.
Pretreatment intraoral photographs of a 32-year-old woman with 36 and 46 missing. We can note mesial tipping of 37 associated to a mesiolingual rotation. The space of 36 is more closed than that of 46. (a and c) Buccal occlusion views, (b) Frontal occlusion view, (d) Occlusal view of the lower arch.

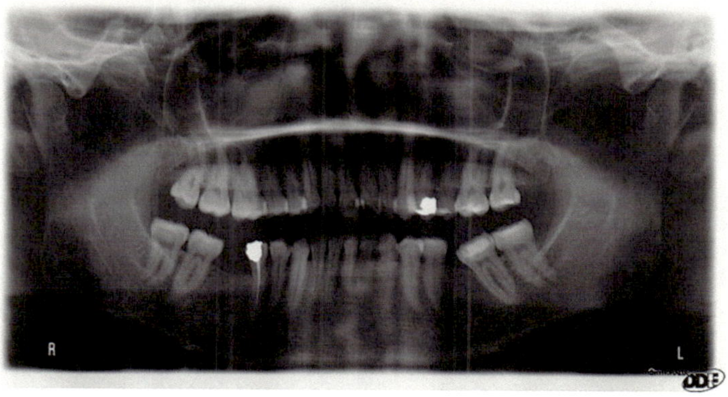

Figure 7.
Radiographic image of the mesial tipping of teeth 37 and 47, after extraction of lower FPM. Pseudo-pocket was formed adjacent to 37. Tooth 28 is absent.

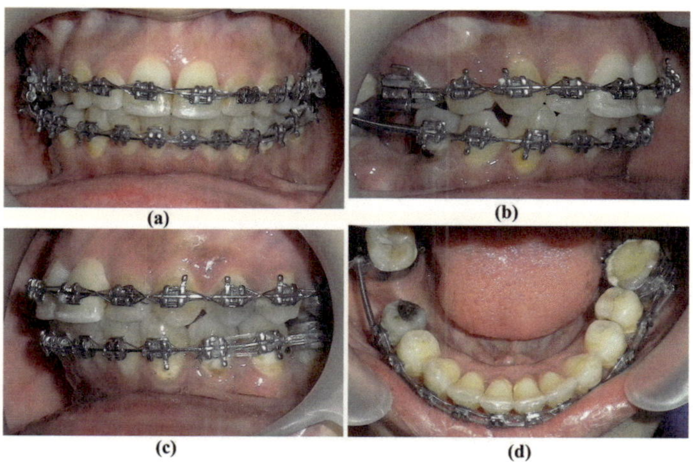

Figure 8.
Intraoral photographs of treatment progress. Extraction site of 36 was closed along with reopening of 46 space. (a) Frontal occlusion view, (b and c) Buccal occlusion views, (d) Occlusal view of the lower arch.

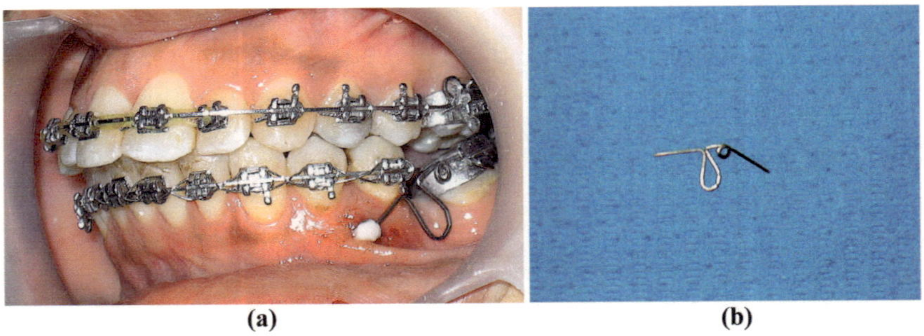

Figure 9.
Root correction and mesializing spring used to close left lower space with miniscrew-reinforced anchorage. (a) Buccal left occlusion view, (b) Design and activation of the spring used.

Case no. 2 (**Figures 10–13**).

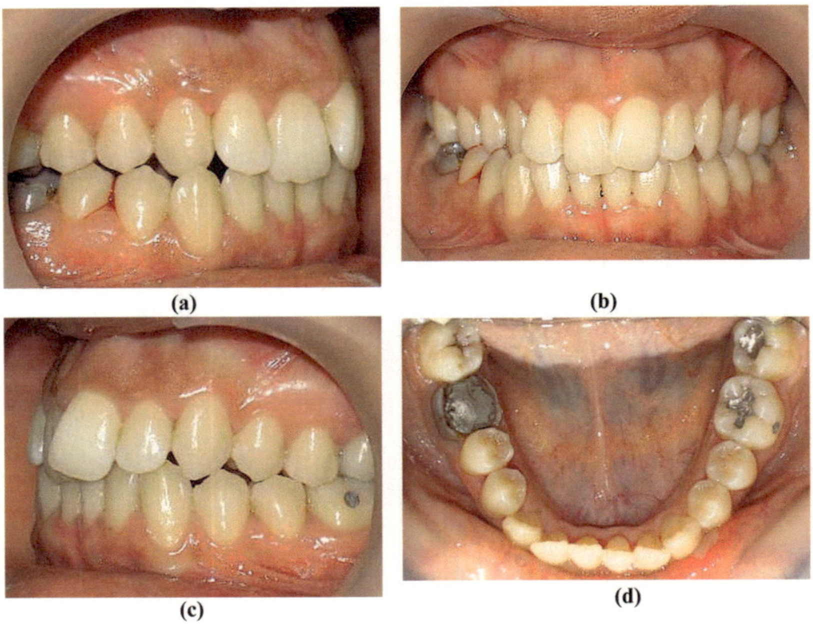

Figure 10.
This case of an adult shows dilapidated 46 with slight over eruption of 16 but not remarkable drifting of 47. (a and c) Buccal occlusion views, (b) Frontal occlusion view, (d) Occlusal view of the lower arch.

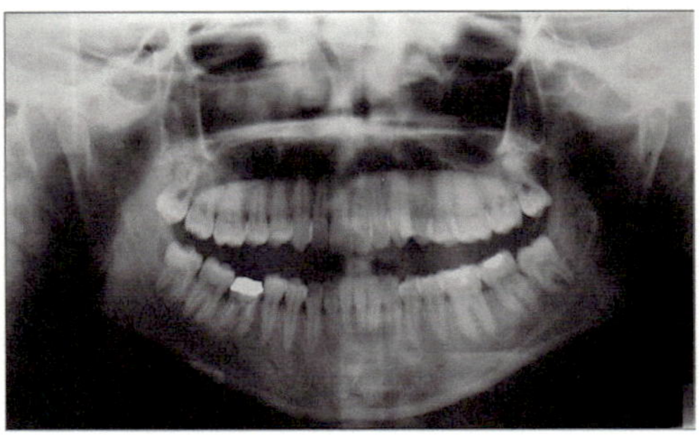

Figure 11.
OPG showing difference in molar level at the upper right side. Tooth 46 was unpreservable and enforced extraction was indicated.

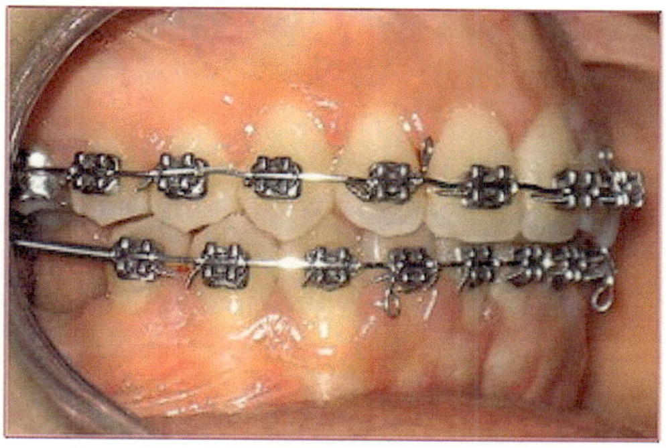

Figure 12.
Orthodontic treatment was undertaken with the objective to correct the malocclusion while keeping the 46 space.

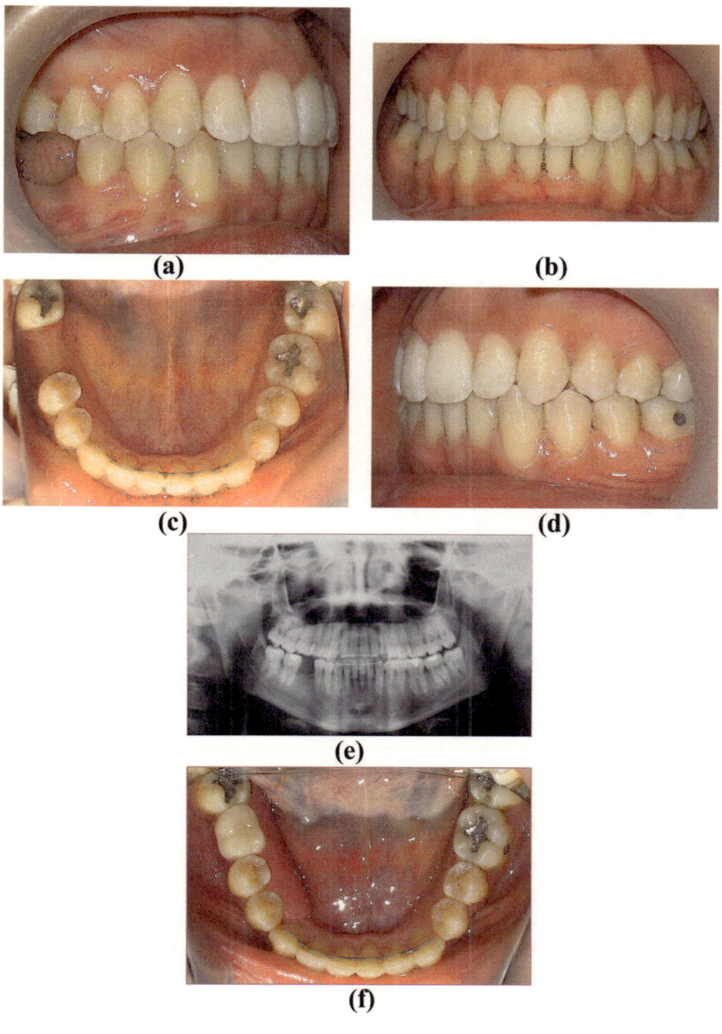

Figure 13.
Posttreatment illustrations. Correction of the dentomaxillary abnormality and prosthetic restoration of missing 46. (a and d) Buccal occlusion views, (b) Frontal occlusion view, (c) Occlusal view of the lower arch, (e) OPG showing the parallelism of the root axes, (f) Occlusal view of the mandibular arch with the provisional prosthesis of 46.

Case no. 3 (**Figures 14** and **15**).

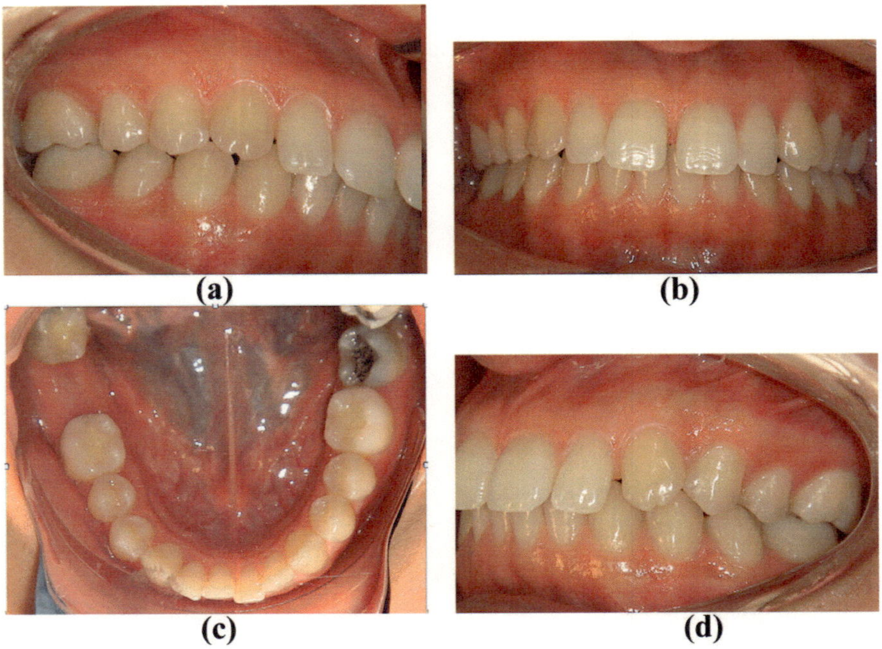

Figure 14.
Case of 47 extraction with large alveolar ridge and no notable migration of opposite and adjacent teeth, except for 48 that slightly drifted mesially. (a and d) Buccal occlusion views, (b) Frontal occlusion view, (c) Occlusal view of the lower arch.

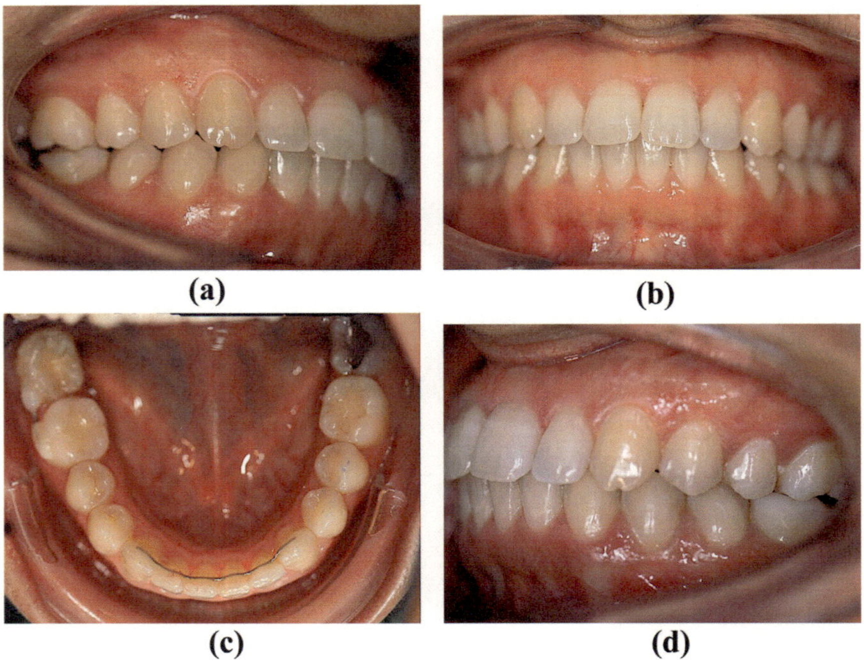

Figure 15.
Lower molar space closure was chosen. After mesializing tooth 48 in place of tooth 47, teeth 46 and 48 have been united to prevent space reopening in waiting for adaptation of periodontal ligament fibers. (a and d) Buccal occlusion views, (b) Frontal occlusion view, (c) Occlusal view of the lower arch.

Case no. 4 (**Figures 16** and **17**).

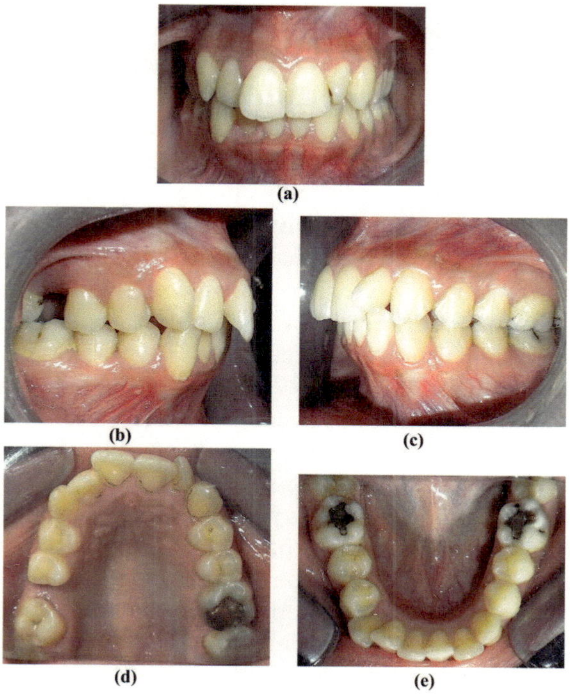

Figure 16.
Case of dentoskeletal class II with absence of 16. We can observe mesial tipping and mesiopalatal rotation of 17. The width of edentulous alveolar ridge was not very narrow. (a) Frontal occlusion view, (b and c) Buccal occlusion views, (d and e) Occlusal views of the upper and lower arches.

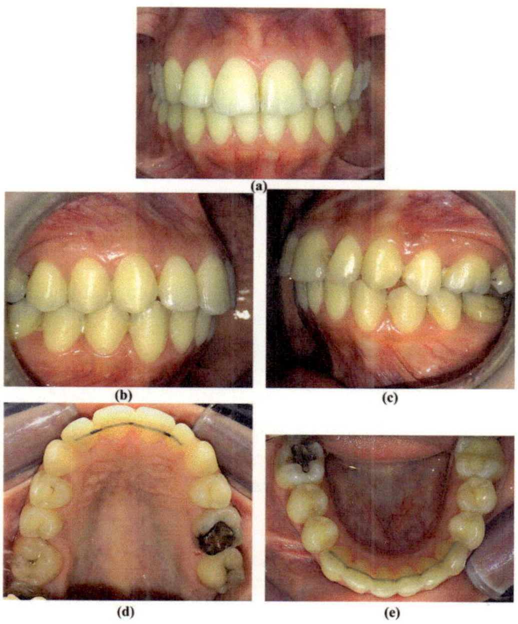

Figure 17.
Posttreatment intraoral photographs. Remaining space was used to correct dental class II relationship and to mesialize 17 in place of 16. In the left side, first bicuspid was extracted. Extraction of 48 was indicated to compensate upper right molars' mesializing. (a) Frontal occlusion view, (b and c) Buccal occlusion views, (d and e) Occlusal views of the upper and lower arches.

5.2 Case discussion

In all the cases presented above, the molar missing was due to dental decay. Indeed, it is the most common infectious disease worldwide [6]. According to the World Health Organization (WHO), 60–90% of school children have dental caries [6]. The molars are the most affected teeth as they evolve early.

When planning orthodontic treatment with molars missing, the patient age correlated to the amount of residual space, even apically, and the wisdom tooth condition are main decision factors described in the literature [1, 9, 16]. Patient wishes and cooperation must also be taken into account.

Case 1 concerns an adult woman who had chief complaints of upper incisors protrusion and smile asymmetry. She also wanted to resolve the residual mandibular spaces of missing 36 and 46 by the same orthodontic treatment. According to some authors [28], the ideal dimensions for the closure of the lower molars' spaces are 6 mm or less for the mesiodistal space and 7 mm for the buccolingual width. In this clinical case, the 36 space was almost closed. Furthermore, since tooth 28 was absent and tooth 18 was in functional occlusion, the treatment plan consisted of reopening the 46 space and completely closing that of 36. Also, due to mesial tipping of teeth 37, the mesializing movement was performed at the same time as the root correction using a miniscrew-supported spring. Temporary anchorage devices were indeed widely described and reported to be efficient in achieving accurate control of anchorage [15, 29] provided that the orthodontists master their biomechanics well. In case 3, as the space of lost 47 was quite large and the orthodontic abnormality not very complicated, the ideal choice was to maintain 47 space and a prosthetic rehabilitation. However, because of the absence of 18 in addition to a low economic profile of the patient, the residual space of 47 was closed at the expense of treatment duration.

In case 2 of an adult patient, all wisdom teeth have evolved and there was no need to extract to correct the anomaly. Thus, orthodontic treatment was undertaken while keeping the 46 space for a subsequent prosthetic restoration. By contrast, in case 4 that required premolars' extraction, remaining space of tooth 16 was used to mesialize 17 in place of 16 and to correct dental class II relationship with retraction of anterior teeth instead of taking out right first bicuspid.

In summary, in case of orthodontic management of molar absence, whether the residual space is closed or maintained, the control of the orthodontic movement including control of anchorage units and vertical forces as well as axial tipping and rotations is crucial to the success of the chosen therapeutic option [28].

6. Conclusion

In case of missing molars, orthodontic solutions consist of either closing or opening the space. A careful case assessment must be undertaken before treatment to ensure that the benefits of treatment will outweigh any potential risk of the treatment decided upon.

Space closure remains the best choice if the suitable conditions, notably in children whose prosthetic rehabilitation is still problematic and should be postponed until the growth and eruption process is completed. In adult patients, biological and psychological characteristics must be taken into account to achieve expected outcomes.

The decision-making process depends also on other factors like concomitant malocclusions, third molar development, absence of other teeth, and patient compliance. An orthodontic treatment based on reasoned biomechanic principles will help accomplishment of initial objectives in accordance with patient expectations.

In the majority of cases, treatment is complicated by all the side effects of the uncompensated absence of molars. Management is sometimes a veritable challenge. Hence, the prevention and early multidisciplinary management are of major importance.

Conflict of interest

The authors declare that they have no conflict of interest.

Author details

Hakima Aghoutan*, Sanaa Alami, Amal El Aouame and Farid El Quars
Department of Orthodontics and Dentofacial Orthopedics, Faculty of Medical Dentistry, Hassan II University, Casablanca, Morocco

*Address all correspondence to: hakimaaghoutan.2014@gmail.com

References

[1] Gupta M, Panda S, Mutawwam FA, Kariri FMM. Diagnosis and management of a patient with congenitally missing maxillary first permanent molars: A rare case report. Case Reports in Dentistry. 2016;**2016**: 3-5. DOI: 10.1155/2016/5891705

[2] American Dental Association (ADA). Tooth eruption—The permanent teeth. Journal of the American Dental Association. 2006;**137**:2006. DOI: 10.14219/JADA.ARCHIVE.2006.0031

[3] Abe R, Endo T, Shimooka S. Maxillary first molar agenesis and other dental anomalies. The Angle Orthodontist. 2010;**80**:1002-1009. DOI: 10.2319/020210-69.1

[4] Bondemark L, Tsiopa J. Prevalence of ectopic eruption, impaction, retention and agenesis of the permanent second molar. The Angle Orthodontist. 2007;**77**:773-778. DOI: 10.2319/072506-306.1

[5] Jamilian A, Darnahal A, Nucci L, D'Apuzzo F, Perillo L. Treatment considerations for missing teeth. In: Kivanç BH, editor. Dental Anatomy. Rijeka: Intech; 2018. pp. 109-120. DOI: 10.5772/intechopen.69543

[6] Saber AM, Altoukhi DH, Horaib MF, El-Housseiny AA, Alamoudi NM, Sabbagh HJ. Consequences of early extraction of compromised first permanent molar: A systematic review. BMC Oral Health. 2018;**18**:1-15. DOI: 10.1186/s12903-018-0516-4

[7] Williams JK, Gowans AJ. Hypomineralised first permanent molars and the orthodontist. European Journal of Paediatric Dentistry. 2003;**4**:129-132

[8] Rai A, Singh A, Menon I, Singh J, Rai V, Aswal GS. Molar incisor hypomineralization: Prevalence and risk factors among 7-9 years old school children in Muradnagar, Ghaziabad. The Open Dentistry Journal. 2018;**12**:714-722. DOI: 10.2174/1745017901814010714

[9] Cobourne MT, Williams A, Harrison M. National clinical guidelines for the extraction of first permanent molars in children. British Dental Journal. 2014;**217**:643-648. DOI: 10.1038/sj.bdj.2014.1053

[10] Eichenberger M, Erb J, Zwahlen M, Schätzle M. The timing of extraction of non-restorable first permanent molars: A systematic review. European Journal of Paediatric Dentistry. 2015;**16**: 272-278

[11] Saga AY, Maruo IT, Maruo H, Guariza Filho O, Camargo ES, Tanaka OM. Treatment of an adult with several missing teeth and atrophic old mandibular first molar extraction sites. American Journal of Orthodontics and Dentofacial Orthopedics. 2011;**140**: 869-878. DOI: 10.1016/j.ajodo.2010.06.027

[12] Yüksel S, Üçem T. The effect of tooth agenesis on dentofacial structures. European Journal of Orthodontics. 1997;**19**:71-78. DOI: 10.1093/ejo/19.1.71

[13] Sandy JR, Hons BDS, Atkinson R. For four sixes. American Journal of Orthodontics and Dentofacial Orthopedics. 2000;**117**:418-434. DOI: 10.1177/00220345420210051101

[14] Thilander B. Orthodontic space closure versus implant placement in subjects with missing teeth. Journal of Oral Rehabilitation. 2008;**35**:64-71. DOI: 10.1111/j.1365-2842.2007.01826.x

[15] Baik UB, Chun YS, Jung MH, Sugawara J. Protraction of mandibular second and third molars into missing first molar spaces for a patient with an anterior open bite and anterior spacing. American Journal of Orthodontics and

Dentofacial Orthopedics. 2012;**141**:783-795. DOI: 10.1016/j.ajodo.2010.07.031

[16] Bassigny F. What to do in case of a dilapidated or already extracted first molar? Justification for orthodontic option. Revue d'Odonto-Stomatologie. 2008;**37**:135-148

[17] Zhao L, Wei Y, Xu T, Zhang B, Hu W, Chung K-H. Changes in alveolar process dimensions following extraction of molars with advanced periodontal disease: A clinical pilot study. Clinical Oral Implants Research. 2019;**30**:324-335. DOI: 10.1111/clr.13418

[18] Cavalcanti MC, Guirado TE, Sapata VM, Costa C, Pannuti CM, Jung RE, et al. Maxillary sinus floor pneumatization and alveolar ridge resorption after tooth loss: A cross-sectional study. Brazilian Oral Research. 2018;**32**:e64. DOI: 10.1590/1807-3107BOR-2018.vol32.0064

[19] Oh H, Herchold K, Hannon S, Heetland K, Ashraf G, Nguyen V, et al. Orthodontic tooth movement through the maxillary sinus in an adult with multiple missing teeth. American Journal of Orthodontics and Dentofacial Orthopedics. 2014;**146**:493-505. DOI: https://doi.org/10.1016/j.ajodo.2014.03.025

[20] Teo TKY, Ashley PF, Parekh S, Noar J. The evaluation of spontaneous space closure after the extraction of first permanent molars. European Archives of Paediatric Dentistry. 2013;**14**:207-212. DOI: 10.1007/s40368-013-0042-7

[21] Teo TKY, Ashley PF, Derrick D. Lower first permanent molars: Developing better predictors of spontaneous space closure. European Journal of Orthodontics. 2016;**38**:90-95. DOI: 10.1093/ejo/cjv029

[22] Sebbar M, Bourzgui F. Predictive factors of third molar eruption. Revue de Stomatologie et de Chirurgie Maxillo-Faciale. 2011;**112**:263-268. DOI: 10.1016/j.stomax.2011.05.003

[23] Baik UB, Kook YA, Bayomec M, Park JU, Park JH. Vertical eruption patterns of impacted mandibular third molars after the mesialization of second molars using miniscrews. The Angle Orthodontist. 2016;**86**:565-570. DOI: 10.2319/061415-399.1

[24] Baik UB, Choi HB, Kim YJ, Lee DY, Sugawara J, Nanda R. Change in alveolar bone level of mandibular second and third molars after second molar protraction into missing first molar or second premolar space. European Journal of Orthodontics. 2019:1-6. DOI: 10.1093/ejo/cjz001

[25] Sayagh M, Maniere-Ezvan A, Vernet C, Muller-Bolla M. Décisions thérapeutiques en présence de premiéres molaires permanentes délabrées chez les sujets jeunes: Enquête descriptive. International Orthodontics. 2012;**10**:318-336. DOI: 10.1016/j.ortho.2012.06.001

[26] Fudalej P, Kokich VG, Leroux B. Determining the cessation of vertical growth of the craniofacial structures to facilitate placement of single-tooth implants. American Journal of Orthodontics and Dentofacial Orthopedics. 2007;**131**:59-67. DOI: 10.1016/j.ajodo.2006.07.022

[27] Baik UB, Kim MR, Yoon KH, Kook YA, Park JH. Orthodontic uprighting of a horizontally impacted third molar and protraction of mandibular second and third molars into the missing first molar space for a patient with posterior crossbites. American Journal of Orthodontics and Dentofacial Orthopedics. 2017;**151**:572-582. DOI: 10.1016/j.ajodo.2016.01.019

[28] Raveli TB, Shintcovsk RL, Knop LAH, Sampaio LP, Raveli DB. Orthodontic replacement of lost permanent molar with neighbor molar:

A six-year follow-up. Case Reports in Dentistry. 2017;**2017**:1-9. DOI: 10.1155/2017/4206435

[29] Raveli TB, Raveli DB, De Mathias Almeida KC, Pinto ADS. Molar uprighting: A considerable and safe decision to avoid prosthetic treatment. The Open Dentistry Journal. 2017;**11**:466-475. DOI: 10.2174/1874210601711010466

Chapter 13

Impacted First and Second Permanent Molars: Overview

Sanaa Alami, Hakima Aghoutan, Meriem Bellamine and Farid El Quars

Abstract

Impaction of a permanent tooth is a relatively common clinical occurrence in the human dentition. First mandibular molars and maxillary second molars are rarely impacted with a reported prevalence of 0–2.3% for second molars, 0.02% for the maxillary first molar, and of less than 0.01% for the mandibular first molar. The failures in their eruption mechanism may occur due to an obstacle such as the presence of a supernumerary tooth or an odontoma, lack of adequate space in the arch, an abnormal eruption path, or with idiopathic etiology. It is an asymptomatic pathology which is usually a casual discovery. Early diagnosis and treatment of permanent molars eruption disturbances contributes to optimal outcomes and favorable long-term prognosis by reduction of complication. The purpose of this is chapter is (1) to define prevalence and etiopathogeny of impacted first and second permanent molars, (2) to pinpoint the needs of earlier diagnosis, and finally (3) to highlight the treatment options.

Keywords: unerupted, impacted teeth, first molars, second molars, permanent molars, retained asymptomatic molars, uprighting molars, orthodontic treatment

1. Introduction

Impaction of a permanent tooth is a relatively common clinical occurrence in the human dentition. It mostly involves the mandibular and maxillary third molars, the maxillary canines or central incisors, and the mandibular second premolars while the first mandibular molars and maxillary second molars are seldom concerned. It deals with an abnormality of position in the wake of the failure of eruption [1].

Raghoebar et al. [2] suggested that teeth of the permanent dentition, of which the first and second molars, may fail to erupt either as a result of mechanical obstruction, such as the presence of a supernumerary tooth or an odontoma, lack of adequate space in the arch, or because of disruption to the eruptive mechanism itself, or idiopathic etiology.

This multifactorial origin disturbance entails various clinical forms. Thereby, a broad range of terms are used so as to illustrate this phenomenon: retention and impaction. In reality, each of these words designates various etiologic factors and involves an accurate diagnostic what leads to the prognosis and the treatment of such a disturbance.

This asymptomatic pathology is most of the time a casual discovery and may incite various pathologic conditions of neighboring and opposing teeth, such as caries, periodontitis or roots resorption, and eventually malocclusions. And so, it is an unpredictable situation dentists have to keep up with through the use of proper clinical and radiological assessment [2–5].

Indeed, optimal outcomes can be reached if both of diagnosis and treatment of such a disturbance are early done. However, multiple local factors are involved in the failure of eruption and influence its prognosis and treatment. Among them are inclination axis, stage of the root formation, and the depth of the molar, although their exact roles have not been established and the age of the patient is probably a key factor in the evolution of the cases [1–3].

The treatment options are based on the type of eruptive abnormality and the age of the patient, including observation, orthodontic or surgical approaches and extraction of the unerupted molar. Each approach has its indications, contraindications, advantages, and disadvantages [1, 2].

This chapter copes with an overview of this pathology and aims (1) to recall the mechanisms of normal and disturbed eruption, (2) to define prevalence and etiopathogeny of impacted first and second permanent molars, (3) to shed light on the needs of earlier diagnosis, and ultimately (4) to bring the limelight on the treatment options.

2. Normal and disturbed eruption of permanent molars

Eruption comes down to a process of biological maturation which involves the axial movement of a tooth from the developmental position within the jaw toward the functional position in the occlusal plane [1, 6]. The grounds of this biological mechanism remain unknown even if several hypotheses have already been argued. Amidst these hypotheses, root growth, hydrostatic pressure, and selective bone deposition and resorption are not sufficiently supported by experimental data.

Moreover, there is no denying that the periodontal ligament and the dental follicle provide the required force to generate this tooth eruption. However, although this theory is widely disregarded because eruption also occurs in its absence, it obviously remains the cogent argument. To sum up the foregoing, eruption is a multifactorial process in which the loss of one factor can be successfully offset by another [7].

The eruption of the first and second permanent molars is especially significant for the coordination of facial growth, and for providing sufficient occlusal support for undisturbed mastication [1, 6]. Their eruption differs from that of other permanent teeth in the sense that [2]:

- They do not have preceding primary teeth.
- Their development is sequentially initiated in the tuberosity of the maxilla and at the junction of the ascending and horizontal ramus of the mandible.
- As a result of the growth of the jaws, the relative position of the first molar shifts anteriorly at the time of the development of the second molar.
- At the beginning, the occlusal surface of the mandibular molars is mesial while that of the maxillary molars is distally inclined.
- During growth of the jaws, the crowns gradually move to an upright position.
- Just after emergence, half of the roots of lower first permanent molars and central incisors have been formed while three quarters of the roots of all other tooth have normally been formed.

Eruption disturbances of teeth are usual and can have a negative sway on the development of the tooth and jaw system. The clinical spectrum of eruption disturbances may vary from delayed eruption to failure of eruption.

Failure of eruption, unlike delayed eruption, is considered as the inability of the tooth to emerge in the oral cavity [1]. It may affect one or several teeth, in either the primary or the permanent dentition, and can be partial or complete. In this case, teeth may be totally covered by bone or soft tissue. In every instance, the failure is contingent on underlying etiology [8].

Average eruption ages have been established for each dental category; however, there is individual variability in the eruption pattern and dental development. First molars emerge on the mean at 6 years of dental age. Eruption of the permanent second molars occurs, typically, few months after primary second molars, and maxillary primary canines are replaced by their successors at dental age 12 [9]. According to Helm and Seidler, it normal emergence was defined as in the maxilla 12.4 and 11.9 years in the mandible, and 11.9 and 11.4 years for boys and girls, respectively [1, 6].

It is important to consider that 6-month delay in eruption of a permanent mandibular second molar compared with its contralateral counterpart or a 1-year delay in eruption of both molars should indicate a need for further radiographic investigation [9]. When eruption of a permanent tooth is at least 2 years behind schedule, disorder eruption should be suspected [3].

3. Epidemiology

Impaction of a permanent tooth most commonly involves the mandibular and maxillary third molars that accounts for more than 80% of all impacted teeth. In [9], the following teeth concerned by the impaction are the maxillary canines or central incisors and the mandibular second premolars themselves followed by first mandibular molars and maxillary second molars.

Failure of first and second permanent molars is rare. Their prevalence has only been reported in a few studies. Baccetti [6] found a prevalence rate of 1.7% failure of eruption of both first and second molars. According to Grover [1], for the first permanent molar, it stands for 0.01 and 0.06% in the case of the second one.

Palma et al. [1] and Valmaseda-Castellón et al. [5] found lower second molars to be the most frequently affected, followed by upper second molars. First permanent molar impaction is seldom, with prevalence rates of 0.02% for the maxillary and of less than 0.01% for the mandibular. As regards Grover and Lorton, they found that the prevalence rate of impaction of upper second molars is 0.08% of the population and 0.06% for lower second molars [5].

Likewise, Bondemark and Tsiopa [6] have determined the frequency of anomalies concerning the position and the eruption affecting the second permanent molar. In a point of fact, there is an overall prevalence of eruption disturbances of 2.3% including 1.5%, for ectopic eruption, 0.6% for primary retention, and 0.2% for impaction.

The findings in South Indian population, with an age range of 15–67 years, brought to the limelight that the prevalence of impacted second mandibular molars was about 0.16% [10].

Such rates explain that earlier studies have focused only on the prevalence of disturbed eruption of the lower second molar.

Furthermore, the prevalence of second lower molar seems to be linked to the age of the patient. The results show the frequency higher as patients are younger. Indeed, the prevalence in Sweden was estimated to be around 0.15% for cases between 10 and 19 years old according to Varpio and Wellfelt, while it accounts for 0.58% for 12-year-old Chinese children according to Davis. Shapira et al. found that the Chinese-American population was representing a higher prevalence (2.3%) of mandibular second molar impaction compared with the Israeli population (1.4%). Likewise, Shiu-yin Cho [9] found higher prevalence of 1% in Chinese schoolchildren.

As regards genders, some studies found a marked prevalence of this abnormality in males [1, 6]. On the contrary, other studies argued that there are more females with impacted lower second molars than males [3, 9, 10]. But in reality, not any significant difference has already been detected [3, 6, 9].

Additionally, the findings of some comparative analysis revealed that the prevalence of eruption has been increasing compared to the previous rates [1, 9, 11]. Evan et al. in their studies aimed to investigate the incidence of lower second molar impaction among two samples of 200 orthodontic patients referred to the Orthodontic Department of Bristol Dental Hospital consecutively in 1976 and 1986. Thereby they concluded in favor of this statement [11].

4. Etiopathogeny

Numerous local factors are involved in the failure of eruption, and they influence its prognosis and treatment. Teeth of the permanent dentition may fail to erupt either as a result of mechanical obstruction which could be idiopathic or pathological or because of the eruptive mechanism disruption [2]. According to Andreasen et al. [4], three main causes have been involved in the eruption disturbances. These causes include ectopic tooth position, obstacles in the eruption path, and failures in the eruption mechanism.

The failures of the eruption mechanism may occur due to the presence of an obstacle such as a supernumerary tooth or an odontoma, lack of adequate space in the arch, an abnormal eruption path, or an idiopathic etiology.

As a whole, causes of eruption disturbances, particularly failure of tooth eruption, could be categorized into general and local factors. It may depend on syndromic and non-syndromic problems for both kinds of factors [4, 6, 12].

- Systemic factors are present in patients with certain syndromes. Usually, multiple teeth are affected. However, eruption failure in the permanent dentition is associated with small number of syndromes [8] (**Figure 1**).

- In cases with local eruption disturbance, only one or a few teeth are affected. Local factors related to the failure of eruption include malocclusion disturbances of the deciduous dentition, the position of the adjacent teeth, lack of space in the dental arch, idiopathic factors, supernumerary teeth, odontomas, or cysts.

- Heredity is also mentioned as an etiological factor. Recently, mutations in parathyroid hormone receptor 1 have been identified in several familial cases of primary failure of eruption. Nevertheless, on occasion, the failure of eruption of first and second permanent molars is not associated with any systemic conditions or genetic alterations.

Differential diagnosis for these abnormal eruption patterns was not easy to identify either clinically or radiographically before starting the treatment.

We may conclude that the eruption disturbances of permanent molars may occur due to an impaction, primary retention, or secondary retention [1, 2].

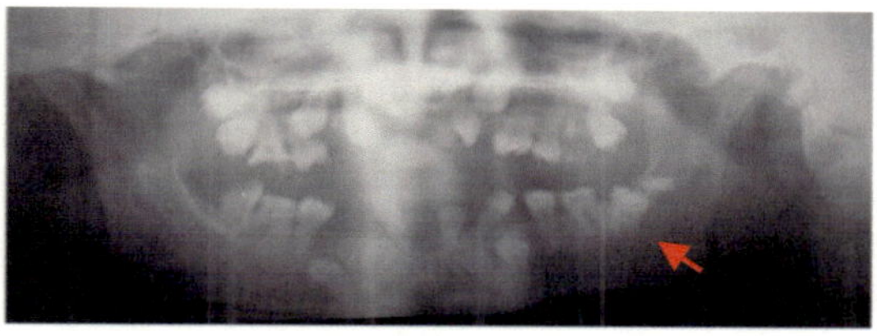

Figure 1.
Panoramic radiograph of a 17-year-old patient with mental and growth retardation. We can note the agenesis of 15, 31, and 48, as well as multiple retentions including 37 inclined distally and overlapped by the germ of 38.

These terms are used indifferently and often synonymously. The etiology of the three disorders is, however, different as is their diagnosis and treatment approach [13].

4.1 Etiology of impaction

Impaction is the cessation of the eruption of a tooth. Tooth was deemed to be impacted when its complete eruption to occlusal height was prevented by an abnormal contact with another tooth in the same arch [11].

The majority of cases are caused by a clinically or radiographically detectable physical barrier in the eruption path, which is independent of the eruption process. It may be supernumerary teeth and odontogenic tumors or cysts. Impaction may also due to an unusual orientation of the tooth germ [1, 2]. Idiopathic factors was also mentioned as other factor that cause impaction.

In most cases, the impaction of maxillary first molars is usually associated with an ectopic eruption path at a mesial angle to the normal path of eruption. It may be the result of failure of the molar to upright from its mesial inclination during eruption [2].

Insufficient space in the dental arches has been also considered as an etiological factor for impaction of second lower molar. It could be explained by the fact that the increase in arch length does not synchronize with the eruption of the second molar, more commonly in the mandible than in the maxilla [1, 11, 12, 14]. The erupting mandibular second premolar and second molar may quite often compete for space in the posterior area of the arch. When this space is inadequate, the earlier erupting second premolar may result in the impaction of the second molar [15].

In addition, the developing third molar may also compete for space behind and above the second molar, resulting in its impaction. Its potential involvement in the second lower molar impaction was suggested, due to its altered position caused by dento-alveolar disproportion. As a result, many authors recommended to extract the third molars, as prophylactic measure, to allow for correct eruption of the second molars in teenagers. However, the relationship between impaction of lower second molars and ectopic third molars is often a controversial subject. All the more so, at the usual age of eruption of the second molar, the third molar cannot constitute a barrier in the eruption path [1, 5].

4.2 Etiology of primary retention

Primary retention is synonymous of "unerupted" and "embedded." It is defined as cessation of eruption before gingival emergence, with neither a physical barrier in the eruption path nor being the result of (or and not due to) an abnormal position. The arrest of the eruption process occurs before the crown has penetrated the oral mucosa, and the non-resorbing bone occlusally of a primarily retained molar should be considered as a normal barrier in the eruption path [2, 16].

According to Raghoebar [8], primary retention is an isolated condition associated with a localized failure of eruption but no other identifiable local or systemic involvement. It may be caused by a defect in the eruption mechanism and is associated with a disturbance in the resorption of overlying bone. It is not due to an abnormality of the periodontal ligament; but the disturbance in the dental follicle constitutes the main etiological factor that fails to initiate the metabolic events responsible for bone resorption in the eruption trajectory. According to Raghoebar et al. [8], primary retention of permanent teeth is an isolated condition associated with a localized failure of eruption but no other identifiable local or systemic involvement.

4.3 Etiology of secondary retention

Secondary retention is synonymous of "submerged," "reimpaction," and "reinclusion." It refers to unexplained cessation of eruption after emergence, precisely after a tooth has penetrated the oral mucosa as reported by Raghoebar [8]. This abnormality occurs without the evidence of a physical barrier in the eruption path ectopic position, and it affects less frequently permanent molars than primary molars [2, 13, 16].

The etiology of secondary retention is not well understood. Trauma, infection, disturbed local metabolism, and genetic factors have been suggested as etiological factors. However, ankylosis is probably the main factor in its development. Raghoebar et al. [13] examined 26 secondary retained lower second molars, and they found that all of them had ankylosed areas. However, it is still not clear whether the state of ankyloses was a result of arrested eruption or if it was the primary cause resulting in arrested eruption.

All these factors present something of a diagnostic challenge to the clinician. It is important to distinguish between these three phenomena in order to understand the clinical features and to choose an adequate treatment.

5. Diagnostic approach

The failure of eruption is an asymptomatic pathology. That means that it is usually a casual discovery and its diagnosis is generally made late. It may incite various pathologic conditions on the permanent dentition such as caries, periodontitis, pericoronitis, and risk of root resorption of adjacent teeth as well as the situations leading to the loss of permanent teeth, incomplete development of the alveolar process, shortening of the facial height, and occlusal disturbances. Thus, it is suggested that these abnormalities should be diagnosed and treated at an early age [3, 5].

Indeed, prompt diagnosis is essential in order to improve prognosis and to palliate the consequences of the failure of eruption of permanent molars. It involves full medical history, and it appropriates clinical and radiographic examinations which are sufficient to distinguish clearly between impaction, primary, and secondary retention [1, 2, 17]. As eruption time may vary between individuals, an appropriate follow-up of children with mixed dentition is required at 6-month intervals to manage their eruption pattern and dental development, especially in cases of posterior crowding and when molar retention is suspected [9].

5.1 Clinical analysis

This is a crucial step in the management of these abnormalities. It is important to raise the civil age, which must be correlated with dental age in order to claim a possible eruption delay. A child is considered to be late toothed when the dental and civil ages differ by more than 2 years from the average values for permanent teeth.

In addition, it is imperative to note on questioning a history of trauma or infection as well as a possible notion of heredity, emphasizing a family history of eruption failure or ankylosis affecting at least one primary tooth [8]. This facilitates the identification of the clinical form of the abnormality according to possible etiological factors.

The clinical examination cannot claim to make a reliable diagnosis of dental impaction or retention. Only radiographic analysis will make it possible to conclude this and above all to decide between the three clinical forms, namely, impaction, primary, or secondary retention.

Some signs, although rare, could be characteristic of particularly secondary dental retention. Indeed, clinically secondary retention is usually suspected on the one hand when a molar is in infra-occlusion at an age when the tooth would normally be in occlusion (**Figures** 2 and 3) This is because the adjacent teeth continue to erupt but the growth of the alveolar process in the affected area stops. On the other hand, the involvement of ankylosis might be detected with the percussion test [3].

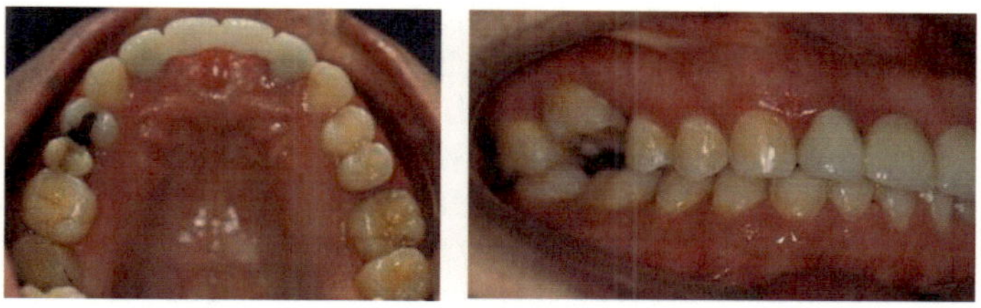

Figure 2.
Intraoral photographs showing arrested eruption of the tooth 16 after gingival rupture associated with an infraocclusion in this side and growth cessation of the alveolar process.

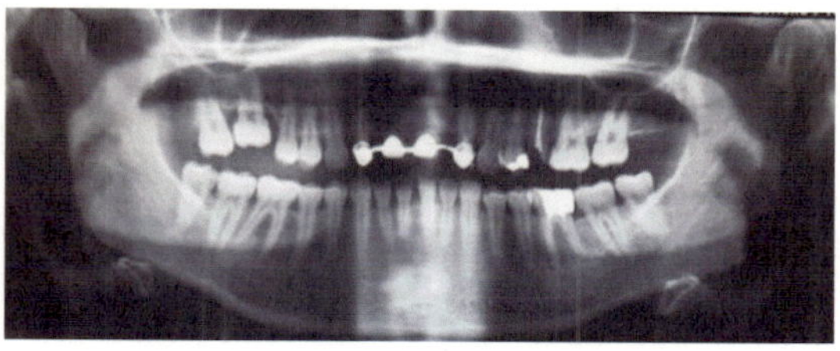

Figure 3.
The orthopantomogram revealed the absence of a physical obstacle and a vertical position of the tooth 16 related to secondary retention.

However, particular attention should be focused on the number of teeth with delayed eruption, referring to the contralateral tooth. A 6-month delay in eruption of a permanent mandibular second molar compared with its contralateral or a 1-year delay in eruption of both molars should justify suspicion of molar retention and should indicate a need for further radiographic investigation [9].

The involvement of ankylosis might be detected with the percussion test and radiographic evidence of the periodontal ligament obliteration. The scanner or the cone beam computed tomography are the only tools which may identify the ankylosis' diagnosis [3].

5.2 Radiographic analysis

Unerupted molar is often detected in a routine panoramic radiograph during pedodontic or orthodontic evaluation and treatment planning. But, it is usually not the main reason for referral to the orthodontist. Early detection and treatment is imperative to avoid possible complications and to eliminate the need for advanced orthodontic and surgical treatment [15].

The radiological examination must first conclude that the germs of unerupted molars are present. Also, as reported by Vedtofte [12, 18], it should also focus on registration of dental abnormalities in tooth retained and dentition in general such as:

- Root deflection dilacerations
- Taurodontism
- Invagination
- Resorption or tooth decay in adjacent primary or permanent teeth (primary molar or second premolar in case of impacted first molars, and first molar in case of impacted second molar)

Vedtofte and Andreasen [18] found a high prevalence of dens invagination and taurodontic in second lower molars with arrested eruption (**Figure 4**). They suggested that there was an association between morphological deviations and periodontal membrane malfunction, the latter causing eruption disturbances. Root dilacerations were also observed in arrested eruption upper and lower molars but they are not related to a particularly deep bony position of the molar. It could explain the association between root abnormalities and eruptive disorders in permanent molars [12].

In addition, some measurements must be recorded on the orthopantomogram as the angulation of impacted tooth and depth of retention. The inclination axis of the molars is measured from tracing long axis of unerupted teeth and adjacent teeth, perpendicular to the tangent to the tips of the cusps. The angle between these lines is measured for each side of the jaw in order to conclude an average value [9, 11, 12] (**Figure 5**).

The degree of non-eruption could be evaluated radiographically in millimeters of bone, from the alveolar ridge to the central fossa of the unerupted molar or vertical distance between distal marginal ridge of the first molar and mesial marginal ridge of the impacted second molar [1, 3] (**Figure 6**).

Because permanent teeth may fail to erupt either as a result of mechanical obstruction or disruption to the eruptive mechanism itself [2], both clinical and radiographical diagnosis approach should conclude in an impaction, primary, or secondary retention on the basis of the various etiological factors, which are as follows:

- The detection of mechanical obstruction and posterior crowding typical of molar impaction;
- The root growth stage;
- The signs of ankylosis characteristic of secondary retention.

5.2.1 Radiological characteristics of impaction

The orthopantomograph reveals, in this specific case, odontogenic cysts, odontoma, supernumerary teeth, or signs of insufficient space in the posterior side

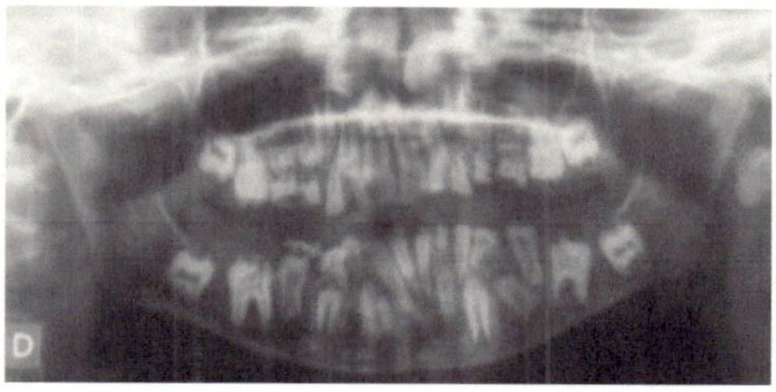

Figure 4.
Panoramic radiograph of a 13-year-old patient showing a delayed eruption of first and second permanent molars with intrapulpal calcifications and taurodontism of the first lower permanent molars and second lower premolars. We also note the reinclusions of the second temporary molars.

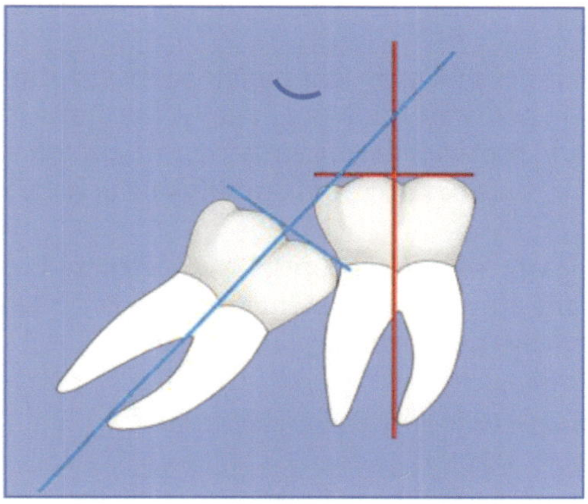

Figure 5.
Readapted from [11, 12]. Registration of angulation of impacted teeth from the angle between long axis of first and second lower molars. Angle greater than 40° means mesial inclination. Angle between 40 and −20° means vertical position. Angle less than −20° means distal inclination.

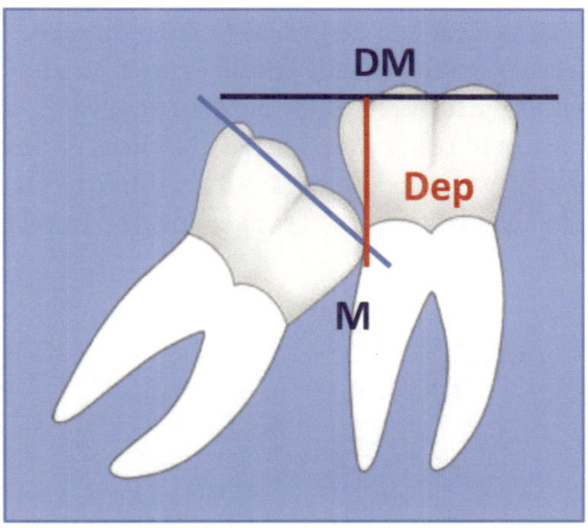

Figure 6.
Readapted from [3]. Registration of impacted teeth depth from distal marginal ridge of the first molar (DM1) to the mesial marginal ridge of the impacted second molar.

of dental arch as malposition of the tooth germs of the third molars overlapping with lower second molar.

The great majority of mandibular second molar impaction was associated with a degree of mesial angulation which could be radiographically seen as an oblique or even horizontal position of the tooth. A very rare case of an inverted impacted second molar where its crown was directed toward the lower border of the mandible was reported [15].

Nevertheless, when the first molar is affected, the radiographs show a mesial inclination and atypical resorption of the distal surface of the adjacent primary second molar. The main sign is the long axis which is not parallel to the normal eruption path [2].

5.2.2 Radiological characteristics of primary retention

Because the arrest of the eruption process occurs before the crown has penetrated the oral mucosa, the crown is often covered by bone and mucosa. Thus, the non-resorbing bone occlusally should be considered as a normal barrier in the eruption path [2, 16].

Primary retention is defined as an incomplete tooth eruption despite the presence of a clear eruption pathway. Radiographically, the molar is normally oriented in its eruption path, and roots are deeply situated and sometimes completely formed. The growth of roots has occurred apically due to bone resorption around the radicular portion [4, 16].

A follow-up of at least 6 months is necessary to detect radiographically whether the tooth is showing any eruptive movement or not, in order to make a differential diagnosis between primary and secondary retention.

5.2.3 Radiological characteristics of secondary retention

Ankylosis was suggested to be the main etiological factor in secondary retained permanent teeth. Histological study conducted by Raghoebar compared 26 secondarily retained molars removed in children group (mean age = 16.2 ± 3.9 years), with six normally erupted molars which were removed for orthodontic or prosthetic reasons [13]. The author found areas of ankylosis along the roots of all secondary retained molars located at the bifurcation and interradicular root surface in 81% of the cases.

Thus, it is difficult to specify the diagnosis of such disturbance only from orthopantomographs. Intraoral periapical radiographs allows to identify a periodontal obliteration and hypercementosis. The computed tomography scan represents supplemental examination to bring a definitive diagnosis of ankylosis [3].

Another factor in favor with the diagnosis of secondary retention is tooth position. Wellfelt maintains that ankylosis is often suspected in vertically positioned teeth (**Figures** 7 and **8**).

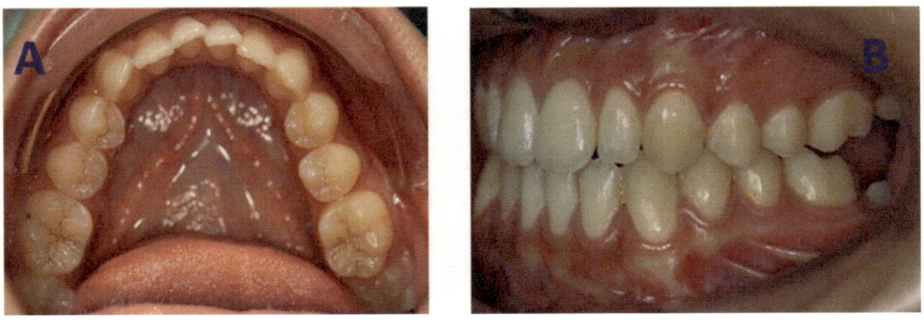

Figure 7.
Intraoral photographs (A) before treatment and (B) 2 years after orthodontic and surgical treatment, showing arrested eruption of 37 after gingival rupture, with no movement of this tooth related to secondary retention.

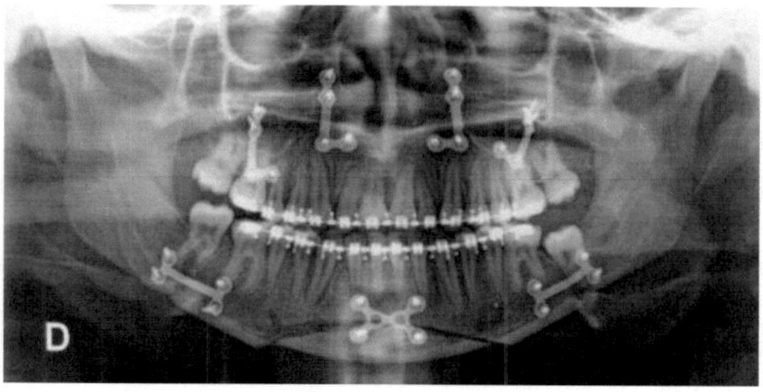

Figure 8.
Post-treatment panoramic radiograph revealed vertical position of retained tooth.

Finally, primary and secondary retention could be differentiated considering the stage during which the molar stops the eruption process [2]. In addition, the mesial angulation of the molars is characteristic of the impaction, whereas in the primary and secondary retention, tooth is rather vertical.

6. Treatment

The diagnosis characteristics of eruption disorders are different but the treatment approaches are identical in some cases. Primary and secondary retention of permanent molars reflects disturbances in a particular stage of the eruptive process, while impaction is due to a physical barrier or an abnormal tooth position and thus not directly related to a particular eruptive stage. It is important to distinguish between these three phenomena in order to understand the clinical features and to choose a suitable treatment [2, 8].

6.1 Decision-making factors of treatment

Multiple local factors are involved in the failure of eruption and influence its prognosis and treatment. We cite lack of space in the arch, dental anatomy, inclination axis, stage of the root formation, and the depth of the molar. Although their exact roles have not been yet established. The age of the patient is probably a key factor in the evolution of the case.

Several entities are an indicator of retention's severity and could influence the prognosis and treatment protocol of unerupted permanent molars. The following variables could be mentioned [1, 3]:

- Dental inclination,
- Degree of non- eruption,
- Stage of root formation,
- Age.

The inclination axis of the molars has certainly an impact on clinical treatment results [1]. Wellfelt [1] reported that the mesioangular inclination was most successfully treated because the ankylosis is often suspected in vertically positioned teeth, thus in secondary retention.

The degree of non-eruption or depth of the impaction seems to be a less decisive factor in the evolution than the stage of root formation. In fact, it was reported that when roots of the unerupted tooth are completely formed, the chances of successful treatment decrease [1]. Furthermore, Fu et al. found, in their study conducted on a Taiwanese population, that the impacted depth was highly and positively correlated with the initial uprighting period [3].

This could explain that patient's age is considered as a key factor in the prognosis of this disorder. Most pediatric population studies show that resulting malocclusions and abnormalities in adjacent and opposing teeth are frequent and start at very early ages. [5] Furthermore, we have mentioned that the age affects certainly the initial uprighting period, but it has a small impact on the performance and outcomes of the technique. Thus, these teeth malposition should be diagnosed and treated at an early age. Fu et al. suggested that there was a statistically significant relationship between poor evolution of the unerupted molar and the following factors: age over 14 and root formation of the unerupted molar in its last stages [3].

Finally, both diagnosis and treatment planning should be placed into the perspective of the patient's age, the stage of eruption, as well as of factors like the patient's needs and self-image [2]. Even if the disturbances do not occur frequently, it is important to develop an early diagnosis in order to start the treatment at the optimal time, between 11 and 14 years, when root formation is incomplete [3, 6].

6.2 Treatment modalities

Eruption disturbances may manifest clinically and radiographically as impaction, primary retention, or secondary retention. The treatment protocol for its management is based on the type of eruptive abnormality and the age of the patient. Treatment options include observation, surgical exposure or repositioning, orthodontic uprighting, and extraction of the unerupted molar. Each modality has its indications, contra-indications, advantages, and disadvantages.

Generally, as stated by Andreasen [8], the active orthodontic and/or surgical treatment is indicated in cases of impacted ectopic erupting teeth and primary retention. However, a primary observation period seems to be required before any intervention to confirm diagnosis through a radiographical follow-up. Spontaneous eruption into normal occlusion could occur in rare cases. Abstention is recommended in cases of secondary retention due to ankylosis, or deeply impacted lower second molars. Extraction may be the norm in case of failure of teeth repositioning.

Due to low frequency of impacted first molars, numerous studies and case reports are available regarding the clinical management of second molar disturbed eruption. All approaches and techniques can also be applied to unerupted first molars despite their low incidence.

6.2.1 Observation

Kavadia and others underline the importance of tight control of impacted lower second molars. They suggest that active treatment should only be considered after an observation period of at least 12 months exclude the possibility of self-correction [9].

So when the identified etiology is an obstacle, the early removal of the barrier usually allows the molar to erupt spontaneously.

Furthermore, abnormal position of the germ of a third molar may form a barrier causing impaction of the second molar. The recommended treatment is removal of the third molar at the age of 11–14 years in combination with a thorough follow-up of the eruption of the second molar [2]. In other cases, some clinicians advocate removal of the second molar allowing eruption of the third molar at its position [14].

Once the chance of self-correction has been ruled out, dentists should discuss with patients and parents the various treatment options for the impacted molars, which may include [9]:

- Orthodontic uprighting
- Surgical repositioning
- Extraction of the impacted second molar to allow the third molar to drive mesially
- Extraction of the impacted second molar and transplant of the third molar into the extraction site.

6.2.2 Orthodontic uprighting

Generally, as stated by Andreasen [8], the active orthodontic treatment is indicated in cases of impacted ectopic erupting teeth and primary retention. Orthodontic approach is important to provide a good occlusion and to reduce the risk of caries and periodontal disease and can be performed with or without extraction of the adjacent third molar. However, in cases of extreme horizontal impaction or widely diverging roots, orthodontic uprighting of permanent molars is contraindicated [2, 15].

The optimal moment for uprighting is when two-thirds of the roots have been formed, between 11 and 14 years old for second molar. Molars with fully formed roots have a poor prognosis [2].

Beyond age, orthodontic modalities are depending of mesial tipping and depth of concerned teeth. So, when orthodontics is indicated, an efficient mechanics plan is required [13]. Numerous methods can be considered:

- Conventional appliances
- Distalization segment wire
- Temporary skeletal anchorage.

All of these methods, however, have limitations, especially in the approach of deeply impacted teeth.

6.2.2.1 Conventional appliances

When a second molar is slightly mesially angulated with a sufficient emerging area, several devices have been suggested in the literature to correct simply this malposition such as separating elastic or brass ligature wire between tipped teeth and neighboring one. These artifices operate as a spring, relieving contact between the teeth and allowing "self-correction" and eruption [15].

Interarch vertical elastics and a removable appliance with an uprighting spring have been also reported [4].

The correction of this abnormality can also be done simply by including the impacted molar in the orthodontic treatment from the first stage of alignment and leveling of the orthodontic treatment. A tube is then bonded to the vestibular surface of the molar, which will be engaged in the continuous arch. Alignment and distalization will be ensured by superelastic arches and a push coil spring

(**Figure 9**). A variant of the same device can be proposed; the superelastic wire used for alignment and leveling of the teeth is curved distally of impacted molar which is engaged in the tube and bended on mesial (**Figure 10**).

Such methods might require considerable treatment time with the risk of extending the overall duration of orthodontic treatment. Indeed, since the arch sections cannot change, the leveling of the dental arches is delayed. This widely justifies the use of fixed auxiliaries as an efficient alternative.

6.2.2.2 Distalization segment wire/auxiliary spring fixed

A button, mini tube, or eyelet button is usually bonded on the visible area of the tooth. An auxiliary segment is constructed of flexible wire nickel titanium, copper Ni Ti, or titanium molybdenum alloy (TMA) with loop. This cantilever is generally placed after leveling of the dental arch, which is then used as stabile unity for distalization of impacted tooth. In fact, molar uprighting requires good anchorage control, and subsequently, a full-arch fixed appliance is necessary to protect from undesirable tooth movements [19]. Continuous 0.019 × 0.025 stainless steel wire from first molar to second premolar or first molar is recommended as an anchorage unit.

Then, NiTi wire can be used to upright the tooth. Finally, the tube is bonded to introduce the tooth into the conventional wire to complete leveling and finish treatment [14, 15, 20].

Various patterns have been revealed in the literature, from the simplest to the most complex, taking advantage of the elastic properties of wire alloys.

The 0.016 × 0.022 Ni-Ti or 0.016 × 0.025 Cu Ni-Ti may be used to distalize angulated molar. The segment wire is inserted between the retained molar and the neighboring tooth on the arch. Due to its superelasticity, the wire is curved and then bonded to the occlusal face of the adjacent tooth. A moment of force is generated resulting in move of the molar to the distal (**Figures 11** and **12**).

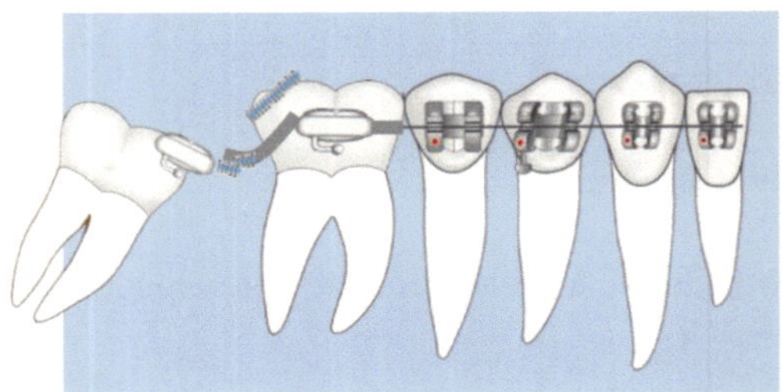

Figure 9.
Association of superelastic wire and coil spring between first and second lower molars.

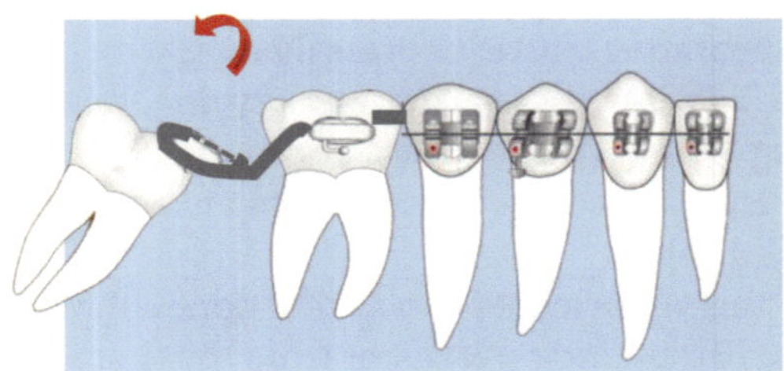

Figure 10.
Continuous superelastic wire curved in distal of second lower molar then introduced into the tube to achieve its distalization.

Like Fu et al. [4], the same sections of Ni-Ti or copper Ni-Ti can be used to upright orthodontically the mandibular second molar. The sectional wire is here ligated on the continuous wire that served to align and level the dental arch (**Figure 13**).

In other retrospective study, Fu et al. [3] described the pole arm appliance as an effective treatment modality and success predictable for impacted second lower molar.

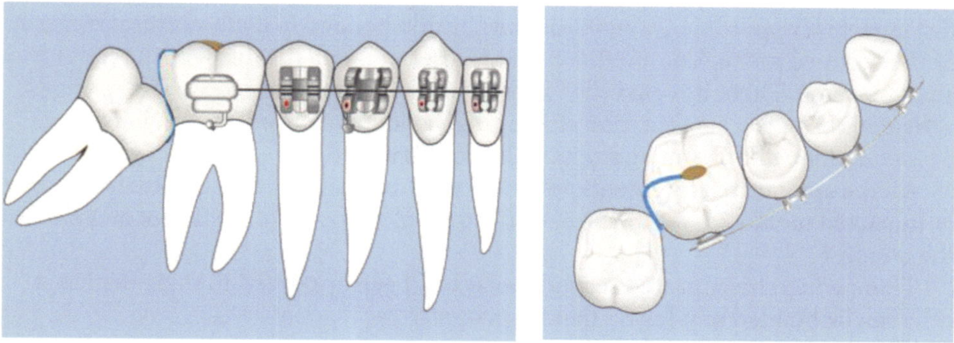

Figure 11.
0.016 × 0.022 Ni-Ti or 0.016 × 0.025 Cu Ni-Ti sectional wire, placed between first and second retained molars, is occlusally curved and bonded on occlusal face of first molar aligned on the arch.

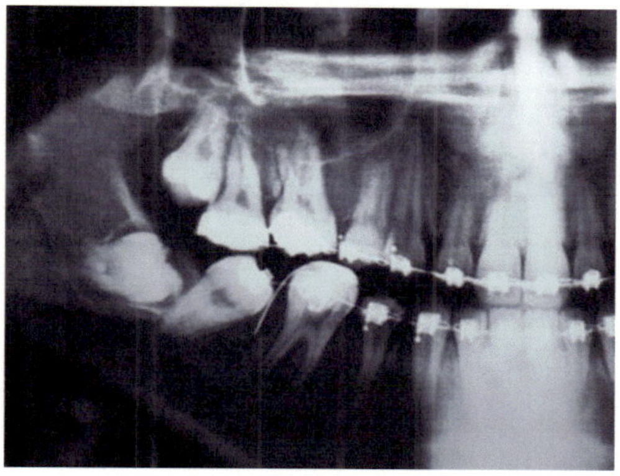

Figure 12.
Right quadrant of a panoramic radiograph illustrating the placement of the 0.016 × 0.022 Ni-Ti sectional wire between first molar (46) and lower retained second molar (47).

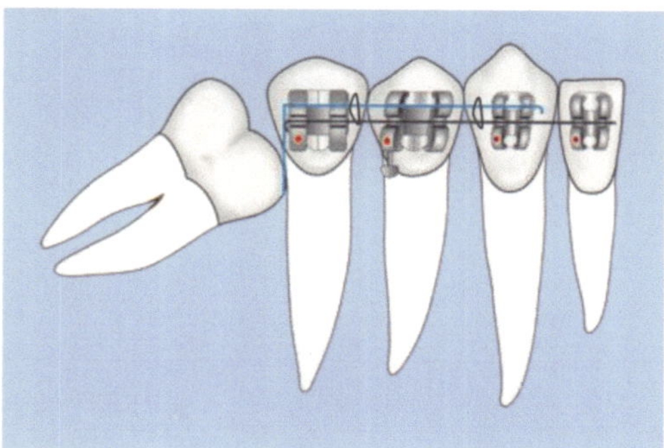

Figure 13.
0.016 × 0.022 Ni-Ti or 0.016 × 0.025 Cu Ni-Ti sectional wire, ligated to stainless steel continuous arch wire and then introduced between second premolars and impacted first molar, produces a sufficient moment to distalize the impacted tooth.

The pole arm is constructed of 0.016 × 0.022 inch titanium molybdenum alloy (TMA) wire (**Figure 14**). The distal part is inserted from lingual side under the contact point, between first molar and second angulated molar, then it is pushed buccally. The uprighting spring is curved to the mesial dental arch and ligated to the anchor wire. Finally, the lingual extremity is fixed with composite resin on the occlusal surface of the first molar (**Figure 15**). The reactivation of the pole arm is recommended every 6 weeks, simply by lifting the buccal arm occlusally.

Majourau et al. [14] proposed 0.017 × 0.025 TMA "cemented springs" whose distal part is supported by a stainless steel button bonded to disto-occlusal surface of the retained molar. The auxiliary wire is inserted from the distal of the first molar auxiliary tube. Then, it is curved to give it the configuration of loop. The spring is activated through a combination of the gingival loop form and open coil inserted between a loop and the auxiliary molar tube (**Figure 16**).

All the appliances aforementioned have the advantage of avoiding early bonding of impacted molars as well as the need of surgical exposure of sufficient surface for the bonding.

Then, when the impacted second molar had been uprighted to some degree, a tube can be bonded to it for further alignment.

TMA uprighting spring, with or without helical loop is needed to finish distal displacement of molar and to produce eruptive force to bring teeth into occlusion with their upper opponents.

Majourau [14] reports using 0.017 × 0.025 TMA cantilever spring, which is engaged in the second molar tube and hooked distally to the canine. The intrusive

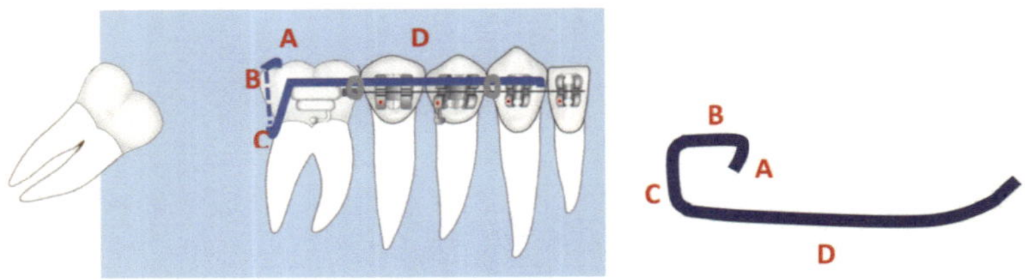

Figure 14.
The pole arm uprighting spring of 0.016 × 0.022 TMA is used. The lingual extremity is bonded on occlusal surface of adjacent tooth; then, the arm is introduced from lingual under contact point. The buccal part is curved and ligated to anchor continuous arch wire (readapted from [3]).

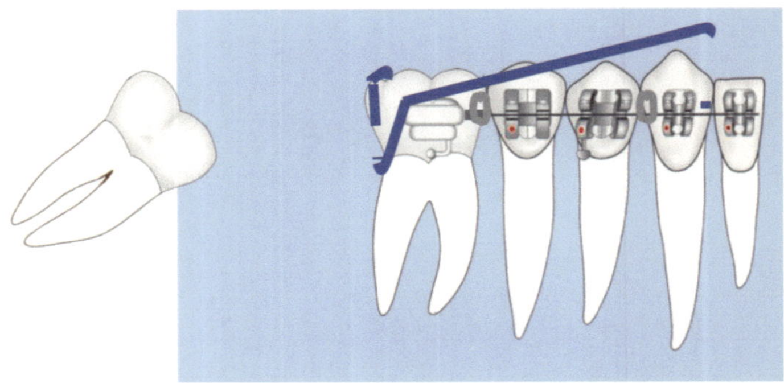

Figure 15.
The activation of pole arm uprighting spring is ensured by a plicature leading the mesial arm occlusally (readapted from [3]).

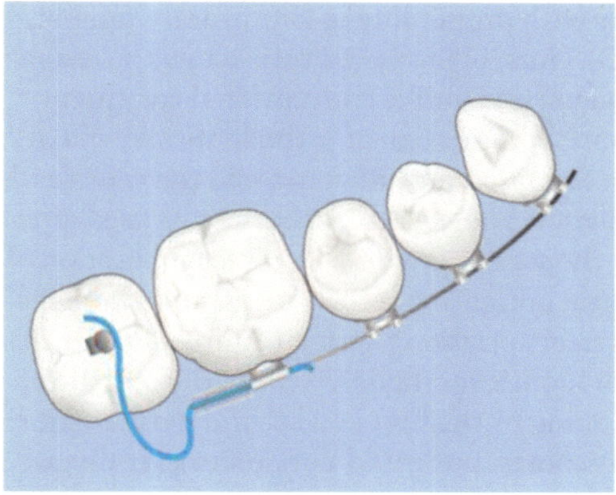

Figure 16.
Illustrative diagram of 0.017 × 0.025 TMA sectional wire associated with open coil to upright impacted the second lower molar. TMA spring is bent around the button, then configured as loop, and finally inserted from distal in accessory tube of the first molar. Continuous 0.019 × 0.025 stainless steel wire from first molar to first molar is used as an anchorage unit (readapted from [14]).

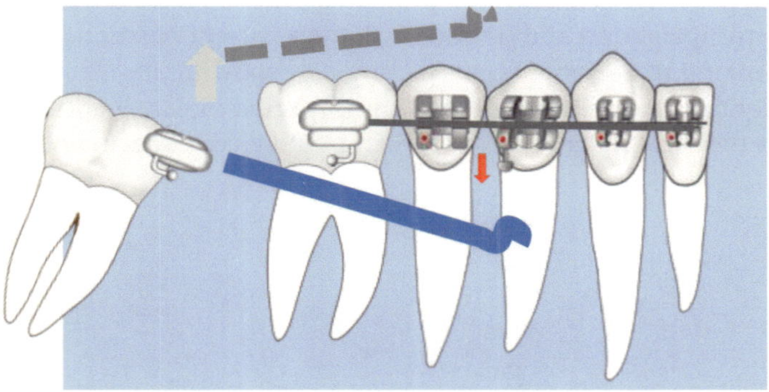

Figure 17.
Illustration of eruptive force produced by TMA cantilever spring without loop. This sectional wire is required to achieve impacted molar repositioning in correct occlusion (readapted from [14]).

force was negligible since a continuous stiff stainless steel wire consolidated the lower arch from first molar to first molar (**Figure 17**).

Many others suggested the use of tip back cantilever of 0.017 × 0.025 TMA wire with loop [15, 21, 22]. It is a long cantilever which gives a high moment-to-force ratio and produces effects on the tooth in three planes, mainly in the mesiodistal direction and the vertical direction providing both distal crown tipping and molar extrusion (**Figure 18**).

6.2.2.3 Temporary skeletal anchorage

Orthodontic treatment methods, with continuous or segment wire, for molar uprighting have some disadvantages, including extrusion of the target molar, unwanted reciprocal movement of the anchorage units, need for bulky appliances, and longer treatment time. The development of orthodontic miniscrew implants provided solutions to most of these problems [19].

Skeletal anchorages have some advantages in that they reduce the side effects formerly associated with dental anchorage and provide vertical and distal traction forces simultaneously with proper line of action and moment. It is also beneficial for obtaining [19] [23] Thus, orthodontic miniscrews have a major impact on reducing the overall treatment time unlike conventional treatment.

Moreover, they simplify the design of orthodontic devices. All the abovementioned devices can be used in combination with it to avoid the need for dental anchoring. Depending on the situation, the skeletal anchor can be used directly; the minivis serves as a docking point for the sectional wire with direct application of an appropriate force system. Lee et al. suggest uprighting second molar into two steps, using an open coil spring and a stainless steel uprighting spring (**Figures 19** and **20**) [19].

Conventional orthodontic methods are often the best alternative to extraction or surgically repositioning of the first and second permanent molars. It produces certainly excellent outcomes, but could not be successfully predicted or may be contraindicated for horizontally position, deeply impaction or molars with gross displacement [9, 15, 19]. In such challenging cases, a combination of surgical and orthodontic treatment is appropriate [2, 4].

6.2.3 Surgical approaches

Surgical approaches of unerupted permanent molars included surgical exposure for orthodontic uprighting and traction into their correct position in the arch, as well as challenging treatment options of surgical repositioning. It consists essentially of uprighting and repositioning of the impacted molar, eventually including extraction of the third molar [15] [20]. Posterior available space should be analyzed

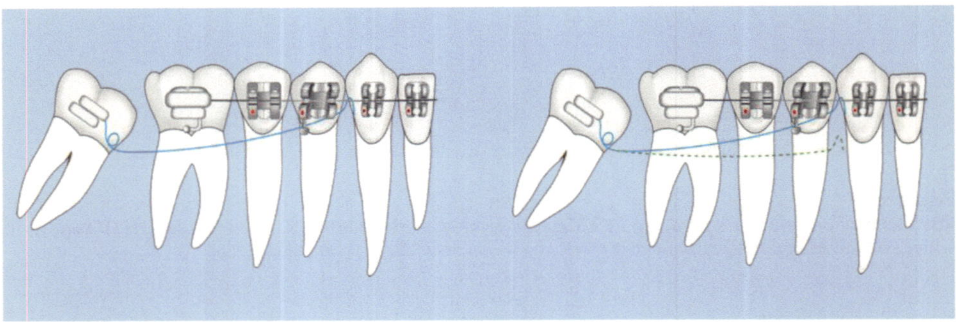

Figure 18.
Diagram of tip back cantilever: It is a long uprighting spring of 0.017 × 0.025 TMA. The activation force is directed to the occlusal (readapted from [15, 21, 22]).

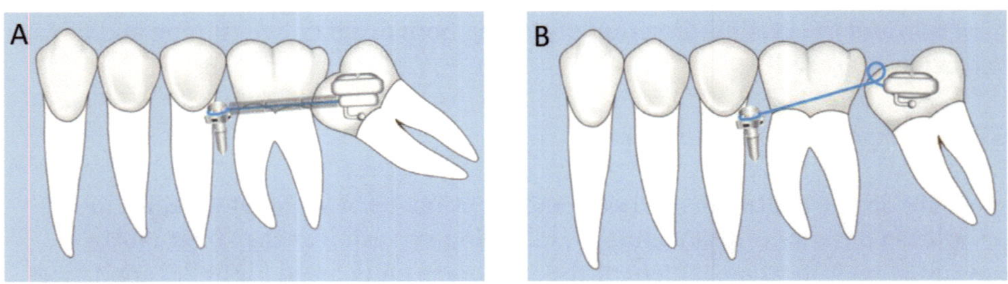

Figure 19.
Miniscrews used as direct anchor with segmental wire and coil spring to distalize and extrude the second lower molar. In the first step (A), the distalization is ensured by 0.016 stainless steel wire and open coil spring. In the second step (B), tip back moment is delivered from 0.016 × 0.022 in. Stainless steel wire spring to upright impacted molar (from Lee et al., readapted from [19]).

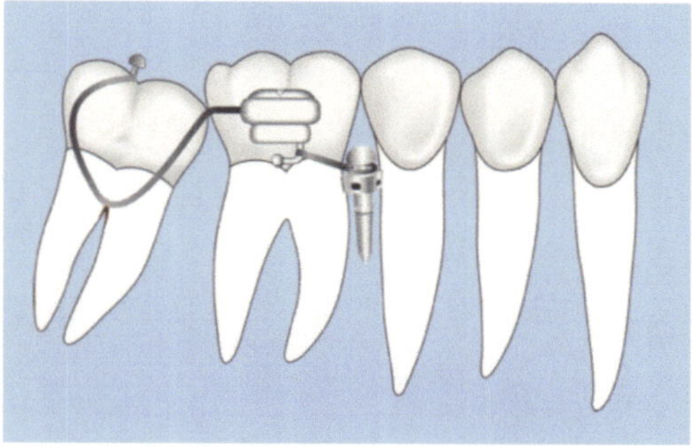

Figure 20.
Miniscrews used as indirect anchor to reinforce dental stabile unit then with tip back cantilever to extrude it.

before planning orthodontic and surgical traction, to prevent periodontal risks. Removal of the third molar often completes this procedure, and more rarely, the second molar when the first one is impacted. Undoubtedly, analysis of anatomic location, desired eruption path, and available space should proceed the uprighting process for a favorable outcome [19].

6.2.3.1 Surgical exposure

In cases of horizontally or deeply impaction, orthodontics alone cannot straighten the molar because of the limited access. A surgical exposure is required following by orthodontic traction or luxation.

Magnusson et al. in their study found that [24]:

- Surgical exposure was the most successful treatment and the best choice of treatment, with a success rate of 70%.
- The success rate was 50% when surgical exposure was combined with extraction of the third molar and/or luxation of the second molar.
- Surgical exposure of the second molar, with or without extraction of the third molar and/or luxation of the second molar, seems to result in the most successful treatment in both jaws.

6.2.3.1.1 Surgical exposure and orthodontic traction

It consists of exposure and uncovering the crown, followed by bonding an orthodontic attachment. Temporary skeletal anchorage is the appropriate and efficient means to upright and tract the tooth in its ideal position [15, 23].

Kim [23] suggested the use of 1.3–1.2 mm × 8 mm mini screws in the retromolar area following extraction of the third molar. Traction is initiated on the day of surgery with elastic threads that were replaced every 4 weeks.

Chang [25] reported a simple, effective, and expedient mechanics for managing horizontally and deeply impaction of second lower molar in only 4 months. 2 × 14 mm stainless steel bone screw is positioned superiorly in ramus under local anesthesia. He proposed to (**Figure 21**):

- First, remove all obstructions to eruption, as ectopic position of the third molar follicle

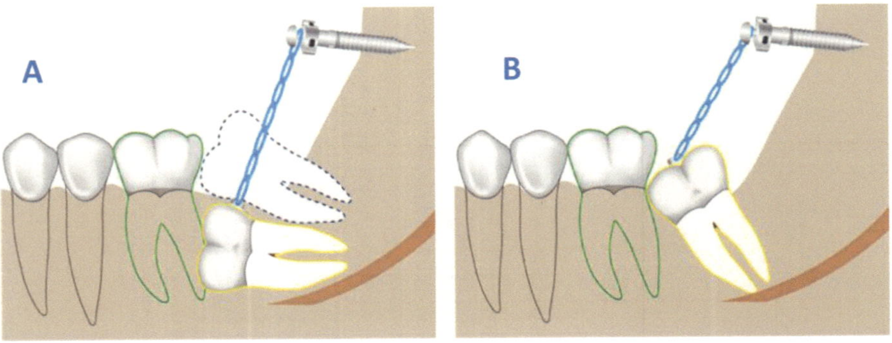

Figure 21.
Illustration of surgical exposure and traction of second lower molar through bone screw. The button is bonded to the accessible surface (A) and then moved if necessary (B) so as to obtain a sufficient amplitude of traction on the minivis. 2 × 14 mm stainless steel bone screw is inserted into the ascending ramus, and power chain is connected between attachment and screw (readapted from [25]).

- Expose surgically and luxate the lower second molars to rule out an eventual ankylosis. The covered bone is removed down to the level of the cementoenamel junction for optimal molar uprighting.

- Bond button or eyelet on distal surface and then connect elastic chain from attachment to bone screw before closing soft tissue with interrupted sutures to control blending.

6.2.3.1.2 Surgical exposure and luxation

Luxation is an effective technique with good long-term prognosis. Such approach finds its major indication in favorable impacted molars before complete apical root edification. Indeed, it has been reported that molars luxated prior to complete root formation erupted spontaneously and continued their normal root development.

The potential risks of luxation include pulpal devitalization and root fracture, although a prophylactic endodontic treatment of the luxated molar is not recommended.

During the 1916s, luxation has been described to be used successfully in ankylosed permanent molars that are typical of secondary retention, although luxation seems to promote new areas of ankylosis rather than breaking bony connections [2].

The prognosis seems to be better than that of dental transplant because the tooth is not removed from its socket and the apical blood vessels are not damaged.

6.2.3.2 Surgical repositioning

It is a simple technique which produces fast results; it seems to be the most convenient procedure when patient compliance is minimal, when impacted teeth have limited access or failed to respond to orthodontics methods, or for angle of inclination of less than 75° [9, 15, 26]. Nevertheless, there is a risk of pulp necrosis, root resorption, and ankylosis [9].

Several authors suggested that this procedure usually lead to predictable successful results if root formation is not completed, usually between the ages of 11 and 14. According to Botton [17], if surgery is performed too soon, then the tooth may be unstable and may shift from its position. If performed too late, then there is risk of root fracture and possible disruption of blood supply leading to pulpal necrosis [17] [24].

Removal of the third adjacent molar is often necessary to make surgical uprighting easier. In addition to that, surgically tipped molar should be stabilized for few weeks.

Boyton et al. [17] Kravitz et al. [26] describe the stages of surgical uprighting of second lower molar. After intrasulcular incision from the distobuccal line angle of the first molar to posteriorly the external oblique ridge, a full-thickness mucoperiosteal flap is raised to expose the second and third molars if it is present. Then, distal and buccal bone of molar is removed to expose the cement-enamel junction avoiding any contact with the cementum and periodontal ligament fibers that may cause external root resorption.

The surgeon uses steady and gentle force with straight elevator to elevate the tooth distally and prevent root fracture. Sometimes, the surgeon removes additional distal bone to perform the molar uprighting. When the occlusal surface of impacted molar is approximately level with the occlusal plane, the patient is instructed to bite down gently to ensure that the molar is just below the occlusal plane to prevent occlusal trauma. The site should be irrigated with copious amounts of normal saline and then closed with sutures. The attached gingiva should be kept intact and positioned appropriately to ensure a healthy periodontal environment for the newly positioned second molar.

Some recommended bonding a tube to the molar as soon as it is repositioned. For others, an intact lingual and buccal plate or a periodontal dressing prevents the tooth from migrating bucally or lingually [17, 26].

According to Boyton, no additional autogenous bone or bone substitutes are needed to stabilize the tooth. Other authors [27] advocate the use of absorbable gelatin sponge or autogenous alveolar bone to stabilize the repositioned second molars.

An immediate postoperative Panorex is recommended. The follow-up includes a 1-week postoperative appointment and then another appointment in 6 months for a repeated Panorex. Orthodontic treatment should begin 1–2 weeks after surgery, with a mandibular arch-wire extended through the second-molar bracket for stabilization.

7. Extraction

Surgical extraction of unerupted permanent molar is indicated when exposure, luxation, and orthodontics treatment fail, in the presence of a pathological process, or when prognosis is poor because of fully formed roots or extremely unfavorable position [2, 15].

Extraction as an alternative procedure of retention treatment can be considered in two different approaches as follows:

- Extraction of retained or impacted second molar with the intention of replacing it with the third molar. The third molar drift mesially when it is at low Nolla stage from 5 to 8. Nevertheless, success of this treatment depends on the eruption path of the third molar which could be unpredictable [5, 9, 15]. Magnusson et al., in their study evaluating the outcome after treatment and without treatment of retained second molars, found that treatment with removal impacted molar replaced with the third molar was the least successful both in the maxilla and mandible. They reported that few molars that did erupt were all malpositioned with a risk for elongation of the antagonist because of the delayed eruption of third molar [24].

- Extraction of the impacted second molar followed by immediate transplantation of retained molar or third molar into the extraction site. It is technically demanding and carries a risk of pulp necrosis, root resorption, and ankylosis [9, 15, 24].
- Both transplantation and surgical repositioning were suggested as invasive techniques because of the deeply impacted positions with high risk of neurovascular damage, mandibular fracture, or the deep infrabony defect on the distal surface of adjacent teeth [24].

8. Conclusion

The eruption failure of first and second permanent molars is rare and asymptomatic. This disturbance is often detected in a routine panoramic radiograph during pedodontic or orthodontic evaluation and represents a real diagnostic and therapeutic challenge for the practitioner.

Considering the main etiological factors, three clinical forms can be distinguished: impaction, primary, and secondary retention. Therefore, it is crucial to diagnose this abnormality early for an optimal treatment time and outcomes, as well as reduction of dental and periodontal complications.

Its management is considered difficult and unpredictable, and there is no clear standard solution. Despite observation, abstention, or extraction of unerupted permanent molars, several orthodontic and surgical methods for uprighting impacted molars was reported. All of the methods have specific indications, advantages, and disadvantages depending of clinical form, retention depth, stage of root formation, and age of patient.

If the prognosis of orthodontic and/or surgery repositioning of impacted and primary retained molars is favorable, the treatment of secondary retention seems to depend on the age of the patient and the extent of infraocclusion and malocclusion.

The major treatment concern of secondarily retained molars is that these molars cannot be moved orthodontically due to an abnormal periodontal ligament. By contrast, orthodontics or combined surgical-orthodontic approach is a major modality in treatment of impacted teeth as these molars often have an abnormal position in the eruption path. Primarily retained molars can also be moved orthodontically, but this is often not necessary because of the normal position in the eruption tract.

Acknowledgements

The authors would like to express their gratitude to all the specialists in the orthodontics and pedodontics department at the Ibn Rochd University Hospital of Casablanca for their kind contribution to the work. Their special thanks go especially to Dr. N. Falah, Z. El Jalil, S. El Kaki, A. Moutawakil, and L. Bouchghel.

Conflict of interest

The authors declare that they have no conflict of interest.

Author details

Sanaa Alami[1]*, Hakima Aghoutan[1], Meriem Bellamine[2] and Farid El Quars[1]

1 Faculty of Dental Medicine, Department of Dento-facial Orthopedic, Hassan II University of Casablanca, Morocco

2 Department of Orthodontics, Casablanca Hospital center, Morocco

*Address all correspondence to: sanalami1@yahoo.fr

References

[1] Palma C, Coelho A, González Y, Cahuana A. Failure of eruption of first and second permanent molars. Journal of Clinical Pediatric Dentistry. 2015;**27**:239-245. DOI: 10.17796/jcpd.27.3.dm4v13441p161928

[2] Raghoebar GM, Boering G, Vissink A, Stegenga B. Eruption disturbances of permanent molars: A review. Journal of Oral Pathology and Medicine. 1991;**20**:159-166. DOI: 10.1111/j.1600-0714.1991.tb00913.x

[3] Fu PS, Wang JC, Wu YM, Huang TK, Chen WC, Tseng YC, et al. Impacted mandibular second molars. A retrospective study of prevalence and treatment outcome. The Angle Orthodontist. 2012;**82**:670-675. DOI: 10.2319/102111-656.1

[4] Fu PS, Wang JC, Chen CH, Huang TK, Tseng CH, Hung CC. Management of unilaterally deep impacted first, second, and third mandibular molars. The Angle Orthodontist. 2012;**82**:565-571. DOI: 10.2319/062411-409.1

[5] Valmaseda-Castellón E, De-la-Rosa-Gay C, Gay-Escoda C. Eruption disturbances of the first and second permanent molars: Results of treatment in 43 cases. American Journal of Orthodontics and Dentofacial Orthopedics. 1999;**116**:651-658. DOI: 10.1016/S0889-5406(99)70200-3

[6] Bondemark L, Tsiopa J. Prevalence of ectopic eruption, impaction, retention and agenesis of the permanent second molar. The Angle Orthodontist. 2007;**77**:773-778. DOI: 10.2319/072506-306.1

[7] Cassetta M, Altieri F, di Mambro A, Galluccio G, Barbato E. Impaction of permanent mandibular second molar: A retrospective study. Medicina Oral, Patología Oral y Cirugía Bucal. 2013;**18**:564-568. DOI: 10.4317/medoral.18869

[8] Ahmad S, Bister D, Cobourne MT. The clinical features and aetiological basis of primary eruption failure. European Journal of Orthodontics. 2006;**28**:535-540. DOI: 10.1093/ejo/cjl033

[9] Cho SY, Ki Y, Chu V, Chan J. Impaction of permanent mandibular second molars in ethnic Chinese school children. Journal of the Canadian Dental Association. 2008;**74**(6):521. Available from: www.cda-adc.ca/jcda/vol-74/issue-6/521.html

[10] Srinivasan MR, Poorni S, Venkatesh A, Vasanthi B. Prevalence of impacted permanent mandibular second molars in south Indian population: A cross-sectional study. Indian Journal of Dental Research. 2016;**27**:540-543. DOI: 10.4103/0970-9290.195645

[11] Evans R. Incidence of lower second permanent molar impaction. British Journal of Orthodontics. 2014;**15**:199-203. DOI: 10.1179/bjo.15.3.199

[12] Cassetta M, Altieri F, Calasso S. Etiological factors in second mandibular molar impaction. Journal of Clinical and Experimental Dentistry. 2014;**6**:150-154. DOI: 10.4317/jced.51382

[13] Raghoebar GM, Boering G, Jansen H, Vissink A. Secondary retention of permanent molars: A histologic study. 1989;**18**:427-431. DOI: 10.1111/j.1600-0714.1989.tb01338.x

[14] Majourau A, Norton LA. Uprighting impacted second molars with segmented springs. American Journal of Orthodontics and Dentofacial Orthopedics. 1995;**107**:235-238. DOI: 10.1016/S0889-5406(95)70137-0

[15] Shpack N, Finkelstein T, Lai YH, Kuftinec MM, Vardimon A, Shapira Y. Mandibular permanent second molar impaction treatment options and outcome. Open Journal of Dentistry and Oral Medicine. 2013;**1**:9-14. DOI: 10.13189/ojdom.2013.010103

[16] Hanisch M, Hanisch L, Kleinheinz J, Jung S. Primary failure of eruption (PFE): A systematic review. Head and Face Medicine. 2018;**14**:2-9. DOI: 10.1186/s13005-018-0163-7

[17] Boynton T, Lieblich SE. Surgical uprighting of second molars. Atlas of the Oral and Maxillofacial Surgery Clinics of North America. 2013;**21**: 235-237. DOI: 10.1016/j.cxom.2013.05.001

[18] Vedtofte H, Andreasen JO, Kjær I. Arrested eruption of the permanent lower second molar. European Journal of Orthodontics. 1999;**21**:31-40. DOI: 10.1093/ejo/21.1.31

[19] Magkavali-Trikka P, Emmanouilidis G, Papadopoulos MA. Mandibular molar uprighting using orthodontic miniscrew implants: A systematic review. Progress in Orthodontics. 2018;**19**:1-12. DOI: 10.1186/s40510-017-0200-2

[20] Yordanova G. Treatment of impacted lower left second molar and over erupted upper second molar. Journal of Dental Health, Oral Disorders and Therapy. 2018;**9**:106-108. DOI: 10.15406/jdhodt.2018.09.00338

[21] Sawicka M, Racka-pilszak B, Rosnowska-Mazurkiewicz A. Uprighting partially impacted permanent second molars. The Angle Orthodontist. 2007;**77**:148-154. DOI: 10.2319/010206-461

[22] Shapira Y, Borell G, Nahlieli O, Kuftinek MM. Uprighrting mesialy impacted mandibular permanent second molars. The Angle Orthodontist. 1998;**68**:173-178

[23] Kim K-J, Park JH, Kim M-J, Jang H-I, Chae J-M. Posterior available space for uprighting horizontally impacted mandibular second molars using orthodontic microimplant anchorage. Journal of Clinical Pediatric Dentistry. 2018;**43**:56-63. DOI: 10.17796/1053-4625-43.1.11

[24] Magnusson C, Kjellberg H. Impaction and retention of second molars: Diagnosis, treatment and outcome. The Angle Orthodontist. 2008; **79**:422-427. DOI: 10.2319/0003-3219 (2009)079[0422:iarosm]2.0.co;2

[25] Lin S-Y, Chang C, Roberts WE. Simple mechanics to upright horizontally impacted molars with ramus screws. Orthodontic Journal of Nepal. 2016;**5**:42-47. DOI: 10.3126/ojn.v5i2.15231

[26] Kravitz ND. Surgical uprighting of lower second molars. Journal of Clinical Orthodontics. 2016;**50**(1):33-40. Available from: www.jco-online.com

[27] Johnson JV, Quirk GP. Surgical repositioning of impacted mandibular second molar teeth. American Journal of Orthodontics and Dentofacial Orthopedics. 1987;**91**:242-251. DOI: 10.1016/0889-5406(87)90454-9

Chapter 14

Evolution of Dental Implant Shapes and Today's Custom Root Analogue Implants

Ayse Sumeyye Akay

Abstract

Native tooth has a unique design to serve perfect stomatognathic function and esthetics which could never be replaced with another material or apparatus if it is lost. Over the past few decades, screw-type endosseous implants have been considered to be as the gold standard for the rehabilitation of edentulism owing to the similarity with the anatomical root shape and location inside the alveolar bone. They have been widely investigated so as to find out the ideal characteristics. Further researches have focused on the cervical region of the dental implant because the maximum stress is pronounced around the implant neck. The ideal characteristics indicate that a wide implant neck for better stress distribution, and a large surface area with a minimal thread geometry for a better long term crestal bone stability. Along with the growing clinical knowledge and digital technology, an innovative and noteworthy approach for implant dentistry, custom root analogue implant (RAI), has evolved. With the computer aided design and manufacturing (CAD/CAM) methods, original and optimized characteristics could be transferred to the custom dental implants just as performing an original root replacement.

Keywords: dental implant, custom root-shaped implant, anatomically shaped implant, root analogue implant, CAD/CAM, digital dentistry

1. Introduction

Natural teeth have unique design which serve complex stomatognathic functions and fulfill distinctive biomechanical needs. The anatomy of the natural tooth eventuates after a complex biological process which is moderated by epithelial-mesenchymal collaboration [1]. The morphological features in each type of tooth are variable, and several classifications have been proposed to define the diversity of root forms and potential anomalies regarding the number and shape of the roots [2–5]. Basically, the natural root has conical shape with a smaller width towards to the apex and often with longitudinal grooves. The root of the maxillary central incisors is wider mesiodistally in vestibular part, and both maxillary and mandibular canines have wider and longer root forms in order to compensate the lateral and oblique forces whereas maxillary lateral and mandibular incisors present a modest shape. Premolars generally have single root with a slight curve at the apex except from the maxillary first premolar which has probably two roots at vestibular and lingual aspects of the alveolus. In the posterior region that corresponds the great occlusal forces, molars have multi roots. Maxillary first and second molars have three roots, mandibular first and second molars have two roots, and third molars tend to have fused complex roots [2, 3]. Some of the anomalies of the roots excluding the aforementioned common variations are supernumerary roots such as maxillary molars with four roots, distolingual root in mandibular molars, mandibulary canine with two roots [2, 6, 7]. All of the diversity is originated from the distinctive biomechanical requirements and functions. Therefore, understanding the original root anatomy is a precondition for all kind of surgical interventions and functional rehabilitations in dental practice from the preventive and regenerative surgeries to the indispensable tooth extraction [4, 8, 9]. Additionally, tooth loss has not been literally replaced regarding both biomechanically and physiologically yet.

Screw-type endosseous implants have been the most preferable rehabilitation of tooth loss for decades, and have demonstrated highly successful survival rates and clinical outcomes [10]. Numerous experimental studies demonstrated successful osseointegration for immediately placed and loaded dental implants into the fresh extraction socket. It has been suggested that immediate procedures could minimize the alveolar bone and soft tissue resorption, thus, provide better cosmetic results [11]. However, there still have been some obstacles for immediate placement procedures of screw-type dental implants. The foremost deficit is a remained void between the implant and the alveolar socket due to the incongruent geometry of these two. Many grafting or barrier techniques have been studied extensively to overcome this problem [12], yet no approach does literally meet the clinical needs.

While searching new solutions for recovering the fresh socket with immediate screw-type implants, a philosophy of custom root formed implant fabrication had come along. The philosophy of custom made dental implant started in 1960s as an idea of replacing the extracted tooth with eligible dental materials such as composites or polymers [13]. It was realized that if the implant had the same design of the extracted root and was congruent with the socket geometry, no residual voids hereby would remain [14]. Thus, a better recovering and esthetics would be achieved.

Starting with the plastic materials and primitive techniques, the custom root analogue implant production evolved up to the digital rapid prototyping [15] technology. Both milling and additive manufacturing techniques have already been utilized with both titanium and zirconia materials in order to fabricate custom root analogue dental implants [15–17]. Thus, a new perspective to be investigated for the dental practice is upon the stage.

2. The evolution and the fabrication procedures of root shaped dental implants

The first attempt of custom root shaped implant was described by Hodosh et al. in 1968 which was called 'Tooth Replica Polymer Implant Concept' [13, 18]. According to this attempt, a plaster mold of the extracted tooth was made right after the extraction. Then, autopolymerizing heat processed polymethacrylate was used alone or with freezed dried cancellous (anorganic) calf bone for creating a 'plastic' or 'plastic-bone mixture' implant material. After the polymer was processed in a flask, and then zephirin chloride washing, the plastic implant was inserted into the alveolar socket. It was the only immediate replacement of lost natural teeth at that time. However, because it resulted in fibrointegration instead of osseointegration, the polymer dental implant was not used for years in clinical practice [19].

In 1992, the root shaped implant idea was revived by using titanium material instead of any polymer by Lundgren and colleagues, and resulted in 88% of bone-to-implant contact [20]. This novelty was inspired by Andersson's method of spark erosion combined with milling machine duplication which was developed for titanium crown fabrication [21]. The milling machine had a tool system that held a stone die of the extracted tooth, and a milling unit integrated with a detection needle and a hydraulic servo-unit which transferred and copied the outer surface of the stone die to a titanium blank.

Following the elementary attempts of creating a dental root analogue, a computer milled anatomical implant system (ReImplant® System, Hagen, Germany) was presented by Kohal et al. [22]. This system was the first computer aided manufacturing of dental implant carrying the original root contours of the extracted tooth. The procedure yet again started after the extraction. The space between the tooth and the socket wall was measured by repositioning the extracted tooth into the socket again for compensating the lost periodontal width. The cervical width was transferred to the computer unit subsequently the data of the laser scanned tooth. Finally, the milling unit with integrated laser camera and computer control station fabricated the root analogue implant out of prefabricated Grade II titanium blank according to the computer data. After polishing the extraosseous cervical part and sandblasting the intraosseous part with Al_2O_3 powder, implant was ultrasonically cleaned with alkaline and autoclaved, and tapped into the respective socket [14, 22]. Similarly, zirconia material was also studied with the computer numerical control (CNC) milling method by Kohal and colleagues first [23].

Another idea for immediate placement of prefabricated anatomically shaped dental implants was suggested by Coatoam [24, 25]. The proper one of the series of anatomically shaped implants in varying lengths (PACE, CAL-Form Inc., Longwood, Fla) was inserted into the healed socket after a waiting period of 6–8 weeks. They asserted that a moldable osteoid which was formed in the early healing socket would readily accept the implant integration and could also facilitate indirect sinus lifting [24, 25]. However, relevant studies have been very limited to state an inference for clinical practice.

In the last decade, growing computer based digital technologies guided the contemporary approaches up to custom root analogue implants, which were called RAI. The clinical procedures were shifted prior to the tooth extraction. Instead of copying or laser-scanning of the extracted tooth, literally computer aided designing (CAD) on the preoperative radiographic data was included to the procedure in addition to the computer aided manufacturing (CAM) methods.

One of the first CAD/CAM combined high-resolution computed tomography based RAI methods was described and commercially available (REPLICATE Immediate Tooth Replacement System, Natural Dental Implants). According to the system, digital imaging and communications in medicine (DICOM) data from a high-resolution cone beam computed tomography (CBCT) or a digital volume tomography (DVT) was obtained. Besides, a digital or two-stage elastomeric impressions with bite registrations were taken preoperatively. Master stone cast models were created and optically scanned. Then, the standardized triangulation language (STL) data of the digitalized master models and the DICOM data of three-dimensional (3D) visualization were offered to compose a 3D envelope that constitutes the digital environment for RAI planning. On 3D envelope, endosseous titanium root-implant portion, zirconia abutment to be glass-soldered onto the titanium root, root analogue implant try-in, provisional crown etc. could be designed [15, 19, 26]. After CAD data was transferred to a five-axis rapid manufacturing machine, the titanium root part out of a medical grade IV solid titanium workpiece and the zirconia parts out of presintered yttria-stabilized tetragonal zirconia material (Y-TZP) were milled, subsequently, the titanium and zirconia parts of implant were glass-soldered to form a one-piece implant. The zirconia parts remained machined surface, and the titanium root was sandblasted and acid-etched. Finally, the implant was delivered in sterile packaging and tapped into the socket [15, 26].

Another digital root analogue implant approach evolved with the help of 3D additive manufacturing technology which was a procedure to fabricate 3D metallic objects from metal powders on the basis of 3D data. The main powder bed fusion methods have been known as direct metal laser sintering (DMLS) or selective laser sintering (SLS) and selective laser melting (SLM) or direct laser metal forming (DLMF). According to the procedures, metal powder microparticles were formed layer by layer with a focused laser-induced fusion in order to create complex solid objects [27]. RAI fabrication out of Ti-6Al-4V alloy material by a high-end SLM method was first proposed by Moin and colleagues [16]. A high-resolution computed tomography (CT) was performed and the datasets were transferred in the DICOM format. The 3D reconstruction software simulated the virtual extraction of the tooth on 3D projection, and the implant with prosthetic components was designed on a reverse engineering software. Processing was carried out in ytterbium (YB) fiber laser in argon atmosphere, and implants were delivered sterile packaged after ultrasonically cleaned [27].

After titanium, zirconia material was also employed for RAI fabrication with the rapid prototyping technology. Dispersion of a zirconium oxide powder into a liquid solution of polyacrylate was used to form a solidified ceramic object by high-end digital light processing 3D printing method as similar with the powder bed fusion technique [17].

3. The evaluation and clinical predictability of root shaped implants

Considering the early attempts, it could be noticed that root analogue implant fabrication required exhausted and complex clinical and laboratory procedures and had some drawbacks formerly. Hodosh's polymer implant resulted in fibrointegration. The proposal method of Lundgren required a long surgical time which could be regarded as a disadvantage. The computer milled anatomical implant system suggested by Coatoam also required a long time and additional complex procedures. Besides, insufficient primary stability was another matter for these trials because of the periodontal space and the enlargement of the socket during the extraction. ReImplant system tried to compensate this problem by integrating an extra measurement and data transfer onto the laser scanned root. This measurement was obtained on the cervical part of the root, and then applied to the whole root surface. An experimental study in monkeys, regarding the root analogue implants of upper central and lateral incisors showed a mean bone-to-implant contact of 41.2% after 6 months of healing, and the study also reported a common clinical complication, –the fracture of the buccal plate during the implant placement [22]. In accordance with this finding, it could be considered that the extra measurement and the width enlargement of socket could also act as another incongruence for achieving the appropriate passive fit into the fresh socket.

Though, ReImplant and PACE system could serve a similar role for the treatment of convex root form. On the other hand, in cases with unfavorable root shape such as concave contours or complex morphology, original root shaped implant could jeopardize the placement and the hygienic maintenance. However, PACE system could be used to eliminate the disadvantages of unfavorable root form, and it would also take less time to perform in clinical practice because it was totally prefabricated [25].

REPLICATE system was first introduced for single tooth replacement. After revealing the clinical advantages in an animal study [28], a 35-year-old woman was subjected to replacement of a maxillary left central incisor [19]. After the implantation with an approximately 1.4 mm of reduced buccal design, a mixture of platelet-rich plasma (PRP) and osteoconductive bovine bone substitute was inserted in the buccal space for the purpose of stabilizing the buccal tissue architecture. After 6 months of healing with immediate provisional crown, the final zirconia restoration was delivered. At almost 1 year of loading, good esthetics and functional stability of surrounding tissues were reported. Simultaneously, in a dog study, the usage of multi-rooted single tooth implant with a custom shaped lingual splint which is bonded by a self-curing luting cement onto the surrounding teeth was tested. Some of the splints were debonded, but no sign of infection was observed within the 16 months of healing. Bone-to-implant contact and mineral apposition rates yielded no significant change, however, the vertical bone loss was significantly lower (0.35 mm for root analogue implant, 0.79 mm for the control implant) compared to the threaded control implants [15]. In another subsequent human study which reported the clinical and radiographic observations within the 1-year of functional loading, one single premolar out of the five had peri-implant infection with mobility after 4 weeks, and the other two of them were identified in the absence of buccal bone around the implant [26]. The implants of this system were roughened, large-grit sandblasted, and acid-etched (SLA) surface characteristics similar to the conventional threaded implants as an advantage for clinical predictability. On the other hand, considering the poor clinical findings, it should be further investigated to reassure tangible results.

Rapid manufacturing techniques also seem promising for fabricating modern root analogue implants. The accuracy of root analogue implant fabricated by powder bed fusion methods revealed acceptable discrepancy. The volumetric measurement of the 3D surface model of the tooth was 0.27% of greater than the optical scanned original root while the RAI was 6.33% of smaller than optical scanned original root [16] and was 0.6–5.9% of smaller than the socket [29]. The local disparity of RAI was more pronounced at the incisal area and the root apex, with a maximum of 0.15 and 1.86 mm, respectively [29]. In a prospective clinical study, 1-year survival revealed 100% of stable with a confirmed good condition of the peri-implant tissue, and no prosthetic complications was observed [30]. In addition to the favorable results, it was suggested that a perfect fit of RAI on the buccal cortical bone could be accused for esthetic failure and also pressure-induced bone loss or fracture of the buccal plate. Therefore, reducing the diameter about 0.1–0.3 mm was offered as a useful strategy [27].

Pirker and Kocher reported the clinical results of computer milled zirconia RAI. Zirconia was used because of its well-known improved biomechanics and esthetic results. The diameter of the implant next to the thin cortical bone was reduced for avoiding fracture and pressure-induced bone loss. The implant with a surface of only sandblasting failed within 2 months, but the other implant surface strategy which added macroretentions on entire root surface showed 92% survival after 2-year follow-up [31]. Nevertheless, CNC milling zirconia was reported to have some disadvantages such as being time-consuming, substantial waste of raw material, and limited accuracy [17, 32] whereas the 3D printed zirconia RAI was a faster procedure as against, and demonstrated a disparity less than 1 mm [17].

4. Advantages of the root shaped implants for immediate placement and future considerations

Owing to the 3D additive manufacturing technology, remarkable characteristics such as functionally graded titanium material, and 3D interconnected controlled porous structure could be delivered to the custom root shaped dental implants [33–35]. Thus, minimizing the stress-shielding effects, providing a long-term stable fixation, and improving bone ingrowth could be possible [36]. Additionally, lower risk of implant surface contamination is another advantage of laser metal sintering method since minimal postprocessing treatment is required [35].

Regarding these knowledge and available clinical results, it could be suggested that combining the root analogue implant strategy with digital technology provide a number of advantages over the previous procedures such as faster preoperative preparation, relatively easier surgical procedures, simpler fabrication of esthetic restoration, and improved biomechanics. Also it would be a cheaper alternative for immediate implant and prosthetic requirements in compromised clinical conditions.

As another matter of fact, comprehensive experimental and clinical studies indicate the importance of the cervical region of the dental implant because the maximum stress is pronounced around the implant neck [37]. The ideal characteristics of dental implant is suggested that a wider neck for a better stress distribution [38], and a large surface area as well as possible with a minimal thread geometry for a better long term crestal bone stability [39]. Therefore, the original root shaped dental implant would be a plausible strategy to achieve better crestal bone stability and supporting esthetics. In addition to that, optimized surface roughness and chemical factors should be taken into account for a good long term biological health. In the literature, the micro-nano hybrid surface topography of titanium alloy was mentioned beneficial on biological responses of osteoblasts [40]. Alkaline phosphatase activity of the cells was greater onto nanotextured rough surfaces, and calcium deposition was higher on microtextured rough surfaces rather than nanotextured surfaces [41]. With the guidance of this knowledge, custom root analogue implants could be better designed with optimized macro and micro surface features in the future.

5. Conclusion

As a brief, considering the prevalent knowledge of clinical dental implant practice, screw-type dental implant has been the most plausible and predictable approach for replacing edentulous alveolar sites. However, it seems not so convenient and could not meet the clinical needs for immediately restoring the fresh extraction socket. Custom root shaped implant strategies emerged as the only realistic implementation and the prospective preference of immediate implant placement for both single- and multi-rooted teeth.

Contemporary computer aided digital technologies assist to overcome the hazardous anatomical drawbacks of jaws, and also to eliminate the excessive surgical augmenting procedures and compromise healing. On the contrary, the CAD/CAM root analogue implant strategies would simplify the immediate tooth replacement and improve the reliability.

Lastly, it should be noted that there are scarce number of objective clinical data regarding 3D planned and manufactured root analogue dental implant methods, and further clinical studies are required to conclude significant results.

Acknowledgements

The author reported no external funding.

Conflict of interest

The author reported no declaration of interest.

Author details

Ayse Sumeyye Akay
Department of Oral and Maxillofacial Surgery, Faculty of Dentistry,
Istanbul Medeniyet University, Istanbul, Turkey

Address all correspondence to: ayse.akay@medeniyet.edu.tr

References

[1] Shrestha A, Marla V, Shrestha S, Maharjan IK. Developmental anomalies affecting the morphology of teeth—A review. Revista Sul-Brasileira de Odontología. 2015;**12**(1):68-78

[2] Nelson SJ, Ash MM. Wheeler's Dental Anatomy, Physiology, and Occlusion. 9th ed. St. Louis: Saunders Elsevier; 2010

[3] Fuller JL, Denehy GE, Hall SA. Concise Dental Anatomy and Morphology. Year Book Medical Publishers, Chicago; 1984

[4] Ahmed H, Versiani M, De-Deus G, Dummer P. A new system for classifying root and root canal morphology. International Endodontic Journal. 2017;**50**(8):761-770

[5] Ahmed HM, Dummer PM. A new system for classifying tooth, root and canal anomalies. International Endodontic Journal. 2018;**51**(4):389-404

[6] Versiani MA, Pécora JD, de Sousa-Neto MD. Root and root canal morphology of four-rooted maxillary second molars: A micro–computed tomography study. Journal of Endodontics. 2012;**38**(7):977-982

[7] Song JS, Choi H-J, Jung I-Y, Jung H-S, Kim S-O. The prevalence and morphologic classification of distolingual roots in the mandibular molars in a Korean population. Journal of Endodontics. 2010;**36**(4):653-657

[8] Gher ME, Vernino AR. Root morphology—Clinical significance in pathogenesis and treatment of periodontal disease. The Journal of the American Dental Association. 1980;**101**(4):627-633

[9] Alvira-González J, Figueiredo R, Valmaseda-Castellón E, Quesada-Gómez C, Gay-Escoda C. Predictive factors of difficulty in lower third molar extraction: A prospective cohort study. Medicina Oral, Patologia Oral y Cirugia Bucal. 2017;**22**(1):e108

[10] Doornewaard R, Christiaens V, De Bruyn H, Jacobsson M, Cosyn J, Vervaeke S, et al. Long-term effect of surface roughness and patients' factors on crestal bone loss at dental implants. A systematic review and meta-analysis. Clinical Implant Dentistry and Related Research. 2017;**19**(2):372-399

[11] Ebenezer V, Balakrishnan K, Asir RVD, Sragunar B. Immediate placement of endosseous implants into the extraction sockets. Journal of Pharmacy & Bioallied Sciences. 2015;**7**(Suppl 1):S234

[12] Masaki C, Nakamoto T, Mukaibo T, Kondo Y, Hosokawa R. Strategies for alveolar ridge reconstruction and preservation for implant therapy. Journal of Prosthodontic Research. 2015;**59**(4):220-228

[13] Hodosh M, Povar M, Shklar G. The anatomic anorganic bone—Polymethacrylate endosteal dental implant. Oral Surgery, Oral Medicine, Oral Pathology. 1968;**25**(6):883-888

[14] Strub JR, Kohal RJ, Klaus G, Ferraresso F. The ReImplant® System for immediate implant placement. Journal of Esthetic and Restorative Dentistry. 1997;**9**(4):187-196

[15] Kontogiorgos ED, Gharpure P, Iheanacho EO, Gonzales CJ, Opperman LA. Preclinical evaluation of a crown-splinted custom root-shaped implant. International Journal of Oral & Maxillofacial Implants. 2017;**32**(5):1023-1032

[16] Moin DA, Hassan B, Mercelis P, Wismeijer D. Designing a novel dental

root analogue implant using cone beam computed tomography and CAD/CAM technology. Clinical Oral Implants Research. 2013;**24**:25-27

[17] Anssari Moin D, Hassan B, Wismeijer D. A novel approach for custom three-dimensional printing of a zirconia root analogue implant by digital light processing. Clinical Oral Implants Research. 2017;**28**(6):668-670

[18] Hodosh M, Povar M, Shklar G. The dental polymer implant concept. Journal of Prosthetic Dentistry. 1969;**22**(3):371-380

[19] Pour RS, Randelzhofer P, Edelhoff D, Prandtner O, Rafael CF, Liebermann A. Innovative single-tooth replacement with an individual root-analog hybrid implant in the esthetic zone: Case report. International Journal of Oral & Maxillofacial Implants. 2017;**32**(3):e153-e160

[20] Lundgren D, Rylander H, Anderssong M, Johansson C, Albrektsson T. Healing-in of root analogue titanium implants placed in extraction sockets. An experimental study in the beagle dog. Clinical Oral Implants Research. 1992;**3**(3):136-144

[21] Andersson M, Bergman B, Bessing C, Ericson G, Lundquist P, Nilson H. Clinical results with titanium crowns fabricated with machine duplication and spark erosion. Acta Odontologica Scandinavica. 1989;**47**(5):279-286

[22] Kohal RJ, Hürzeler MB, Mota LF, Klaus G, Caffesse RG, Strub JR. Custom-made root analogue titanium implants placed into extraction sockets. An experimental study in monkeys. Clinical Oral Implants Research. 1997;**8**(5):386-392

[23] Kohal RJ, Weng D, Bächle M, Strub JR. Loaded custom-made zirconia and titanium implants show similar osseointegration: An animal experiment. Journal of Periodontology. 2004;**75**(9):1262-1268

[24] Coatoam GW. Indirect sinus augmentation procedures using one-stage anatomically shaped root-form implants. The Journal of Oral Implantology. 1997;**23**(1-2):25-42

[25] Coatoam GW, Mariotti A. Immediate placement of anatomically shaped dental implants. Journal of Oral Implantology. 2000;**26**(3):170-176

[26] Moin DA, Hassan B, Wismeijer D. Immediate nonsubmerged custom root analog implants: A prospective pilot clinical study. International Journal of Oral & Maxillofacial Implants. 2018;**33**(2):e37-e44

[27] Figliuzzi M, Mangano F, Mangano C. A novel root analogue dental implant using CT scan and CAD/CAM: Selective laser melting technology. International Journal of Oral and Maxillofacial Surgery. 2012;**41**(7):858-862

[28] Schwarz F, Alcoforado G, Nelson K, Schaer A, Taylor T, Beuer F, et al. Impact of implant–abutment connection, positioning of the machined collar/microgap, and platform switching on crestal bone level changes. Camlog foundation consensus report. Clinical Oral Implants Research. 2014;**25**(11):1301-1303

[29] Moin DA, Hassan B, Parsa A, Mercelis P, Wismeijer D. Accuracy of preemptively constructed, C one B eam CT-, and CAD/CAM technology-based, individual Root Analogue Implant technique: An in vitro pilot investigation. Clinical Oral Implants Research. 2014;**25**(5):598-602

[30] Mangano FG, De Franco M, Caprioglio A, Macchi A, Piattelli A, Mangano C. Immediate, non-submerged, root-analogue direct laser metal sintering (DLMS) implants:

A 1-year prospective study on 15 patients. Lasers in Medical Science. 2014;**29**(4):1321-1328

[31] Pirker W, Kocher A. Immediate, non-submerged, root-analogue zirconia implants placed into single-rooted extraction sockets: 2-year follow-up of a clinical study. International Journal of Oral and Maxillofacial Surgery. 2009;**38**(11):1127-1132

[32] Klocke F, Gerent O, Schippers C, editors. Machining of advanced ceramics in the green state. In: Ceramic Forum International. Baden-Germany: Göller Verlag GmbH; 1997

[33] Xue W, Krishna BV, Bandyopadhyay A, Bose S. Processing and biocompatibility evaluation of laser processed porous titanium. Acta Biomaterialia. 2007;**3**(6):1007-1018

[34] Traini T, Mangano C, Sammons R, Mangano F, Macchi A, Piattelli A. Direct laser metal sintering as a new approach to fabrication of an isoelastic functionally graded material for manufacture of porous titanium dental implants. Dental Materials. 2008;**24**(11):1525-1533

[35] Mangano C, Mangano F, Shibli JA, Luongo G, De Franco M, Briguglio F, et al. Prospective clinical evaluation of 201 direct laser metal forming implants: Results from a 1-year multicenter study. Lasers in Medical Science. 2012;**27**(1):181-189

[36] Peng W, Xu L, You J, Fang L, Zhang Q. Selective laser melting of titanium alloy enables osseointegration of porous multi-rooted implants in a rabbit model. Biomedical Engineering Online. 2016;**15**(1):85

[37] Anitua E, Tapia R, Luzuriaga F, Orive G. Influence of implant length, diameter, and geometry on stress distribution: A finite element analysis. International Journal of Periodontics & Restorative Dentistry. 2010;**30**(1):89-95

[38] Eazhil R, Swaminathan SV, Gunaseelan M, Kannan GV, Alagesan C. Impact of implant diameter and length on stress distribution in osseointegrated implants: A 3D FEA study. Journal of International Society of Preventive & Community Dentistry. 2016;**6**(6):590

[39] Ryu H-S, Namgung C, Lee J-H, Lim Y-J. The influence of thread geometry on implant osseointegration under immediate loading: A literature review. The Journal of Advanced Prosthodontics. 2014;**6**(6):547-554

[40] Yin C, Zhang Y, Cai Q, Li B, Yang H, Wang H, et al. Effects of the micro-nano surface topography of titanium alloy on the biological responses of osteoblast. Journal of Biomedical Materials Research Part A. 2017;**105**(3):757-769

[41] Wimmers Ferreira MR, Rodrigo Fernandes R, Freire Assis A, Dernowsek JA, Passos GA, Variola F, et al. Oxidative nanopatterning of titanium surface influences mRNA and MicroRNA expression in human alveolar bone osteoblastic cells. International Journal of Biomaterials. 2016;**2016**:9169371